International Association of Fire Chiefs
International Society of Fire Service Instructors
National Fire Protection Association

Foundations of Instructional Delivery

Fire and Emergency Services Instructor I

THIRD EDITION

Forest F. Reeder
Alan E. Joos

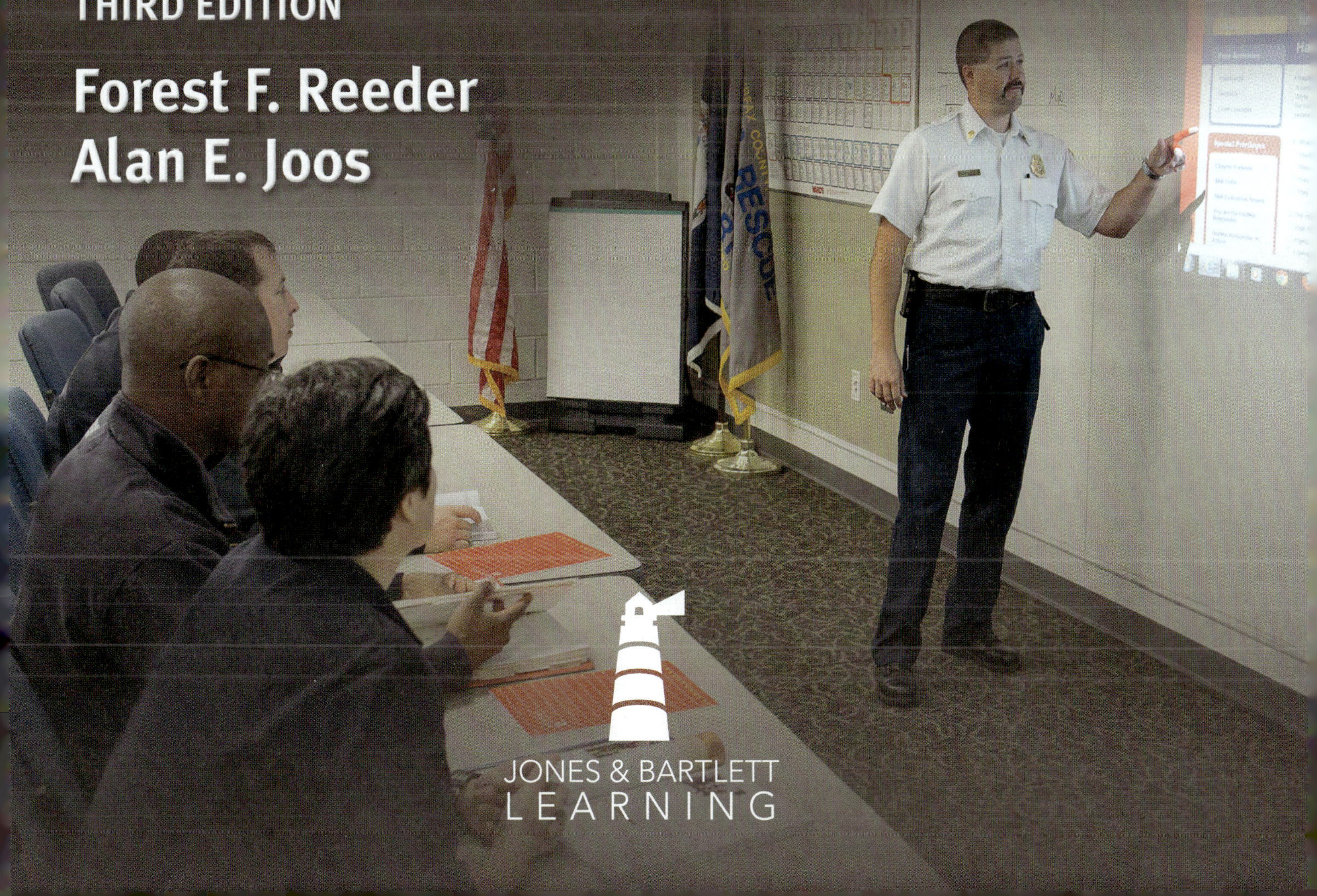

JONES & BARTLETT LEARNING

Jones & Bartlett Learning
World Headquarters
Jones & Bartlett Learning
5 Wall Street
Burlington, MA 01803
978-443-5000
info@jblearning.com
www.jblearning.com

International Society of Fire Service Instructors
14001C Saint Germain Drive
Suite 128
Centreville, Virginia 20121
www.isfsi.org

National Fire Protection Association
1 Batterymarch Park
Quincy, MA 02169-7471
www.NFPA.org

International Association of Fire Chiefs
4025 Fair Ridge Drive
Fairfax, VA 22033
www.IAFC.org

Jones & Bartlett Learning books and products are available through most bookstores and online booksellers. To contact Jones & Bartlett Learning directly, call 800-832-0034, fax 978-443-8000, or visit our website, www.jblearning.com.

Substantial discounts on bulk quantities of Jones & Bartlett Learning publications are available to corporations, professional associations, and other qualified organizations. For details and specific discount information, contact the special sales department at Jones & Bartlett Learning via the above contact information or send an email to specialsales@jblearning.com.

18978-0

Production Credits
General Manager and Executive Publisher: Kimberly Brophy
VP, Product Development: Christine Emerton
Senior Managing Editor: Donna Gridley
Executive Editor: William Larkin
Senior Development Editor: Janet Morris
VP, Sales: Phil Charland
Director of Marketing Operations: Brian Rooney
Director of Production: Jenny L. Corriveau
Director, Relationship Management: Carolyn Rogers Pershouse
Project Manager: Kristen Rogers
Digital Products Manager: Jordan McKenzie
Digital Project Specialist: Rachel Reyes
Production Services Manager: Colleen Lamy
VP, Manufacturing and Inventory Control: Therese Connell
Composition: S4Carlisle Publishing Services
Cover Design: Kristin E. Parker
Text Design: Scott Moden
Director, Content Services and Licensing: Joanna Gallant
Rights & Media Manager: Shannon Sheehan
Rights & Media Specialist: Thais Miller
Cover and Title Page Image: © Jones & Bartlett Learning. Photographed by Glen E. Ellman.
Printing and Binding: LSC Communications
Cover Printing: LSC Communications

Library of Congress Cataloging-in-Publication Data

Library of Congress Cataloging-in-Publication Data unavailable at time of printing.

6048

Printed in the United States of America
22 21 20 19 18 10 9 8 7 6 5 4 3 2 1

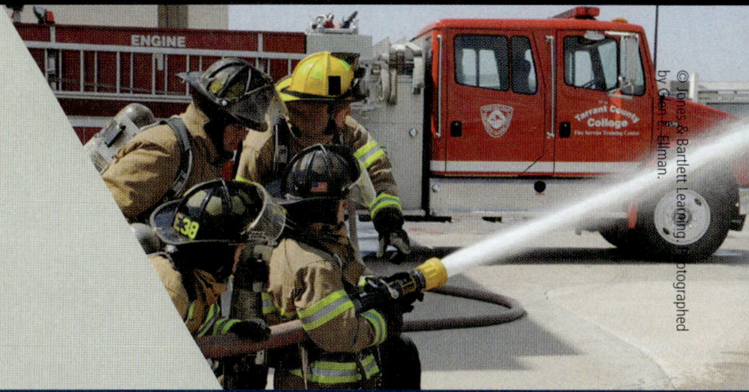

Brief Contents

Contents

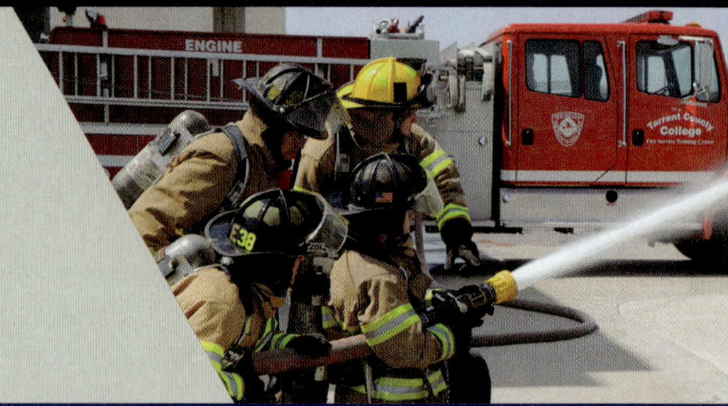

CHAPTER 4

Communication Skills 99

CHAPTER 5

Using Lesson Plans 119

CHAPTER 6

Technology in Training 139

Acknowledgments

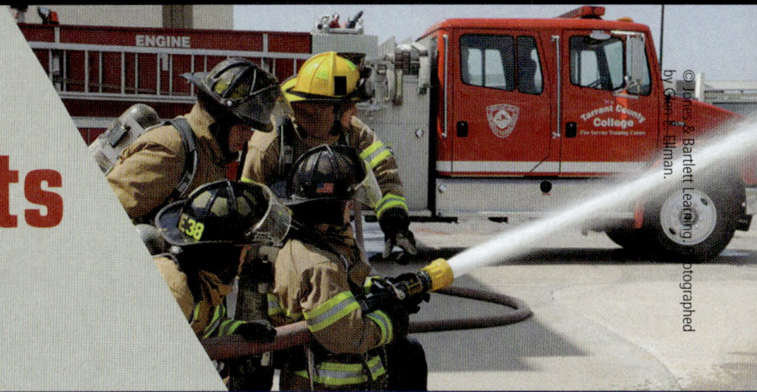

Authors

Forest F. Reeder, MS

Forest Reeder began his fire service career in 1978. He serves as fire chief of the Tinley Park (IL) Fire Department. Forest is the fire officer training coordinator for the Illinois Fire Chiefs Association Educational and Research Foundation and has served as the chairman of many Illinois State Fire Marshal certification committees. He is the author of the weekly drill features at www.firefighterclosecalls.com and at www.fireengineering.com. He has instructed at FDIC for nearly 20 years and trains both locally and nationally on fire service training, safety, and officer development related topics. Several articles on these programs have been published in major trade publications.

Forest holds many Illinois fire service certifications including Fire Officer 3, Training Program Manager, and Fire Department Safety Officer. He has an associate of applied science degree in fire science technology, a bachelor's degree in fire science management, and a master's degree in public safety administration from Lewis University. He was awarded the George D. Post Instructor of the Year by the International Society of Fire Service Instructors at FDIC in 2008.

Alan E. Joos, MS, EFO, CFO, FIFireE

Alan E. Joos currently serves as the chief of firefighter training within the State Fire Marshal's Office of Nebraska. Prior to his appointment in Nebraska he was an assistant director at LSU/FETI. Prior to FETI, he worked at the Utah Fire and Rescue Academy for 12 years as assistant director of the certification system and assistant director of the training division.

Mr. Joos received associate's and bachelor's degrees from Utah Valley University in fire science and business technology management and a master's degree from Grand Canyon University in Phoenix. He is currently a doctoral candidate in human resource education/workforce development at Louisiana State University. He is also a graduate of the Executive Fire Officer's Program at the National Fire Academy, has received Chief Fire Officer Designation from the Commission on Professional Credentialing, and is a fellow with the Institution of Fire Engineers.

Alan's fire service background began in 1985 as a career fire fighter in a combination fire department and then as an on-call fire fighter/EMT-I in Utah. He has continued his fire service involvement with the City of Gonzales, Louisiana, as a contract fire fighter. During his fire service career, he has served as a training officer, driver, shift officer, and EMT.

Alan has been involved with several national organizations, including the International Fire Service Accreditation Congress (IFSAC) and the ProBoard, and has previously served on the NFPA Technical Committee for the Professional Qualification Standards.

Alan is married to Carla Joos, and their family includes Nathan and his wife Shauntelle, Jordan (deceased), and Dallan, and granddaughter Chloe and grandson Gavin.

Contributors and Reviewers

Roderick Armstrong

WVPST (West Virginia Public Service Training) and WVFSE (West Virginia Fire Service Extension)
WVPST, Region 5, Currently Dunbar, West Virginia
WVUFSE, WV State Fire Academy, Jackson Mills, West Virginia

Angela L. Bennett

Manager, Institute Development Section
Maryland Fire and Rescue Institute
University of Maryland

Kendal E. Bortisser

Miramar College Fire Technology Program
San Diego, California

Dave Burgess

Program Manager
Justice Institute of British Columbia

Troy Cailler

Fire Fighter/Co-Owner
Tri-County Training Association, LLC
Litchfield, Maine

Shea Chwialkowski

Richfield Fire Department
Richfield, Minnesota

Mike Consie

Captain
Duluth Fire Department
Duluth, Minnesota

Nathaniel Contreras

Operations Captain
Scarborough Fire Department
Scarborough, Maine

Brent Cowx
Instructor
Justice Institute of British Columbia

Michael Dade
Instructor
Illinois Fire Service Institute
Champaign, Illinois

Leo DeBobes
Associate Professor and Fire Protection Technology Program Coordinator
Suffolk County Community College, Fire Protection Technology
Selden, New York

Jason Decremer
Director of Certification
CT Commission on Fire Prevention and Control
Windsor Locks, Connecticut

Michael F. Dunlap
South Carolina State Fire Academy
Columbia, South Carolina

E. Brene Duggins
Fire Prevention Coordinator/Technology Specialist
Holly Grove Fire Department
Lexington, North Carolina

Doug Eggiman
Fire Chief
Midway Fire Rescue
Pawleys Island, South Carolina

J. Michael Freeman
Director
WV Public Service Training
Clarksburg, West Virginia

Christopher L. Gilbert
Paramedic/Hazmat Specialist
Alachua County
Gainesville, Florida

Casey Hall
Kentucky Fire Commission
Greenville, Kentucky

Shawn Kelley
International Association of Fire Chiefs
Fairfax, Virginia

Steve Knight
Coordinator / Professor
Lambton College
Sarnia, Ontario

Jason Loeb
Program Manager
Illinois Fire Service Institute
Champaign, Illinois

Patrick McArdle
Chief of Training
Fayetteville Technical Community College
Fayetteville, North Carolina

Michael C. Mire
Assistant Fire Chief
Houston Fire Department
Houston, Texas

Nick Morgan
Captain
St. Louis Fire Department
St. Louis, Missouri

Keith Padgett
Director, College of Safety and Emergency Services
Columbia Southern University
Orange Beach, Alabama

Ian Pleet
Senior Exercise Planner
Leidos
Life Member, Manassas Volunteer Fire Company
Reston, Virginia

Joseph Ramsey
Battalion Chief
Winston-Salem Fire Department
Winston-Salem, North Carolina

Steven L Riley Jr.
Lieutenant
Columbus Fire Department
Columbus, Ohio

Lt. John W. Ross, Jr.
City of Aurora Fire Department
Aurora, Illinois

Mike Rutkowski
Battalion Chief
Grayslake Fire Protection District
Grayslake, Illinois

Kelli J. Scarlett, J.D.
Adjunct Professor
University of Maryland University College
Adelphi, Maryland

Timothy Smith
District Fire Chief
Boston Fire Department
Boston, Massachusetts

Jeremy Souza
National Fire Protection Association
Quincy, Massachusetts

Larry Straffin
Deputy Chief/Training Officer
North Berwick Fire Department
Fire Instructor
Maine Fire Service Institute and New Hampshire Fire Academy and EMS
Brunswick, Maine

Bobby Strozier
LSU Fire and Emergency Training Institute
Baton Rouge, Louisiana

Robert Taggart
Training Officer
Shreveport Fire Department
Shreveport, Louisiana

Luis F. Videgaray
Captain/Training Officer
Natchez Fire Department Training Center
Natchez, Mississippi

Chris Walker
Captain
Fort Wayne Fire Department
Fort Wayne, Indiana

Laura Walker
Associate Professor
Montezuma Fire Department
Sinclair Community College Fire Academy
Dayton, Ohio

Devon Wells
International Society of Fire Service Instructors
Hood River, Oregon

John West
Oregon Department of Public Safety Standards & Training
Salem, Oregon

Angela White
Education Director - Fire Service Training
Wisconsin Technical College System
Madison, Wisconsin

Becki White
Eden Prairie Fire Department
Eden Prairie, Minnesota

Kim Williams
Deputy Director
Fire and Rescue Commission
Raleigh, North Carolina

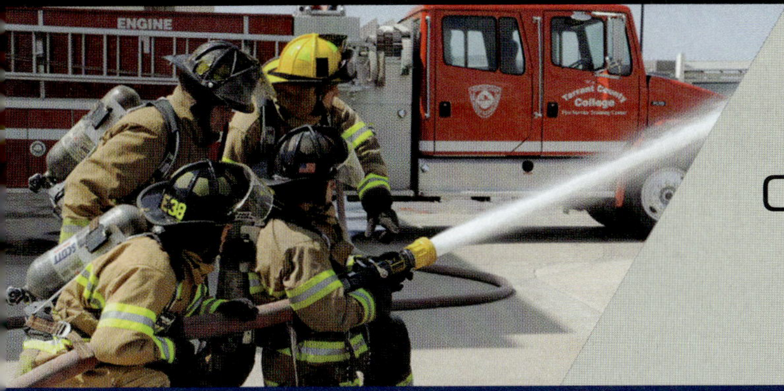

CHAPTER 1

Today's Fire and Emergency Services Instructor

NFPA 1041 JOB PERFORMANCE REQUIREMENTS

4.1.1 The Fire and Emergency Services Instructor I shall meet the JPRs defined in Sections 4.2 through 4.5 of this standard.

4.2.5 Complete training records and reports, given policies and procedures, so that required reports are accurate and submitted in accordance with the procedures.

(A) Requisite Knowledge.

Types of records and reports required, and policies and procedures for processing records and reports.

(B) Requisite Skills.

Report writing and record completion.

4.4.2 Organize the learning environment, given a facility and an assignment, so that lighting, distractions, climate control or weather, noise control, seating, audiovisual equipment, teaching aids, and safety are addressed.

(A) Requisite Knowledge.

Learning environment management and safety, advantages and limitations of audiovisual equipment and teaching aids, classroom arrangement, and methods and techniques of instruction.

(B) Requisite Skills.

Use of instructional media and teaching aids.

KNOWLEDGE OBJECTIVES

After studying this chapter, participating in a structured learning environment, and completing assigned assessments, you will be able to:

- Define the roles and responsibilities of the Fire and Emergency Services Instructor I. (**NFPA 1041: 4.1.1**, pp 4–5)
- Identify the physical elements of the learning environment. (**NFPA 1041: 4.4.2**, pp 9–10)
- Explain the importance of succession planning for the instructor. (pp 11–12)
- Identify issues of ethics for the instructor. (p 13)
- Explain the importance of continuing learning for the instructor. (p 13)
- Describe how laws and standards apply to the instructor. (pp 15–19)
- Explain the importance of proper recordkeeping. (**NFPA 1041: 4.2.5**, pp 14–15)
- Identify three methods instructors can use to manage multiple priorities. (pp 19–21)
- Identify professional organizations that will help in the professional development of the instructor. (pp 22–23)
- Identify and discuss the value and importance of coaching and mentoring the next generation of instructors. (p 27)

SKILLS OBJECTIVES

After studying this chapter, participating in a structured learning environment, and completing assigned assessments, you will be able to:

- Complete a record of a training event. (**NFPA 1041: 4.2.5**, pp 14–19)
- Prepare a report following a training event. (**NFPA 1041: 4.2.5**, pp 18–19)

You Are the Fire and Emergency Services Instructor

As the only Fire Instructor I assigned to your shift, your company officer has asked you to lead a training session with your company. Because this is your first assignment of this nature, ask yourself the following questions:

1. What are the roles and responsibilities of the Fire Instructor 1?
2. What are four ethical issues an instructor must be aware of?
3. Which laws and standards, particularly NFPA standards, apply to the instructor in your jurisdiction?

JONES & BARTLETT LEARNING NAVIGATE 2 *Access Navigate for more practice activities.*

Introduction

Remember when you began your career in the fire service? Somewhere in your memory is probably an outstanding fire and emergency services instructor. He or she even may be the person who introduced you to your career. Instructors are the guardians of knowledge, skills, and ability in the fire service; their knowledge is wrapped up in a long tradition that has served many generations of fire fighters well. As protectors of that tradition, instructors look to and rely on innovation and creativity while constantly striving for perfect training.

In years past, firefighting training was often left to on-the-job education. New recruits would be handed coats, boots, helmets, and gloves and told to jump on the back of the rig as it rushed to the scene of the emergency. In those days, the fire ground was the recruit's training ground—and the title of "fire and emergency services instructor" may have been handed out too generously. Formal instructors and, in some cases, formal instruction were left to the larger departments that had budgets large enough to hire specialized personnel and build training facilities.

Clearly, times have changed. The fire service is now being pushed to the limit by communities that expect more out of the types of services provided. Retired Phoenix Fire Chief Alan Brunacini often referred to today's recipient of that service as "Mrs. Smith." As a pioneer of customer service, Chief Brunacini knew the value of the instructor in preparing the troops to meet Mrs. Smith's demands. Today, fire departments rely on their instructors both to train new recruits and to maintain the skill levels of existing fire fighters.

Qualities of an Instructor

What does it take to join this elite group of fire fighters on whose shoulders rest the success and safety of emergency operations? Although excellent instructors possess many attributes, a few important qualities come to mind and rise to the top of the list. First, there

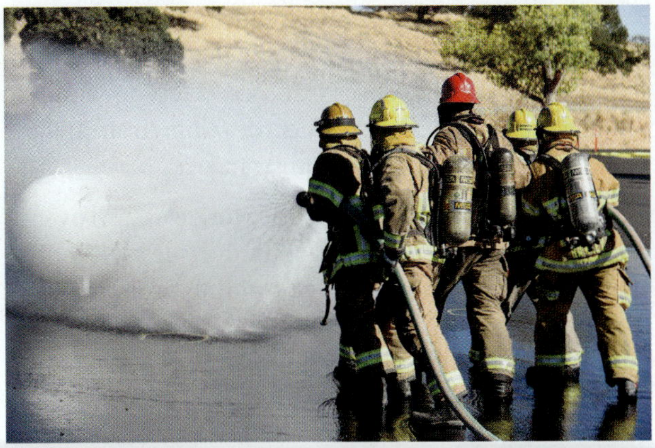

FIGURE 1-1 The instructor brings a blend of experience and education to every training opportunity.

is desire—a desire to be of assistance to those in need. In this case, we are not referring to those persons who require our assistance during times of trouble or emergency, but rather to those individuals who would require the knowledge needed to assist those in trouble. These fire fighters must be trained so that they will gain the knowledge, skills, and abilities necessary to serve and respond to those in need of assistance. The instructor gives freely without hesitation in the pursuit of excellence (**FIGURE 1-1**). He or she should certainly have experience in the subject matter taught. Students have more confidence in instructors who have demonstrated competence in the subject matter through experience; in turn, experience opens the door for the instructor to reach the minds of the students. Even so, good instructors understand that they cannot rely on experience alone. They must remain vigilant to their dynamic environment and gather the newest information, technology, and skills to remain out front and stay current with an ever-changing work and instructional environment.

Good instructors also demonstrate flexibility. They are able to work in a variety of environments while offering instruction on a variety of topics to a class full of students with a variety of talents, backgrounds, and experience levels. Instructing the adult learner can be challenging, and the instructor must be willing to alter the approaches to education used to reach all students. In some cases, the fire department's schedule provides the greatest challenge, as instruction time is often interrupted by calls for assistance. In other fire departments, it is the fire fighters' personal schedules that present the challenge, as training time competes with family time and full-time work schedules.

Motivation is one of the keys to bringing excitement to the training environment. Nothing breeds fire fighter motivation like a motivated instructor. The right kind of motivation leads to the attitude, "I can't wait to teach," and, just as important, "I can't wait to learn." Motivation is contagious; it can spread from the learning environment to the station floor, and ultimately it can drive the quality of the service provided to the community. Motivated instructors bring creativity and ingenuity to the learning environment as a means of creating excitement about the learning process.

The skills to be an effective instructor can be learned by a person who has the desire to develop and perfect them. The ability to use these skills at the correct time and in a manner that helps others learn a topic is developed by teaching courses and being mentored, coached, and supervised by experienced trainers. The learning process never ends for those who desire to improve their knowledge and skills. All instructors start out at the Instructor I level; with additional training and professional development, they may reach the top of the qualification set owing to their desire to learn and develop their skills. Desire matched with knowledge creates great instructors.

In addition to being motivated and skilled, instructors will benefit from a sense of ethics. Ethics can be broken down into personal beliefs, interpersonal actions, and professional ethics. Instructors should recognize the interrelated aspects of personal, interpersonal, and professional ethics.

Are you up for the challenge? Can you accept the responsibility? Can you be a steward of tradition while remaining open to teaching new ideas? Can you strive to maintain desire, experience, flexibility, and motivation as you pursue operational excellence? If your answers to these questions are all "yes," then you are on your way to joining the ranks of the greatest profession. Ideally, your curriculum will serve as the launching pad for excellent fire fighters and serve them well as a critical resource for years to come.

This text provides information to meet the job performance requirements (JPRs) outlined in National Fire Protection Association (NFPA) NFPA 1041: *Standard for Fire and Emergency Service Instructor Professional Qualifications*. These definitions resulted from a task analysis intended to validate these levels and to create specific requirements that would apply to each level. Although the levels are identified as instructor qualifications, in many states they may become certification levels, with candidate prerequisites to be completed before a certification is granted.

Levels of Fire and Emergency Services Instructors

According to NFPA 1041, the duties performed by specific instructors are broken down into three distinct levels. These three classifications build on one another and progressively give the instructor additional skills, duties, and responsibilities.

Instructor I is defined as follows (**NFPA 1041, Section 3.3.2.1**):

> A fire and emergency services instructor who has demonstrated the knowledge and ability to deliver instruction effectively from a prepared lesson plan, including instructional aids and evaluation instruments; adapt lesson plans to the unique requirements of the students and authority having jurisdiction; organize the learning environment so that learning and safety are maximized; and meet the record-keeping requirements of the authority having jurisdiction.

Stated in the most basic terms, the Instructor I delivers instruction from prepared materials at the direction, and often under the supervision, of an Instructor II or higher. Emphasis of this level of instructor is on the ability to communicate effectively and to use various methods of instruction, including hands-on training and lecture. In many cases, the Instructor I will deliver the majority of the fire department company training.

The Instructor II is an instructor who, in addition to meeting the Instructor I qualifications, satisfies the following criteria (**NFPA 1041, Section 3.3.2.2**):

> Has demonstrated the knowledge and ability to develop individual lesson plans for a specific topic including learning objectives, instructional aids, and evaluation instruments; schedule training sessions based on overall training plan of authority having jurisdiction; and supervise and coordinate the activities of other instructors.

The Instructor II functions at a higher level of authority and responsibility than the Instructor I; he or she is responsible for all duty areas of the Instructor I, and is also able to create the training materials. In the purest sense, the Instructor II will create the training materials for distribution to the Instructor I to present to the students. In reality, both tasks may be completed by the same person.

An Instructor III is defined as follows (**NFPA 1041, Section 3.3.2.3**):

> A fire and emergency services instructor who, in addition to meeting Instructor II qualifications, has demonstrated the knowledge and ability to develop comprehensive training curricula and programs for use by single or multiple organizations; conduct organization needs analysis; design record keeping and scheduling systems; and develop training goals and implementation strategies.

The Instructor III typically works as an overall training program manager and oversees the entire spectrum of a comprehensive training program. This includes the planning, development, and implementation of curricula and development of an evaluation plan and training program budget.

Roles and Responsibilities of the Fire and Emergency Services Instructor I

Throughout our lives, we are asked to conform to someone else's idea of how we should act or behave. Child, adolescent, adult, parent, spouse, employee, supervisor, owner, citizen—all are examples of roles that we fill while negotiating through life. With each of these roles, expectations direct our actions and allow us to evaluate our success or failure at that role.

The fire service mirrors life in that it also contains various roles, each with its own expectations and responsibilities. At every step along the fire service path, from recruit to fire chief, we strive to meet these expectations and responsibilities. The instructor is one of those important roles in the fire service that requires dedicated and competent individuals who can positively influence the entire fire department.

The roles and responsibilities of a fire instructor vary greatly by fire department according to the size, make-up, and delivery system used. Understanding the responsibilities for the Instructors I, II, and III is essential for success in these key positions.

The role of the Instructor I includes the following:

- Manage the basic resources and the records and reports essential to the instructional process.
- Assemble course materials.
- Prepare training records and reports.
- Prepare requests for training resources.
- Schedule instructional sessions.
- Review and adapt prepared instructional materials.
- Deliver instructional sessions using prepared course materials.

- Organize the learning environment, laboratory, or outdoor learning environments.
- Use instructional media and materials to present prepared lesson plans.
- Adjust presentations to students' different learner characteristics, abilities, and behaviors.
- Operate and use audiovisual equipment and demonstration devices.
- Administer and grade student evaluation instruments.
- Deliver oral, written, or performance tests.
- Grade students' oral, written, or performance tests.
- Report test results.
- Provide examination feedback to students.

The relationship between training and education is often confusing. Education is the process of imparting knowledge or skill through systematic instruction. Education programs are conducted through academic institutions and are primarily directed toward an individual's comprehension of the subject matter. Training is directed toward the practical application of education to produce an action, which can be an individual or a group activity. There is an important distinction between these two types of learning.

Within the fire service, training has been considered essential for many years. In contrast, the emphasis on fire fighter education is a much more recent development. The first Wingspread Conference on Fire Service Administration, Education and Research was sponsored by the Johnson Foundation and held in Racine, Wisconsin, in 1966. This conference brought together a group of leaders from the fire service to identify needs and priorities. They agreed that a broad knowledge base was needed and that an educational program was necessary to deliver that knowledge base. Their conclusions became the blueprint for the development of community college fire science and fire administration programs, as well as the degrees-at-a-distance program. The transition from training to education had begun.

In 1998, the U.S. Fire Administration hosted the first Fire and Emergency Services Higher Education (FESHE) conference. That conference produced a document, "The Fire Service and Education: A Blueprint for the 21st Century," that initiated a national effort to address and update the academic needs of the fire service. Participants at the 2000 FESHE conference began work to develop a model fire science curriculum that would span from the community college through graduate school levels. At the 2002 conference, U.S. Fire Administration Education Specialist Edward Kaplan compared the results of the FESHE effort with the Wingspread higher education curriculum. The FESHE work affirmed the soundness of the original Wingspread model, with information technology being the only new knowledge item added to the curriculum.

Where Do I Fit In?

Much has been written about the responsibilities of positions within various types of organizations, and the fire service is no different. Fire chiefs have their role, rooted in visions of leadership, as the commander-in-chief of the organization. They have a defined responsibility that not only allows them to assume this role but also gives them the authority to shape their own destiny.

Within the fire service's remaining command structure lie the positions of supervision, including frontline lieutenants, captains, and various chief officers. These ranks have had their roles defined through a history of developed policies and job descriptions created by necessity, the chief's vision, and, yes, tradition. These positions are often referred to as middle management, as they are created and reside in the middle of the chain of command. They are pushed and tested by fire fighters at the bottom and by fire chiefs at the top.

As tough as these positions are, there is one job that still finds itself in a somewhat more precarious spot: the instructor. All too often, an instructor may ask, "Where do I fit in?" Is the instructor a line officer, a training officer, a fire fighter, or someone with a specific specialty? In some fire departments, line officers are assigned to the training division as part of their duties. In volunteer organizations, the training officer often volunteers for the job; alternatively, he or she may be assigned to it. Regardless of how you come to be assigned to training, you may feel challenged if you are not given the proper authority to carry out that job.

In examining fire departments' **organizational charts**, you will find positions identified for operational activities, clearly outlining the chain of command and the corresponding responsibilities for firefighting personnel and their fire officer counterparts. Instructors, if shown at all, are usually found off to the side on the organizational chart, preferably within a training division. This disconnect may create a sense of isolation from the fire fighters whom instructors are expected to train. It may leave the instructor with a void, feeling unfulfilled in terms of a

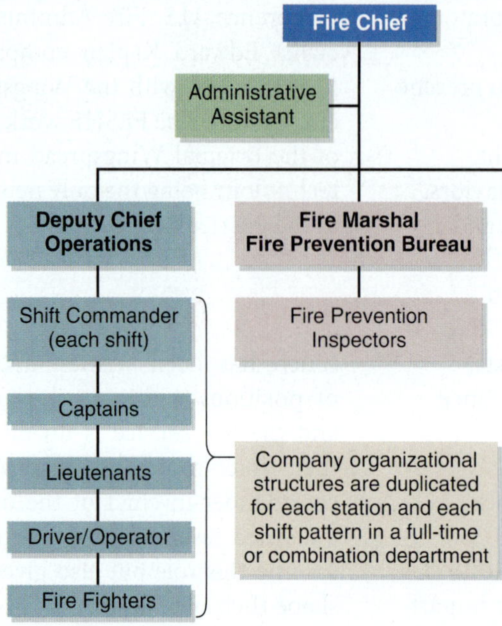

FIGURE 1-2 A sample organizational chart for a fire department.

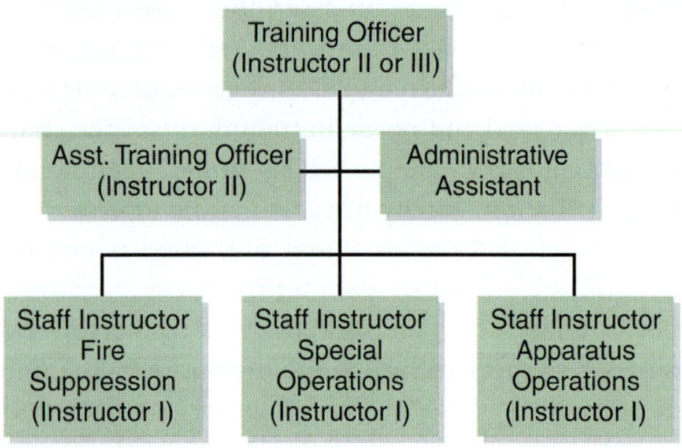

FIGURE 1-3 A training division organizational chart for a typical fire department. The size and make-up of the department will dictate the instructor certification levels for the various positions.

management role that demonstrates the fire department's lack of respect for the role (**FIGURE 1-2**). Fire fighters and even some fire officers are often seen as resisting or even obstructing the training process, because all too often those within the operations staff do not view training as a high priority.

As an instructor, you must remain focused, upbeat, positive, proactive, and true to your role (**FIGURE 1-3**). You must remind yourself that you hold the power to shape the future fire service. Every member of the fire service—from fire fighter through fire officer—has had an instructor affect their careers. That fact demonstrates the importance of your position within the fire department.

The Roles of an Effective Instructor

As a fire and emergency services instructor, you must look beyond charts and titles and instead focus on those important, yet sometimes invisible, roles that produce lasting contributions to overall fire department organizational health and success. Today's instructor is asked to fulfill these roles. These roles are not unique to the fire service; indeed, examples of each can be found in many different professions. Each role is important, however, and will help you develop the talents found within the organization. Understanding each of these roles can assist you in creating and building your own tradition within the fire department.

Fire instructors at all levels must learn to manage the following roles to be effective in carrying out their duties in a department (**FIGURE 1-4**):

- Leader
- Mentor
- Coach
- Evaluator
- Teacher

The Fire and Emergency Services Instructor as a Leader

Instructors are often asked to lead fire departments into the future by preparing fire fighters for new missions. Instructors set the example for all fire fighters to follow in terms of performance excellence. As such,

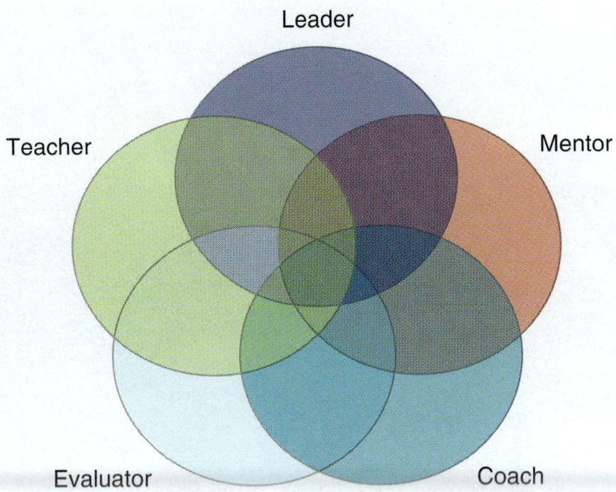

FIGURE 1-4 The five major roles filled by fire instructors.

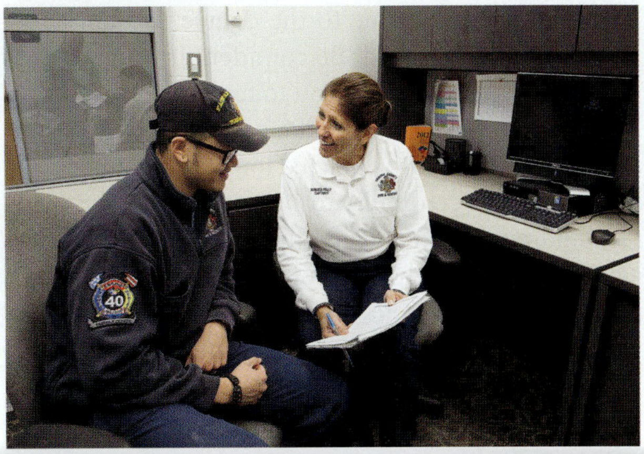

FIGURE 1-5 Mentoring and preparing your successors are both key attributes in quality instruction.

they must remain true to the direction set by upper management and supportive of the mission as defined by the organization.

Your place in front of the classroom puts you in a visible—and sometimes vulnerable—position where you may have to endure the anxieties of an impatient rank and file. Do not waver from the training mission by letting the instructional environment be turned into a debate on issues of management within the fire department. The most powerful leadership tool is the one over which you have the most control: Lead by example. Leading others is a major responsibility. Part of that responsibility is leading in a positive manner. Belittling a new recruit over a mistake may cause the recruit to hide future mistakes, which places both the recruit and others at risk. Instructors should foster an environment that allows for errors and turns mistakes during training into a teaching opportunity.

The Fire and Emergency Services Instructor as a Mentor

Good leaders are also good at identifying future talent. Instructors are in the best position to observe first-hand both the raw talent of recruits and the ongoing growth of department personnel. They can support and enhance the careers of fire fighters by identifying their talents and mentoring them appropriately. Instructors with mentorship abilities enhance the fire department's succession planning by evaluating and developing the talent pool of future instructors and officers. For example, established instructors assist future instructors by showing confidence in their abilities and recommending additional training and opportunities. In short, good instructors mentor future good instructors and leaders (**FIGURE 1-5**).

As an instructor, you must have the respect of the trainees. Respect may come from a title or position, but it can also come from the individual, based on his or her expertise and knowledge. If you find yourself charged with the task of teaching those of higher rank, be prepared to work for their respect.

Earning someone's respect can be done in several ways. Do not wait to begin building credibility until you are asked to teach—be a professional at your job from the first day you join the fire department. Read books, trade magazines, and other material so that you will become well versed in the trade. Take additional courses and training, and learn how to use the internet to research the latest information on topics that you are assigned to teach or that are of interest to you. Get out and practice what you know: For example, organize the medical kit. Demonstrate that you are an avid learner and practitioner of your craft. Other fire fighters will notice and respect your thirst for knowledge, which builds your credibility when you are teaching any topic.

Credibility is a direct result of your knowledge of the subject. Rank does not always equate with knowledge—but hard work does. Go over the material so you can determine the flow of the course. Read the activities carefully so you have the right materials on hand and you understand the intended result. Write notes in the margins of the instructor's guide about comments you want to bring up and examples of the practical application of the material. An ill-prepared instructor is doomed to fall short when it comes to gaining credibility.

In addition to your before-class preparation, be ready to build credibility in the learning environment. Respect the knowledge that the students possess. Take advantage of those individuals with specialized knowledge to add value to the course. Do not allow yourself to be chastised. Be confident in your skills—obviously whoever asked you to teach believes in you. Take control of the class and be a professional. In the long run, you will be respected for your teaching skills if you have the credibility to support them.

Building respect and credibility with students is essential for those who do not have a formal position in the fire department or when teaching those with greater rank. Although it can be more challenging, success can be achieved with proper preparation and implementation.

The Fire and Emergency Services Instructor as a Coach

In their book *A Passion for Excellence*, Tom Peters and Nancy Austin define coaching as follows (Austin and Peters, 1986, 325–326):

> Face-to-face leadership that pulls together people with diverse backgrounds, talents, experiences and interest; encourages them to step up to responsibility and continued achievement; and treats them as full-scale partners and contributors.

In the sports world, the coach receives most of the attention and pressure because he or she is cast in the role of determining the success or failure of the team. In the fire service, we often stress the need for teamwork in all aspects of the job. Teamwork is an important ingredient on the fire ground as the incident commander orchestrates the company's actions through various tactical assignments. Even in the fire station, much of the nonemergency activity is accomplished not by an individual, but rather by a dedicated team of professionals. Whether on the fire ground or in the station, the incident commander acts much like the quarterback of a football team, calling out the formations and plays. In the training environment, the instructor plays a role analogous to that of the football coaching staff: Whereas the coaching staff works on drills to prepare the players for the next game, the instructor works to prepare the fire fighters for the next incident response.

The instructor's job within the fire service corresponds to that of a coach in the sports world in many ways. It is the instructor who must prepare the team for battle. An exterior attack can be as challenging as an interior one; students must be prepared for both equally. The instructor studies the team's opposition (the fire) and prepares the team for what they may face on game day. He or she builds team skills through practice and repetition on the drill ground (**FIGURE 1-6**). The instructor, much like a coach, must enthusiastically encourage fire fighters as they struggle with new ideas and techniques. Finally, the instructor must remember to remain positive, even in tough times, and to support the direction in which the team is headed as determined by the general manager (fire chief) and the owners (residents). Coaches and instructors lead, train, and drive their team's performance.

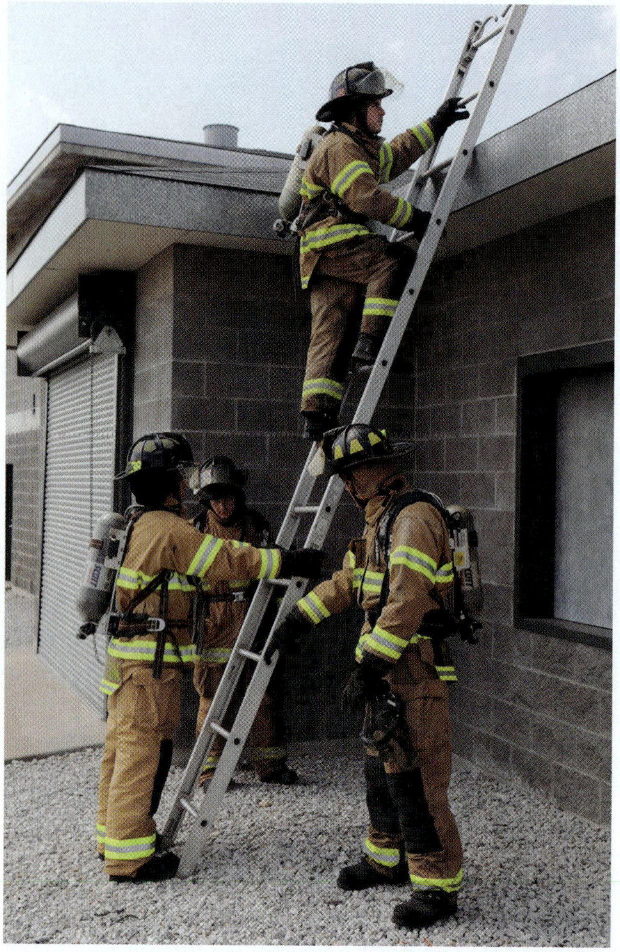

FIGURE 1-6 The instructor builds team skills through practice and repetition on the drill ground.

The Fire and Emergency Services Instructor as an Evaluator

Who is in the best position to evaluate the capabilities of a fire department? The answer is found standing in the front of the classroom: the instructor. As obvious as that answer is, how many fire chiefs have taken advantage of the knowledge fire instructors have assembled through their daily interactions with the troops? Instructors must evaluate students' learning and competencies at many points during the training process. To do so, they must sharpen their skills in evaluating the proficiency and knowledge retained by their students. The ability of the instructor to assess the comprehension of the class or student accurately can determine the pace of the training. Determining the right time to introduce new techniques or to review previously taught topics cannot be done without the ability to evaluate students honestly. Proper evaluations done in the course of training save the department from the heartache of critical evaluations performed by the public at the scene of a mistake.

Instructors are in a unique position to evaluate the capabilities and limitations of fire fighters. In many fire departments, input from the training division and instructors is regularly sought by fire department leadership to help them develop policies and procedures. The instructor can evaluate fire fighters, suggest operational directives, and field-test new standard operating procedures (SOPs).

Instructors should also be evaluators of the learning environment. That is, they must always be able to evaluate their effectiveness, recognizing what the students need and what the students are learning. They must evaluate themselves as well, looking for ways to improve their own teaching techniques. Learning environments and self-evaluations are essential in keeping the training program proactive and on the road to continuous improvement.

The Fire and Emergency Services Instructor as a Teacher

As simple as it sounds, the instructor must be a teacher. What comes to mind as you hear the word *teacher*? Perhaps it is someone you remember from your elementary school days. Why does that name come to mind? Teachers affect students in many ways—many times positively, but unfortunately sometimes negatively. Instructors must teach students new skills and abilities, thereby shaping the abilities of the team. They must remember the potential influence they have with their students. It is not just what the students learn that is important; rather, the shaping of a fire fighter's demeanor, attitudes, and desires ultimately determine how the instructor will be remembered.

Being an effective teacher should be the goal of each instructor. Mastering the interpersonal side of the learning environment goes a long way toward reaching that goal. The best and most remembered teachers shape and mold the total person to become part of the team and contribute the best they have to offer. A true teacher helps others see their potential and develop a path to accomplish those goals.

Setting Up the Learning Environment

Every instructor should understand the effect that the **learning environment** has on the ability of students to grasp the material being presented. You need to take command of that environment and use it to your advantage. The learning environment includes those environmental factors that influence the learning process and can include multiple elements, both physical (e.g., lighting, temperature, furniture configuration) and emotional (e.g., attitudes, comments, learning).

Physically, the classroom and drill ground must provide a safe, comfortable, and distraction-free environment. Emotionally, students' minds must be kept focused on the instructional material in front of them and away from the sometimes-contentious issues found in many fire departments. To make matters even more challenging, some of the factors affecting the learning environment are outside the instructor's control. If you are not careful, you may bring some frustrations into the learning environment, thereby impeding the learning process. To avoid these mistakes, familiarize yourself with the elements that affect the learning environment, including the audience.

COMPANY-LEVEL INSTRUCTOR TIP

One foundational component of ensuring a quality program is paying attention to the learning environment details and arrangement. You can facilitate better learning by eliminating unnecessary distractions and providing a comfortable setting.

Physical Elements Affecting the Learning Environment

Imagine yourself as you walk into a classroom. What do you notice first? Lighting? Cleanliness? Temperature? Or perhaps how far from the front of the room you can sit? Every student who has ever taken a class has evaluated the learning environment. The simple arrangement of tables and chairs can affect how we interact and ultimately learn. The best arrangements

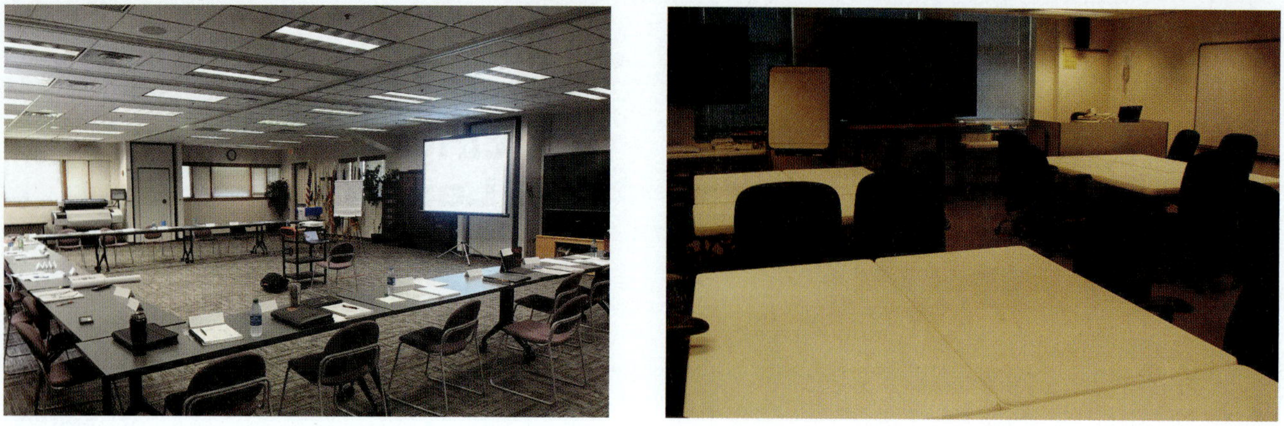

A B

FIGURE 1-7 Tables arrangements such as a U-shape **(A)** or a square **(B)** allow face-to-face interactions.
A: Courtesy of Forest Reeder; **B:** Courtesy of Bill Larkin.

allow for the free exchange of information, both from student to student and from student to instructor.

Traditional school classroom setups can lead to the formation of groups in distinct areas of the room, as students tend to sit next to those with whom they are most comfortable. Both the quiet and the uninterested students vie for the seats farthest from the front, not wanting to become involved in the learning discussion. Tables arrangements such as a U-shape or a square or tables arranged in groups, which allow face-to-face interactions, can sometimes neutralize the hierarchy of traditional settings (**FIGURE 1-7**). These arrangements also allow you to move among the students freely, improving the exchange of information and increasing the attentiveness of students.

In setting up the learning environment, you must also consider both the natural light and the installed lighting. Lighting affects many aspects of the learning environment. If projectors are used in the presentation, lighting becomes critical to the ability of the students to view the projected information. If natural light is a problem, a simple rearrangement of the room may allow the movement of a screen to a better location. If that is not possible, perhaps the addition of window blinds can correct the problem.

You must also evaluate the installed lighting in the room. Improperly installed lights may make it difficult to dim the lights enough to ensure quality projection. Conversely, dimming the lights too much may create reading or note-taking difficulties for students. If installed lighting is causing problems, your supervisor might be able to recommend improvements to the system through the annual department budget process.

Room temperature can also create problems for the learning environment. Take the entire class into account when setting the room temperature. Finding a comfortable compromise for all may turn you into a negotiator. Of course, some classrooms have environmental controls that cannot be changed by those using the facility. In those cases, you may have to alter lecture and break times if temperatures are uncomfortable. You may also have to become a student advocate and seek improvements to the environmental controls. More information on the physical learning environment can be found in Chapter 3, *Methods of Instruction*.

Emotional Elements Affecting the Learning Environment

The instructor has a responsibility to help protect the individual student from the emotional letdown that comes with the inability or difficulty to learn a new task or subject. The fire service training environment includes both rookies and senior personnel, adult learners and students fresh out of school. In addition, it is populated by both students who know what to do and those who think they know what to do. Fast learners and those requiring more individual efforts will challenge even the most seasoned instructors.

The best instructors can present material effectively for all types of learners. Instructors who protect those who struggle by placing them in positions where they can make progress without the embarrassment of failure in front of the greater group will be successful. Good instructors also learn how to use the more talented department members to coach and teach those with lesser skills.

Learning to work within the environment challenges you to be flexible, loyal, confident, and fair. Building a bond of trust with your students will enable you to present new ideas and make needed revisions to old traditions. As the instructor, you are the visionary of the fire service.

The Instructor's Role in the Future of the Department

Have you ever thought about what drives an organization? Why do some survive and others struggle as time forces change?

In examining the structure of a typical fire department, it is easy to point out the formal leader: It is the individual at the top of the pyramid, the chief who provides the formal direction for the troops to follow. The fire chief is responsible for the ultimate success or failure of the fire department. Of course, organizational charts are filled with many other positions as well, each of which has its own responsibility for providing direction in support of organizational objectives. It is within these ranks that you find assistant, deputy, battalion, and division chiefs; line officer positions, including captains and lieutenants; and fire marshals and inspectors.

Where does the instructor fit within this scheme? In many fire departments, the instructor is treated as an operational support assignment more than an official rank or position. The instructor position is often viewed from one of two extremes: as vitally important to the overall operation or as unnecessary by the administration. They may also have a rank, be scene safety officers, or hold other responsibilities in the department. Wise leaders understand that instructors are important members of the team. They use their instructors to maintain their department's state of readiness and prepare their fire fighters for future missions.

It is this role—preparation for future activities—that requires you to keep ahead of the curve. To fulfill it, you must become a visionary force within the fire department. It is vision that drives instructors to keep abreast of the ever-changing world of firefighting. Changes and advancements in firefighting tactics must be reviewed and implemented through revisions in training curriculum. If the fire department desires a change in operations, the instructor and training division will be charged with educating and training fire fighters to make that change. New techniques and advancements must be tested and made applicable to each organization, because many changes are not "one size fits all" measures. You will be challenged as you introduce new ideas that seem to conflict with established traditions.

As the mission of the fire service continues to evolve, you must be able to prepare the troops to carry out the new mission. The history of the fire service is full of pertinent examples, as the instructor has had to evolve to provide training for medical, hazardous materials, and technical rescue services. Today the threats of terrorism, active shooters, and scenes of violence, along with the use of weapons of mass destruction (WMDs), present their own unique challenges for the fire service, with instructors once again being called upon to lead the troops into these new areas of service.

Instructors must monitor the ever-changing learning environment as well. Struggles with budgets and staffing present ongoing problems for instructors, who must continually seek to keep training at the forefront of nonemergency operations. In the instructor role, you must find new and creative ways to reach students and present training. Today, visionary instructors are turning to the cyberworld as online training programs gain a foothold in the instructional world. Technology will continue to advance and, consequently, affect the delivery of training. Instructors with the vision to see how this new technology can be used for training purposes are establishing virtual learning environments and using satellite and video classrooms as effective learning media.

Given the unique challenges apparent in the modern-day fire service, the fire chief would be wise to select the very best personnel for the position of instructor. An instructor with vision can greatly assist the fire chief in meeting the fire department's future challenges.

The Instructor's Role in Succession Planning

Preparing fire fighters for battle is not the only job of the instructor. For any organization to survive and grow, a continuity plan must be in place. Continuity of the organization provides security for the community that the organization serves. The instructor can assist in that regard by becoming involved in **succession planning**.

As trainers of fire fighters, instructors are often in the best position to recognize potential talent and leadership qualities in the fire fighters and officers they train. The instructor's role is to nurture and challenge these fire fighters through the training program. During the course of training, the instructor may use some fire fighters to assist in training other members. By placing fire fighters in leadership positions within the training environment, you allow them to refine, enhance, and demonstrate their leadership qualities.

The instructor may also be in the position of providing input to ranking officers on the performance of fire fighters in training. By recommending high achievers to fire department administrators, you assist in the identification of future fire officers and instructors. You may also be in the best position to identify those fire fighters who do not fit the model fire officer that the fire department has established.

Succession planning also means looking for future instructors who someday will take your place as the lead instructor in your department. As difficult or as uncomfortable as it might seem, identifying, nurturing, and training their replacements is something successful instructors need to learn to do. Another way to approach this goal is to identify someone who is capable of building upon the foundation that you, as an instructor, have established, and can move it to the next level. Because you have worked hard to develop a successful training program, the last thing you would like to see happen is to have the program fail. Herein lies the opportunity to find another fire fighter who is passionate, skilled, and has the desire to train the other members of the department. Succession planning is discussed later in this chapter.

The instructor walks a fine line between operations and training. In organizations with a weak operations leadership, the instructor may become absorbed with setting the operational direction and standards simply because he or she has expertise in specific areas. In other cases, the instructor has a formal role in establishing policy. Of course, you should be careful to ensure that those policies exist to support the direction of the operations division—not the other way around. Although you may not always agree with the standards chosen by the operations chief, you must accept that direction and train fire fighters accordingly.

Instructor Credentials and Qualifications

You've heard it before: "Walk the talk." It's a phrase that can certainly be applied to the instructor. Your best friend is the confidence that your students have in your abilities and knowledge. This is a quality that cannot be learned from a book. Often, instructors are born in the learning environment from energetic students. Others vow to develop their instructional skills after attending a highly charged training session or a lecture delivered by an impassioned instructor. As an instructor, you must be aware that your success or failure might rest with the degree of effort and preparation you put forth at the beginning of your career in the fire service. It is here that dividends are paid.

Laying the Groundwork

Good instructors are born from good students—students who thrive on the knowledge gained through training, and those who actively participate in training activities and are not afraid to learn from their initial failures. These individuals are the fire fighters who understand the value of education and refinement of skills. They continually place themselves in learning situations, looking to upgrade their skills and knowledge.

Think for a moment about the instructors who have influenced you. Students attending any training program immediately focus their attention on the instructor as they begin looking for clues about the quality of the program. They might ask what experience the instructor has in the subject area. What is the instructor's firefighting experience level? If the training is being held in-house, your students might remember the days when you were a student. Your credibility in the learning environment depends on your past behavior. The past always has a way of finding the future, so it is always wise to protect your future by engaging in proper behavior in the present. Laying the groundwork for becoming a good instructor begins the day you join the profession. While some mistakes will be made, you must always guard your credibility and integrity.

Meeting Standards

Standards dictate many things within the fire service. Training programs are not immune from national standards. Standards set the bar for instructors' proficiency and knowledge. They seek to establish uniformity for instructors across the entire profession. NFPA 1041 outlines the instructional levels in the fire service and guides instructor trainer programs; this book is written to be in compliance with this standard. Fire fighters seeking local, state, provincial, or national instructor certifications may be asked to demonstrate compliance with NFPA 1041 as well, though it may not be the only standard that the instructor must meet.

A **degree** is awarded by an institution of higher learning after a person has completed acquisition of the required knowledge in a particular field. A **certificate** is given after attendance at a course. A **certification** is awarded after a person has passed an examination process that is based on a set standard such as an NFPA Professional Qualifications standard.

Fire chiefs and fire departments are free to establish their own set of qualifications for instructors. If the instructor is asked to teach only one class in one department, he or she may not be asked to obtain a formal certification from a certifying agency. Instead, the instructor may simply receive the training that the fire department deems necessary from other in-house instructors. In some cases, instructors may be asked to have a certain number of years of experience prior to taking on an instructional assignment. In other cases, instructor positions might be reserved for those with command authority, holding a line officer's or chief officer's position. Some fire departments set few or no additional requirements in an effort to find a fire fighter willing to take on the extra responsibilities of the instructor.

Whatever the case, it is wise to meet these challenges head on. Becoming an instructor may open doors for future promotions. Meeting the qualifications of this position will also prepare you for future leadership assignments; for example, Fire and Emergency Services Instructor I is a prerequisite for Fire Officer I in the NFPA standards system.

Continuing Education

Meeting requirements, whether set by a national standard or through fire department policy, is just the beginning for the instructor. Working within the dynamic world of the fire service means you need to continue your own professional growth and development. While some individuals dread the idea of **continuing education**, you need to understand the need to improve your knowledge, as it allows you to provide the very best and up-to-date information in the learning environment. The idea of requiring continuing education is not a new one. Many professions, including health care, education, and inspections, require their members to participate in continuing education to remain licensed or certified.

For the instructor, the organization that issues the initial certification decides what, if any, continuing education is necessary. Some states may require only proof of continued instructional activity. Do not rely on the requirements of outside entities as a motivational force to professional growth. You should always strive to be on the cutting edge of the fire service. Attend outside trainings, seminars, and instructional conferences to stay up-to-date with the most current fire-ground tactics, management practices, and instructional techniques available.

Building Confidence

By keeping abreast of the latest information, you demonstrate the very value of education. For learning to occur, students must believe in your knowledge of the subject—which is not to say that you will always know everything about a particular topic.

There is a saying that in the learning environment: "The instructor is always right." Believing in this old adage could be a fatal mistake and result in the eventual loss of your credibility. It does not take many times of being proven wrong in the learning environment to lose the confidence of your students.

Building and maintaining student confidence in both the instructor and the training program go hand-in-hand. Instructors can build high levels of confidence in several ways. For example, you can demonstrate your own commitment to lifelong learning through continuing education. Be willing to admit that you are in doubt about a particular question and seek the answers for the inquisitive student instead of trying to make something up on the fly in an attempt to impress your pupils. Be open to the suggestions and ideas of the students. Because instructors often serve in operational roles as well, be very careful about following all teachings when working the emergency scene or when in the supervision role. One sure-fire way to lose credibility is to project a "do as I say, not as I do" attitude.

Issues of Ethics in the Training Environment

Firefighting is perhaps one of the most respected professions in today's society. The task of maintaining the public's trust in its fire service is held in high regard by all those who wear the uniform.

Ethics reaches beyond laws and standards to define behavior. Codes of ethics spell out what is acceptable and what is unacceptable within a fire department. For many individuals, ethics is rooted in their own personal assessment of right versus wrong (or values), which begins during their early upbringing. Ethics can reflect the attributes of the people we respect and interact with in our own profession. In the end, it is perhaps that feeling in the pit of your stomach—your "gut" instinct—that gives you the best clue about whether a certain behavior is ethical.

The issue of ethical behavior also affects the training program. Instructors are often the ones who are asked to judge which candidates are ready to provide public service. Failing to hold students accountable for their learning objectives or simply passing fire fighters through the training program in the interest of moving on is unacceptable by any standard. This failure to hold to agency standards will affect not only the fire fighter who "slips" through but also those with whom this fire fighter works, and ultimately the instructor who did not maintain the standards of the agency.

Another aspect of ethical conduct from an instructor's point of view is to ensure that your teaching methods and learning environment behavior are acceptable to all students. The fire service has evolved

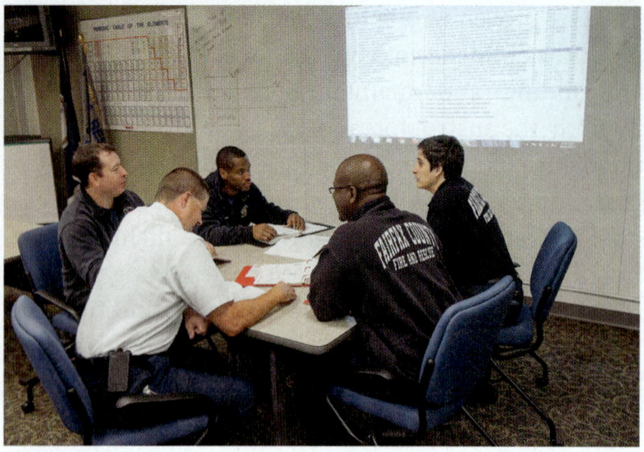

FIGURE 1-8 An effective instructor is aware of who their students are and have a desire for all of them to be successful.

over the years to include members from across all demographics and socioeconomic levels of our society; as an instructor, you have a responsibility to be aware of and sensitive to the diverse backgrounds of your students. This might sound challenging or difficult, but the solution is actually quite simple—treat everyone equally and fairly. It is important to acknowledge the diversity that is found in our learning environments and fire departments. Effective instructors are aware of who their students are and strive to teach all of them with compassion, fairness, and a desire for all of them to be successful in whatever subject is being taught (**FIGURE 1-8**).

Leading by Example: What You Do, You Teach

Ethics in training must begin with the instructor. Instruction must extend beyond the learning environment and into everyday operations. Instructors demonstrate ethical behavior through their "do as I say and as I do" lifestyles. Leading by good example lays the cornerstone for training ethics. If you are responsible for teaching the confidentiality of disciplinary measures in a leadership class but are later seen discussing an employee's behavior around the coffee table, you will lose credibility. Instructors must recognize early on that they are always being watched and their actions are often mimicked by their students.

COMPANY-LEVEL TRAINING TIP

Increasing diversity in the fire service is a major initiative. Instructors at all levels must possess the cultural competencies to provide training to a variety of genders, ethnicities, and generations.

Accountability in Training

Another ethical issue related to the training program is the need to maintain student accountability for training. As an example, if 10 fire fighters attend training on pump operations but only 4 fire fighters actually operate the pump while the remaining 6 chat away, who should receive credit for pump training?

Never put yourself in a position of simply passing a student by rote. It is important to document students who fail to meet training objectives. Because the training program is tasked with preparing fire fighters for critical life-safety operations, you must be dedicated to protecting the program's integrity. The classroom or drill ground is no place for favors and friendship to affect a student's achievement record. At the end of the day, the fire fighter's performance ultimately judges your ability as an instructor.

Recordkeeping

Good records are important to any training program, but only if those records are thorough and accurate. Just as you must maintain accountability in individual training accomplishments, you must also maintain accurate records of program achievements. Training that is not fully completed owing to interruptions should never be recorded as accomplished.

Some instructors have been known to falsify records by simply recording trainings or skill attainments that did not occur for one reason or another. This act of falsification, also known as "pencil whipping an exercise," might look good on paper, but can lead to disastrous consequences once fire fighters have to perform the task under the stress of a true emergency or during a legal issue.

All training sessions must be documented, and accuracy is critical in those records. The records must contain a factual listing of the accomplished objectives. Whenever training records are found to be inaccurate, whether due to negligence or simply because of an error, your credibility will be called into question. Accurate recordkeeping builds confidence in the training program and sets ethical expectations for all to follow.

The accuracy of training records is not only an ethical issue but also a legal issue. In recent court cases dealing with fire fighter fatalities, training records have been used as evidence both for and against the authority having jurisdiction (AHJ). Clearly, accurate and correct training records will have a tremendous influence in the outcome of such lawsuits. Recordkeeping as it pertains to the law is discussed in more detail later in this chapter.

Trust and Confidentiality

Trust and confidentiality go hand-in-hand: Lose one and you risk losing both. Both of these attributes have tremendous influence on how well you are able to lead in the learning environment and maintain an effective teaching ability.

Instructors are often one of the first points of contact fire fighters make when joining the fire department. As such, you are placed in a position where your trust and confidentiality are critical to students. Struggling students may relay personal information referencing problems in their personal lives to explain why they are having difficulty in completing a task. A student might also share information about learning disabilities that require special considerations in the learning environment. Conversations such as these require that you make every effort to maintain confidentiality. If circumstances require that fire department management become involved in the issue, then you should make that fact known first to the student. You may also provide guidance to students about where to go for assistance within the fire department's command structure.

Another area of concern is the need to maintain the confidentiality of student performance in the program. Information dealing with test scores, student evaluations, attendance, and behavioral issues should always be protected. Guidelines for the recording and sharing of this type of information should be written into policy to protect students' rights. Instructors are often required to handle sensitive student information and must consistently demonstrate the ability to do so with professionalism.

The Law as It Applies to Fire and Emergency Service Instructors

In the fire service, training is designed both to keep existing skills sharp and to introduce new skills. Every training session exposes the instructor and the fire department to potential liability. For example, inappropriate comments voiced in a training session based on religion, nationality, gender, or sex—even if made in jest—can subject the instructor and the fire department to liability. A good working knowledge of the law, standard operating guidelines, and the department's own rules and regulations will reduce the potential exposure to liability. An understanding of the legal issues pertaining to training is critical for instructors. You will likely encounter situations during training evolutions, classroom participation, and your daily duties when issues pertaining to federal law will arise. You may face questions about compliance with the Americans with Disabilities Act (ADA), hostile work environment claims, and complaints of sexual harassment. A strong familiarity with these federal laws will prepare you to fulfill your obligations properly. State law could come into play on issues of privacy, indemnification, injuries to training participants, and equipment failures.

It is only through familiarity with the appropriate laws that you can insulate yourself and the fire department from potential liability. Directly associated with familiarity is proper recordkeeping. Maintaining an appropriate documentation system affords you some level of protection; conversely, inadequate or incomplete records may expose you to increased liability.

As an instructor, your conduct is governed by three sources of law:

- Federal law, which is made up of statutory laws
- State law, which is established by each state's legislature
- Policies and procedures crafted by each individual fire department

All three sources set expectations for and restrictions on the conduct of instructors (**FIGURE 1-9**). Nevertheless, federal and state laws differ from a fire department's policies and procedures in an important way. Federal and state laws apply evenly to all citizens and are the standard by which all instructors are measured. The ADA and the Age Discrimination in Employment Act (ADEA) are two examples of federal laws that govern all citizens across the nation. By contrast, policies and procedures are specific to a particular

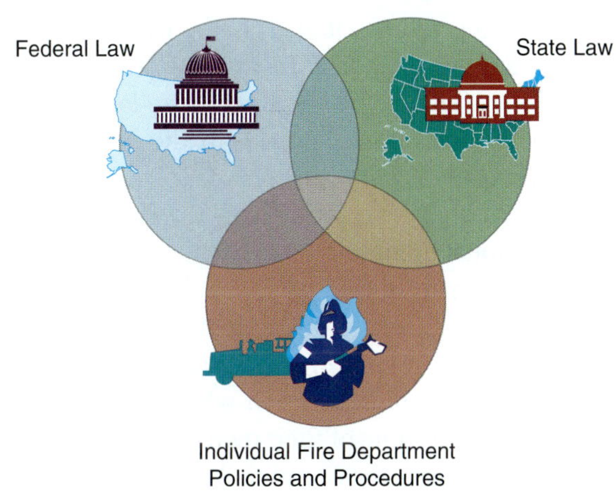

FIGURE 1-9 All three sources of law set expectations for and restrictions on the instructor's conduct.

fire department and vary from region to region within a state, because each fire department must take into consideration numerous variables, such as the size of the community it serves, its locale, and its resources.

A fire department's policies and procedures must not violate any state or federal laws. Indeed, they do not have the same status in the law as state and federal statutes. A fire department's policies and procedures represent the minimum expectations of the fire department and do not necessarily impose a legal duty, as does a state or federal law. The only true benchmark against which the departmental policies and procedures are measured is the national standards or guidelines set within the fire service. Departmental policies and procedures can place obligations upon an instructor that are not otherwise required by federal and state laws. For instance, a fire department's policies and procedures may require the department's instructor to keep all department licenses and permits up-to-date, even though there is no legal requirement for the instructor to do so. The policies and procedures may also specify additional recordkeeping requirements not set forth by state or federal laws.

Federal law is the broadest, in that it applies to all persons and requires the same expectations across the board regardless of your chosen profession or the state in which you live or work. For example, the ADA, the ADEA, and Title VII govern not only fire departments but private employers as well. State laws are somewhat narrower, in that they apply only to the state in which they are enacted. State laws set some expectations for that state, but are not necessarily specific to a profession. The policies and procedures of a fire department have the narrowest scope, being designed specifically for an individual department and the professionals who work in it.

Although the law is designed to set certain standards and expectations, it also can be used to protect instructors from lawsuits. Instructors must have a working knowledge of federal and state laws. In addition, they must be well versed in the policies and procedures of their particular fire department, which requires that they possess a strong working knowledge of national guidelines. Although national guidelines are not legally binding on a fire department, they clearly set out the consensus of the fire service across the United States. The NFPA standards, for example, are the national standards upon which most fire departments model some of their own standards.

Should an instructor's conduct be called into question, the national guidelines serve as the backdrop against which that conduct will be judged. For example, if a live fire training session gets out of control, the instructor's methods will be compared to NFPA 1403: *Standard on Live Fire Training Evolutions* to determine whether the instructor's conduct was reasonable. NFPA 1403 outlines a checklist of safety activities when performing a live fire training session, which includes activities such as ensuring that all utilities are disconnected and that proper permits have been obtained. If an instructor does not follow this checklist, his or her conduct may be considered unreasonable and result in liability.

Instructors have an immense responsibility to conduct, manage, and administer training programs. With that responsibility comes the potential for liability if an injury, accident, fatality, or lawsuit occurs. In our increasingly litigious society, the instructor must be aware of the laws that pertain to each level of instructor responsibility. All certification levels of instructor will have different applications of laws and statutes in the performance of their duty areas, and professional development as an instructor will be necessary throughout your career to review trends and keep up-to-date on cases that have occurred and judgments for and against a fire department and its training program.

COMPANY-LEVEL INSTRUCTOR TIP

Instructors who teach to the national standards, document their instruction, and provide a safe learning environment are not high-risk targets for lawsuits. It is when an instructor does not teach the correct information or does not maintain safety as a top priority that potential liabilities increase.

Federal Employment Laws

As an instructor, you are not expected to know all the laws of the land, but to perform your job correctly you do need to understand three laws: the Americans with Disabilities Act, Title VII, and Section 1983 of the Civil Rights Act of 1964. In all likelihood, you will be called upon to teach or arrange instruction on each of these laws. You will also encounter situations that will require you to act or react to situations involving the practical application of these three laws. Here is a brief summary of their content:

- Americans with Disabilities Act: Prohibits discrimination against a qualified person because of a disability, where discrimination may include hiring, firing, promotions, and compensation
- Civil Rights Act of 1964: Prohibits discrimination based on race, sex, or national origin
- Title VII of the Civil Rights Act: Prohibits discrimination that creates a hostile work environment

Americans with Disabilities Act

The Americans with Disabilities Act of 1990 is designed to protect individuals with disabilities from discrimination in the workplace. A **disability** is a physical or mental impairment that substantially limits one or more major life activities. In 2008, the ADA was amended with the primary purpose of expanding what constitutes a disability. Determining whether an impairment substantially limits a major life activity should not take into account possible mitigating measures. Mitigating measures include medication, medical supplies, prosthetics, hearing aids, mobility devices, and the like. The mitigating measures of ordinary eyeglasses and contact lenses, however, are considered in determining whether an impairment substantially limits a major life activity. While the definition itself did not change with the 2008 revision of the ADA, the amendment added instructions to follow when determining what constitutes a disability. **Major life activities** include functions such as caring for oneself, performing manual tasks, walking, seeing, hearing, speaking, breathing, learning, and working. Conditions that previously would not have qualified as a disability—such as compulsive gambling, kleptomania, pyromania, and current illegal use of drugs—may now be considered a disability. It should also be noted that an impairment that is episodic or on remission is considered a disability if it would limit a major life activity when active.

In the fire service, it is unlikely that you will encounter physical disabilities such as blindness or the inability to walk. Nevertheless, you may encounter many other types of disabilities, including psychological disorders, neurological disorders, cardiac issues, respiratory issues, diabetes, epilepsy, dyslexia, drug and alcohol addiction, and prosthetic devices.

If you are approached by an individual alleging a disability, you should undertake a two-step analysis. First, you must determine whether an actual disability exists. If the answer to that question is yes, then you must determine whether the disability can be reasonably accommodated. The ADA defines **reasonable accommodation** as a modification or adjustment to a job or work environment that will enable a qualified applicant or employee with a disability to perform the essential functions of the job or enjoy the benefits and privileges of employment, and that does not create an undue hardship for the employer. For example, if a fire fighter has diabetes, a reasonable accommodation may be to allow for periodic blood glucose testing during the day or during training (**FIGURE 1-10**).

Examples of reasonable accommodations found to be in compliance with the ADA include modifying facilities to make them accessible to employees with disabilities, restructuring a job, modifying the work schedule, acquiring or modifying equipment, and reassigning a disabled employee to a vacant position for which the individual is qualified. Accommodation is not automatic—that is, you are not required to make an accommodation if it would impose an undue hardship on the operation. An undue hardship exists if the accommodation would require significant difficulty or expense relative to the size, resources, and nature of the employer.

Further, a reasonable accommodation does not have to be provided if doing so would present a **direct threat** to the health or security of others. Four factors are considered when assessing whether a direct threat exists: the duration of the risk, the nature and severity of the potential harm, the likelihood that potential harm will occur, and the imminence of the potential harm.

Like many legal situations, ADA issues are fact driven. There is no "bright line" test; each case must be analyzed based on the particular facts at hand. Courts

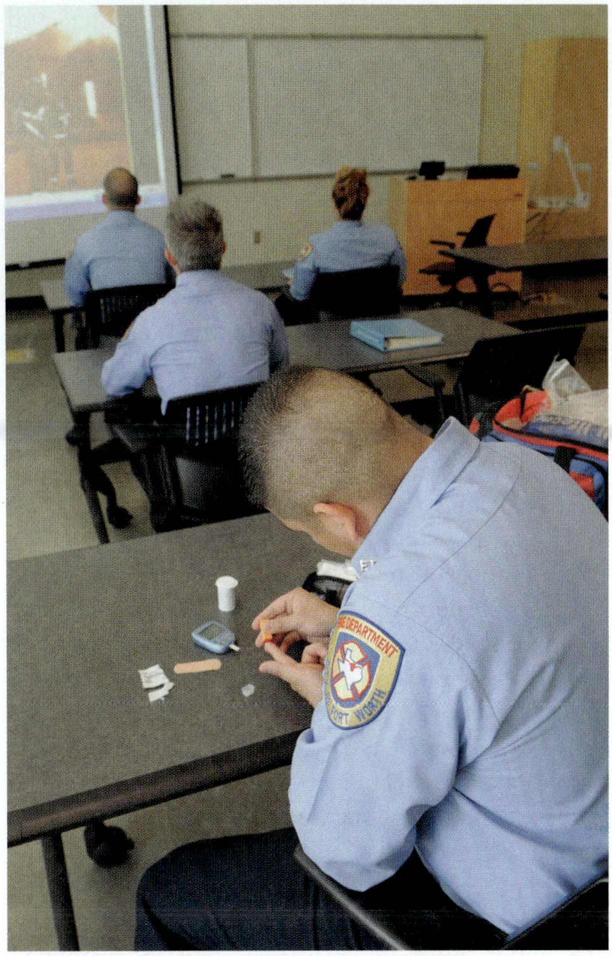

FIGURE 1-10 A reasonable accommodation may include allowing for periodic blood glucose testing during the day or during training.

have ruled on many cases involving fire fighters and the ADA, and those rulings can provide guidance for you in similar situations. For example, the U.S. Court of Appeals for the Fifth Circuit has held that a fire department is not required to accommodate a fire fighter who is unable to perform the essential duties of firefighting owing to a back injury when no light-duty position exists in a small fire department (*Burch v. City of Nacogdoches*, 5th Cir.). In Pennsylvania, a fire department was not required to provide a fire fighter with a second chance at the academy course after he failed due to depression. In Maryland, the court held that it was proper for a fire department to prohibit a fire fighter from using an inhaler when the brand used was highly flammable (*Huber v. Howard County Maryland*, 4th Cir.).

It is important for the instructor and managers up the chain of command to be aware of both the requirements of the ADA and those personnel under their command who qualify for reasonable accommodation under the ADA. In situations when an accommodation is requested during a training evolution, you should take great care to evaluate the request and, if needed, contact a higher authority for advice. Once a decision is made, it should be documented immediately to protect both you and the fire department. Not all medical and psychological issues qualify as disabilities under the ADA. Each issue must be examined separately. Also, any accommodation request must be reasonable.

Freedom of Information Act

Each state has freedom of information laws that govern public access to government records, documents, and other information kept by government bodies. The purpose of the Freedom of Information Act (FOIA) is to promote government accountability and the public's right to know. Although each state has its own variation on FOIA, generally the laws require the following records and information to be made available to the general public upon request:

- Administrative manuals and procedures
- Instructions to staff
- Substantive rules
- Statements and interpretations of policy
- Final planning policies
- Factual reports (such as inspection reports)
- Information about accounts, vouchers, and contracts involving the expenditure of public funds
- Names, salaries, titles, and dates of employment for all employees and public officers
- Meeting notes or recordings
- All records, reports, forms, writings, letters, memoranda, books, and papers (even if in electronic form). This may include training records and reports, such as training rosters.

Generally, members of the public can make a FOIA request through designated public officials. Depending on the applicable state law, there may be exceptions to the disclosure of certain documents or the government body releasing the documents may be required to redact personal information from certain documents. In addition, government entities may be required to retain public records for a specific period of time. In most cases, state record retention laws will dictate the minimum length of time public records must be retained by government entities. Please review your state law and consult with your attorney for more specific information about the requirements of FOIA, the exceptions to FOIA disclosure, and the record retention requirements in your state.

Records, Reports, and Confidentiality

Once you understand the laws that apply to you as an instructor, the next logical question is this: How do you perform your job so that you abide by the law and have protection should a lawsuit be filed? The first line of defense is always proper and thorough recordkeeping. Creating and maintaining records, reports, memoranda, e-mails, and other records in the course of your duties places you in a good position. These records should be constructed contemporaneously and maintained for a reasonable period of time and in accordance with any local law.

The recordkeeping process starts at the outset of each activity. For example, when you are organizing a training evolution, the materials you prepare should set forth the purpose of the training, the activities to be performed, the equipment to be used, and the goals of the training. You should have available any sources that were relied upon in creating the evolution and should confirm that the training complies with all policies and procedures of your fire department.

Lawsuits evolve over long periods of time, which means that the accuracy of your records is vital in mounting a defense against such litigation. Proper recordkeeping is as important as the training you provide to your department. In cases where an injury occurs to a participant in or an observer of a training session, it is crucial to document what occurred, who was present, and what each person observed. The same holds true for claims of sexual harassment: It is necessary for the person who receives the report to document what was said and which actions were taken once the complaint was received.

Proper documentation is essential to the performance of your job, as is storage of the records in an organized and secure setting. Both state and federal laws (Privacy Act of 1979) prohibit the disclosure of certain information. Most likely, your department has a policy or procedure that requires the protection of personal information that is kept in the control of the instructor. Failure to abide by the **confidentiality** provisions required by law or your department could lead to liability or adverse action against you.

Records that should be kept secure and confidential include the following:

- Personnel files: Usually include information such as date of birth, Social Security number, dependent information, and medical information
- Hiring files: Include test scores, pre-employment physical reports, psychological reports, and personal opinions about the candidate
- Disciplinary files: Any report or document about an individual's disciplinary history and related reports

Regardless of the type of training being provided, recordkeeping should be a top priority as part of risk management. Records with sign-in sheets and the topic presented should be maintained for all training sessions for a period of at least 5 years, or longer as required by law. You should also keep copies of the handouts, training outline, and other training materials presented with the sign-in sheet. Records, reports, or memoranda related to any unusual occurrences that happen during training or that are reported to you should be kept for at least 5 years. Because many lawsuits are filed long after the event occurred, the only real protection from this risk for the fire department may be the records kept. Incomplete or missing records often make defending suits more difficult.

Copyright and Public Domain

Many materials you may want to use in training are protected by copyright. More than 3 decades ago, Congress passed the Copyright Act of 1976, which governs copyright issues. The act divides work into two general categories: those protected by the law and those considered to be part of the public domain. Works include written words, photographs, and some artwork. The Copyright Act sets out some specific time frames pertaining to copyrighted material. Any work published before 1923 is considered to be in the public domain. Any works published between 1923 and 1978 have a 95-year copyright protection from the date of actual publication. For any works published after 1978, the author, artist, or photographer has a copyright for life plus 70 years. Violation of the copyright law can result in liability, with the creator of the work being eligible to recover any damages suffered or lost profits.

When providing training materials for fire service employees, many of the handouts used are photocopied from copyrighted materials. The Copyright Act does not prohibit their use outright or require that permission be sought before they are used. Indeed, the fact that some material is protected by a copyright does not necessarily prohibit you from using it in your training, because a "fair use" exception exists relative to the protection afforded by copyrights. Examples of fair use include copying materials for the purpose of criticizing, commenting, news reporting, teaching, and research. Copies for the class in a training session generally fall into this category. Ultimately, fair use depends on the nature of the copyrighted work and how much of the work is copied. For example, it would not be fair use to purchase one copy of a textbook and make copies of the entire book for the class. By contrast, if you want to use an article from a magazine or newspaper for learning environment purposes, that would likely fall within the fair use exception.

If a particular use does not constitute fair use, you may still be able to use the material in a learning environment by contacting the copyright holder and seeking permission in advance to use that material. You should obtain permission in writing prior to using the material.

Whether a work is copied under the fair use exception or with permission, it should include a notice indicating who holds the copyright to the work.

Managing Multiple Priorities as an Instructor

In today's fast-paced world, we are bombarded with many priorities, each demanding our attention and time. As a consequence, success or failure is often determined by the ability to understand and prioritize tasks. Recognition, planning, and delegation are skills that can assist those facing multiple tasks while maneuvering through sometimes hectic and complicated assignments.

Time Management

As an instructor, one of the first skills you need to learn and develop is time management. Several methods or techniques are available to help you make the best use of your time. You should select those techniques that suit your personality and are easy and convenient to use. For example, setting a goal to read one magazine article per shift, or per week, is a good start. Attending one fire service conference per year and earning a new certification are goals that will help in your development.

One helpful method is to set time aside each day to create a "to do" list. Prioritize the items on this list, and then work your way through them, checking off what you have accomplished. Included on this list might be reading an article or reviewing a department SOP. Another method is to set goals for the year and break the goals down into months and weeks. Use whatever method works for you: The key is to develop a system that fits your needs. When creating your personal "to do" list, be mindful of any recertification requirements for your certifications or job position. As a fire fighter and instructor, you might have required hours of continuing education or "recert" hours that must be earned in a set period of time. As you are setting your goals and priorities for the year, make sure that your own credentials do not expire! Budget the time and resources needed to obtain new or renewed certifications, and do not wait until the last moment to complete these requirements.

Regardless of which system you use or develop, perhaps the most important part of successful time management is learning to prioritize your "to do" list. Too often we spend a great deal of time on low-priority items that are easy to handle but distract us from the more important items on our list. Learning how to prioritize your list takes self-discipline and practice. Another challenge to accomplishing the items on your "to do" list is balancing your list against that of your organization. When developing this list, make sure every item supports the mission and goals of your agency. Finding this balance will help you develop both as an individual and as a professional in your organization.

Training Priorities

Managing today's modern fire and emergency services creates multiple priorities for the training program. Deciding what and when to teach is just one of the challenges. The direction that the program takes may be decided at different levels depending on the fire department's organization. In some cases, upper management may choose to lay out the training schedule for the period and then leave it to the instructor to decide how to accomplish it. If the fire chief takes a hands-off approach to training, then the instructor may be asked to develop both the schedule and the training program's objectives.

Training priorities may also reflect specific community characteristics. For example, a community with a heavy chemical industrial presence may place additional emphasis on hazardous materials training. Large cities with high-rise construction may require extra training on high-angle rescue and high-rise fire operations. Rural communities may require training on water supply shuttle operations and farm rescue. Training priorities are driven by mandatory training requirements to maintain certifications or Occupational Safety and Health Administration (OSHA) regulations. Clearly, the task of setting training priorities is not a simple one.

Decisions about how precious training time should be spent must include input from all levels of the fire department. Fire company officers may be able to provide valuable insight into fire-ground performance issues affecting operations; perhaps some problematic issues could be corrected through additional training. Fire chiefs may have knowledge of changes in future missions that will require fire fighters to learn new skills. Training committees may need to be established to provide a broad-based perspective regarding the fire department's training needs, tackling the question, "Should we train more on our most serious hazards or on those hazards we respond to most often?" Both elements deserve consideration in the planning process (**FIGURE 1-11**).

Planning a Program

The level of success of any training program is directly proportional to the planning efforts. In career settings, the schedules of on-duty personnel must be considered when setting up training programs. By contrast, instructors who are dealing with volunteer and part-time fire fighters must take into account the availability of personnel to leave their full-time jobs and to balance family time with the many department requirements. Holidays, vacations, multiple shifts, injuries, and illnesses all affect the need to reschedule or make up lost training opportunities.

The program must also plan for the use of training facilities and equipment. In some cases, outside instructors with special expertise may need to be scheduled.

No employee likes surprises, so consideration of the fire fighter's efforts to be put forth during training and other personal commitments require that training program schedules and completion requirements be established well in advance and communicated clearly to all. Once established, training schedules need to be followed as closely as possible. Although changes will

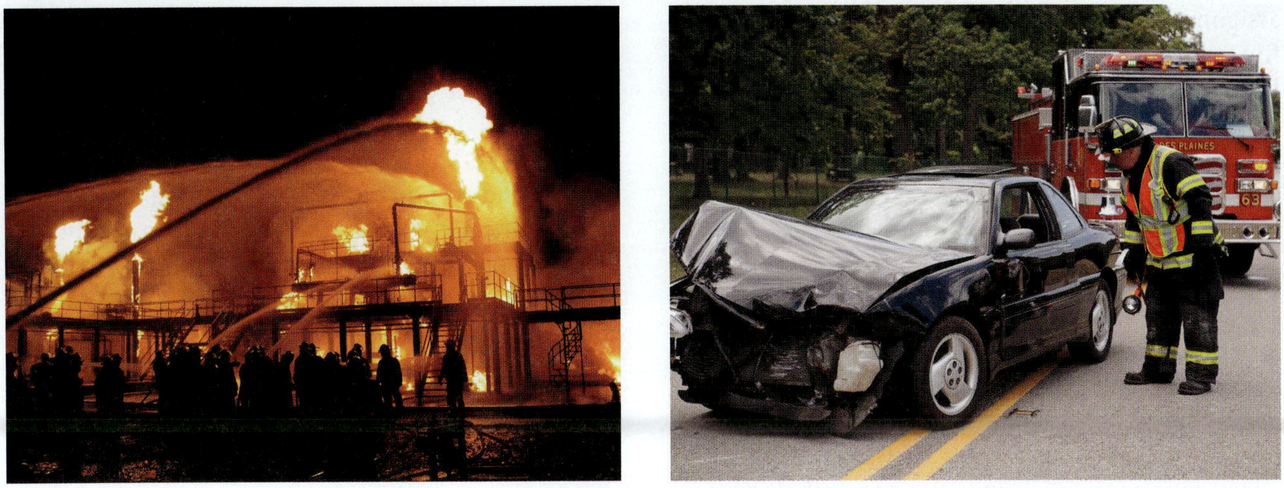

A B

FIGURE 1-11 A refinery or industry fire is an example of a low-frequency-high-risk incident **(A)**. Training committees can identify high-frequency incidents such as a motor vehicle accident and ensure that risk management practices, such as proper apparatus positioning and PPE use, are in place **(B)**.

A: Courtesy of University of Nevada, Reno Fire Science Academy; **B:** © Jones & Bartlett Learning. Photographed by Glen E. Ellman.

inevitably need to be made, any changes should be implemented with as much advance notice as possible and with sufficient time planned for rescheduling of the training to allow fire fighters to readjust their own schedules.

In some locations, a learning environment may be shared by the city government, community access groups, and fire department training programs. Nothing is more frustrating to both fire fighters and instructors than to have an overlap of scheduling or other unforeseen event force a last-minute cancellation or location change of a training session. Given the very nature of emergency services, it is always difficult to schedule training and execute it according to schedule without interruption. In a combination or volunteer organization, conflicting priorities of personal and professional life outside the fire station make the program management portion of fire service training all the more important.

Program management aspects of running a training division and training program include many basic management skills learned in fire officer training, albeit focused in this case on the goals and objectives of the training division. Administration of training policy and procedures, training recordkeeping systems, selection of instructional staff, review of curricula, and design of programs and courses that meet the current and future needs of the organization require a training team to accomplish many tasks.

Instructors also need to plan the content of individual training sessions. Without planning, conflicts among competing groups can arise in the use of facilities and lead to a delay or cancellation of a scheduled training session, further eroding confidence in the instructor's abilities. Contingencies for the use of specialized equipment needed in training evolutions must be built in if dedicated training equipment is not available. The instructor should also plan how a missed training session will be made up and ensure that make-up sessions accomplish the same learning objectives as the original training. Training time should be planned to eliminate distractions and interruptions. This may not always be possible when students attend training while on duty and as part of in-service training, as the need to respond to an emergency can interrupt even the best-laid plans.

Training Through Delegation

Instructors are faced with many tasks in managing the fire department's training program. Planning and scheduling for a multitude of priorities, developing and reviewing curricula, evaluating program effectiveness, coaching and mentoring students, and instructing all place enormous demands on the instructor's time. Without assistance, it is easy to become burned out, even for the most dedicated instructor.

One way to minimize the potential for burnout is through **delegation**. Be alert to those fire fighters who have shown through recognized efforts the ability to handle additional training assignments. Be observant in the learning environment for students who show an interest in instructional activities. It is often said that there is no better way to learn a subject than to have to teach it. Learning can be achieved through delegation, and you can obtain valuable assistance through the assignment of certain instructional tasks to competent fire fighters. Delegate only those tasks where a student has shown competency and where such a hand-off of responsibilities will not jeopardize the safety of other students.

Professional Development

Recall the instructors who shaped and influenced your development (both good and bad). What is the common thread among these individuals who had a positive impact on you? Most likely, they always had a magazine or an article in their hand or their nose in a book. The individuals who actively sought opportunities to learn were often the ones called upon to teach at a moment's notice because they had a wealth of knowledge that others wanted to hear. The same individuals attended conferences to learn and focused on networking with their peers. Eventually, they became presenters after obtaining a thorough knowledge base and developing their own ideas and theories to share with the fire service.

Another way to look at this idea is through an analogy. The speaker who is often heard at various fire service conferences did not start out as the keynote speaker. At one time he or she was just a fire fighter sitting in the audience, taking notes, and listening to every word. This person took what was learned at the conference, returned to the firehouse, and looked for ways to put that new knowledge into practice. As he or she learned more and advanced into higher positions within the department, the instructor had opportunities to teach new concepts and ideas to the next generation. The ideas, concepts, or theories that this individual shared stood the test of time and eventually became the basis for new policies and procedures followed within the department. Soon, word of mouth spread about these new ideas. The fire fighter who once sat in the audience taking notes is now on the stage leading the discussion and is respected by his or her peers as a leader in the profession. All of this came about because of the individual's desire to learn and to develop—because the fire fighter was a true lifelong learner.

An important part of becoming a quality instructor is having the basic desire to always improve and to become a better fire service professional. Who benefits when you develop into a respected instructor? Both you and the fire department benefit, because a good instructor supports the department's goals and, in turn, the department recognizes the instructor's critical value to the fire service.

As grand and interesting as being an instructor sounds, it also carries a great deal of responsibility. A department is often judged by the performance of its fire fighters. When a fire fighter is injured or killed in the line of duty, some of the first items reviewed and scrutinized are the training records and the qualifications of the instructors who taught that fire fighter during recruit school and during his or her time in the department. Keeping up-to-date on all changes and improvements in the fire service is a difficult but critical task. How do you stay informed, do your job effectively, and still maintain your personal life? When teaching a class, title an easel board "Resources." Over the course of the class, add resource information to this list and encourage students to do the same. Typically, this information will include website addresses, books, and names of other instructors.

Staying Current

Subscribe to trade magazines to stay up-to-date on trends and new developments in the fire service. Read other professional magazines in related fields, such as homeland security or business, as well. The benefit from reading trade journals is that this practice helps you stay current in the fire service. The benefit from reading material outside the fire service profession is that it helps you develop into a well-rounded individual and professional.

Another tool for you as an instructor is the internet. The web has opened the door to resources that were difficult to obtain in earlier years, but now are readily available to anyone who has a computer and internet access. The numerous websites hosted by colleges, professional journals, professional organizations, the National Fire Academy (NFA) and state fire academies, and government agencies offer volumes of information at minimal or no cost. Another online resource is the NFPA, which provides a variety of reports, online training, conferences, and workshops. This organization is also the source for the Fire Service Professional Qualifications Standards. Some material on the NFPA website is free, but other access requires a subscription.

One drawback to information found on the internet is the sometimes questionable accuracy of the content presented. If you use material from the internet, you need to verify the authenticity of the source and the accuracy of the information presented. More than one instructor has taken information from the internet and used it in a lesson plan, only to find that it was misleading or completely wrong. This, in turn, hurts the reputation of the instructor and may put students in harm's way. Another challenge when researching content on the internet is that a great deal of information is available at the click of a mouse, and you can easily spend too much time sifting through all you find. The internet is a tool and, just like with any other tool, you need to know how to use it properly.

Higher Education

Another method you can use for personal and professional development is to pursue a degree from an institution of higher education. Most departments require fire fighters to have a high school diploma or a GED as a condition of employment. In addition, many community or state colleges now offer degrees in fire science, emergency management, homeland security, or communication. Although this coursework is within your discipline, colleges also require you to take general education courses such as history and English literature as part of the degree program so that you will become a well-rounded thinker.

Higher education has become more accessible today than ever before, with degrees being offered by traditional colleges as well as online programs offered on the internet. Both of these delivery methods (traditional or online) provide the opportunity to earn an advanced degree and leave you the choice of which methodology you wish to pursue. One big advantage of pursuing an online degree is the convenience and flexibility it offers the student. You can "attend" class on your own schedule, while at the station or at home. Some higher education programs also offer a blended learning format, which combines the use of the internet for much of the classroom work but requires students to meet face-to-face with the instructor during certain points of the course. Check the institute's accreditation before obtaining an online degree. Some programs are not accredited, so your degree will not be recognized by other schools or your employer. Online courses and blended courses are discussed further in Chapter 6, *Technology in Training*.

An increasing number of departments have begun requiring an advanced degree for promotion, such as an associate's degree for the captain's position and a bachelor's degree for the battalion chief's position. Other departments offer financial incentives for engaging in continuing education, paying for college or even giving fire fighters a raise for each college-level course they complete. Attending college can be a time-consuming and expensive proposition. You may be willing to make the time commitment, but your finances may not be flexible enough to handle the entire cost. If so, take some time to investigate the many possible funding sources for which you may qualify. For example, your fire department or city may have a tuition reimbursement program. The federal government provides grants that are awarded to thousands of students every year. If you served in the armed forces, you may qualify for funding as a veteran. Many local charitable organizations also provide scholarships to students, including nontraditional students. Do not automatically assume that you cannot attend college because of money concerns. If you are willing to make the commitment and expend the effort, funding sources are available to support your continuing education.

A major incentive for obtaining a bachelor's degree is the requirement in place at the National Fire Academy that requires an advanced degree to be eligible to enter the Executive Fire Officer Program (EFOP). Beginning October 1, 2009, a bachelor's degree was required for entrance into the EFOP. The EFOP is considered by many to be a key to promotion as a chief officer and is a desirable qualification to add to your toolbox.

Conferences

Attendance at conferences, workshops, or seminars also offers you a chance to increase your skills and knowledge as an instructor (**FIGURE 1-12**). The many professional conferences put on every year provide opportunities for growth and development at all levels. Some conferences provide hands-on training opportunities, whereas others are limited to classroom

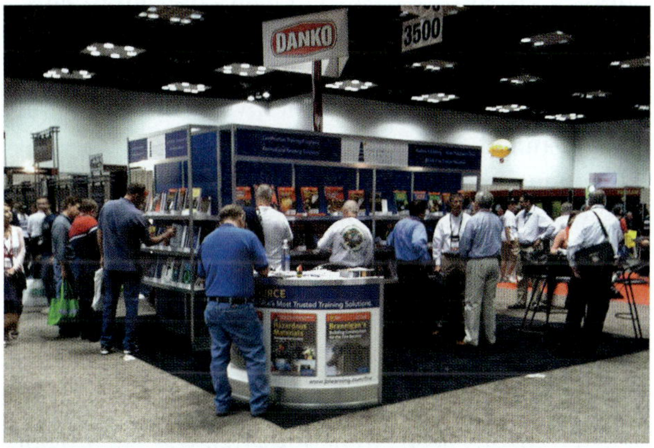

FIGURE 1-12 Attending conferences is an excellent self-improvement activity.
Courtesy of Brian Rooney.

lectures or presentations. One of the largest annual conferences that all instructors should attend if given the opportunity is the Fire Department Instructors Conference (FDIC), which is held each spring in Indianapolis, Indiana. FDIC offers a wide range of courses for everyone in the fire service, from the chief officer to the newest fire fighter. Many courses are directed at the instructor to improve presentation skills and research techniques, and provide new learning tools for instruction and a variety of other skills.

Other instructor conferences are held at the local and regional levels and provide opportunities to learn new skills, enhance your existing teaching skills, and learn from others. Regardless of which type of conference you choose to attend, take advantage of each and every opportunity to learn from your peers. Be willing to look outside the fire service and look for instructional learning opportunities in clubs, community organizations, and community college courses.

Take advantage of the opportunities at these conferences and workshops to network with other instructors from both within and outside the fire service community. Such conferences are great ways to learn new presentation skills that you can add to your own toolbox. **Networking** is a fundamental strategy used by great instructors to learn from others and to bounce an idea off a peer to determine whether it is valid. Networking is a powerful addition to your toolbox that can open the door to sharing or collaborating on an idea and developing a new methodology or course.

A major factor affecting today's fire service is the limited budget that every type of department faces. When an instructor asks the chief permission to attend FDIC or to pursue an advanced degree, the chief is thinking, "How does the department benefit from this investment?" The real benefit comes from instructors who return from the conferences or workshops and improve the way they teach or share new information with their fellow fire fighters and instructors. The relationship between the chief and the instructor is one of respect and trust, and one of investment and return on investment.

Although networking is often associated with politics and "schmoozing," what you are really doing when you network is creating a web of friends. The bigger the web, the more likely you are to have access to the precise resource you need when the time comes. Networking is designed as a give-and-take system.

The best way to create a large web is to be a giver. When someone needs something that you can provide, offer it. If someone has a question, answer it. Helping others be successful creates a powerful network that can work to your benefit. By giving, you become the person who is sought out: The more sought out you are, the more contacts you will have. Develop your network not by schmoozing but by being genuinely interested in helping others succeed.

Lifelong Learning

Lifelong learning is an endless path marked by endless opportunities. For the one person who says he or she has seen it all, there are a hundred other individuals who ask for more. A major career crusher is adopting the attitude that you cannot teach students anything new. Your greatest challenge is to create the desire to learn in all your students.

In your pursuit of becoming a lifelong learner, you need to remember the basics. Your teaching skills got you where you are, so continually brush up on your existing presentation skills and learn new ones. Remember the teacher in high school whom no one liked because he taught as if he was still locked in the past? Remember the high school teacher who stayed current and fresh to students? Those teachers who worked at truly "teaching" a subject and encouraging students to learn were the same teachers whose classes were the first to fill during registration. Learning can be enjoyable. Instructors who are willing to learn new methodologies to present information become valuable assets to the organization because of their willingness to learn and develop themselves into strong instructors.

Keeping your teaching skills sharp and current is just as important as reading magazines, networking, or going to college. If you are the senior instructor in the training division, make a point of teaching one subject once a month so that you keep your teaching skills up-to-date. As your knowledge base about the fire service has grown, have you stayed current with the types of students entering the fire service today? Are you still an effective instructor for the new generation of fire fighters? Test yourself by teaching a class. Be honest with yourself about how effective you were. Great instructors are lifelong teachers who love to teach.

An important skill to add to your toolbox is the acknowledgment and acceptance of the changes we are seeing in the fire service. The new generation of fire fighters is more diverse and has a strong understanding of technology. Effective instructors should recognize that today's students are different and learn how to teach them by using methods that will allow these students to learn the important skills that will save their lives and the lives of others. Perhaps instructional methodology needs to change to assist the new and diverse learners, but what we teach has not changed.

Firefighting is a dangerous profession, and fire will kill either a young or old fire fighter without regard to how they learn. Our job as instructors is to learn whatever methods will enable us to teach life-saving skills to those students whom we are responsible for teaching and training. Part of being an effective instructor is learning to scan the horizon for industry trends and to anticipate which will pan out. Part of this scanning process involves looking for new ways to enhance your skills and abilities. Attending a 1-day skills development program and reading a new book are two ways to stay on the cutting edge of your profession.

Professional Organizations

There are many professional organizations that you can join to help in your professional development. Some organizations operate on the national level, but most are found at the state, local, regional, provincial, or county level. (Among these are state training organizations.) Regardless of the level, these organizations provide many opportunities to network, share resources, and develop contacts. Some are very formal and highly structured, whereas others are more informal and relaxed.

The International Society of Fire Service Instructors (ISFSI) is an organization that is committed to the development of instructors. ISFSI actively supports the professional development of the fire service through its push for qualified instructors teaching quality material. The ISFSI has partnered with UL Firefighter Safety Research Institute (FSRI) and other agencies to develop model curriculums and instructional resources. ISFSI participates in state, local, and national instructor training events, including the FDIC, along with hosting its own national conference. As a member-driven organization, you can participate in many ways by becoming a member. Visit the ISFSI website for information.

The National Fire Academy, which is part of the National Emergency Training Center in Emmitsburg, Maryland, is the nation's "fire university." At the National Fire Academy, you can attend 6-day or 2-week courses that teach you how to develop lesson plans and build courses. In addition, other courses are available to help in all aspects of your professional and educational development. The National Fire Academy also supports two other programs that will help in your professional development: the FESHE initiative and the EFOP.

A key part of what the National Fire Academy is doing to professionalize the fire service can be seen in the FESHE initiative. Across the United States, many different community and state colleges and universities offer degrees in different aspects of fire service management or engineering, but there are no standardized model degree programs. The FESHE initiative is intended to bring together representatives from colleges and universities to develop a standardized degree format and model curricula. If college degree programs follow the same set of rules, students will be able to transfer coursework from one school to another more readily. In addition, courses would present a standard curriculum, which increases the ability to transfer college credits and standardizes the information taught. Another purpose of the FESHE initiative is to develop a career path for those seeking to be chief officers.

Part of this development process has resulted in the National Professional Development Model. This model summarizes the combination of education, training, certification, and experience that leads to the development of a well-rounded and fully developed fire officer who has the skills and ability to lead the fire service into the future.

The EFOP is another program developed by the National Fire Academy that has helped to professionalize the fire service. Its purpose is to provide senior officers with the tools they need to become leaders of the future. Acceptance into the EFOP is by application process only; that criteria can be found on the Federal Emergency Management Agency (FEMA) website. One of the key criteria for application in the EFOP is the individual's "potential for future impact on the fire service." Of the many positions in the fire service, instructors have one of the most crucial roles in influencing the future of their organizations and the fire service in their communities.

The EFOP requires a major time commitment from both the fire officer and the fire department. The program takes 4 years to complete, with attendance at the National Fire Academy for four 2-week courses. At the end of each course, the student is required to submit an applied research project (ARP) within 6 months of the course's ending date. This ARP is evaluated by peer reviewers against a set of criteria established by the National Fire Academy staff. Once the ARP is approved, the student can register for the next course in the series.

Each spring, the National Fire Academy hosts the annual EFOP Graduate Symposium on its campus in Emmitsburg, Maryland. Each year the symposium features a topic of interest to the fire service, and EFOP graduates give presentations on the symposium topic. This symposium serves as an opportunity for EFOP graduates to renew friendships, network, and "charge their batteries" as leaders in their organizations.

The Next Generation

A true mark of a great leader is his or her willingness to plan to be replaced. Succession planning is the process of identifying others within the department who could be mentored and coached to replace you and to carry out the functions you perform.

The concept of training your replacement can be very difficult and challenging to handle on an emotional level. It may be easier if you understand that the process of training another person to take your place usually means that you are also moving up and onward to something new. Another benefit of training your replacement is that you can select someone who shares your own ideals and goals, thereby ensuring that your training program will continue after you leave. Through this legacy, your influence could be felt for many decades in your department (**FIGURE 1-13**).

How do you train your replacement and help him or her to be successful? Four basic concepts will aid you in teaching your replacement:

1. Identifying
2. Mentoring
3. Coaching
4. Sharing

Identifying

Identifying is the process of selecting those whom you would like to mentor, coach, and develop. The identification process almost requires a "crystal ball" approach of looking at individuals—that is, you need to see the person today and forecast who the person could be tomorrow. Look for these qualities:

- The quick learner. Look for those who truly understand how, why, and when (and when not).
- Individuals who expect 110 percent and inspire others by leading by example.
- Individuals who are competent and knowledgeable as fire fighters. This type of fire fighter stands out and is respected by his or her peers.
- Individuals who possess organizational and preparation skills.
- Individuals who understand and exercise time management skills.
- Fire fighters with a passion for the fire service. Passion is contagious and can push a crew or a training division to move to the next level.

There are many important questions to ask the potential instructor. Oral interview questions may include the following:

1. Assume that you are hired to be the training officer and have been approached by members of a fire company who complain that their officer treats training as an unimportant issue and spends as little time as possible on drills. The members respect the officer as a good fire-ground commander, but claim that he has no appreciation for training and does little to support the training program. Which action would you take in this situation?
2. Why are you interested in becoming the training officer? What have you done to prepare for this position?
3. Which personal attributes that you possess will be of the greatest benefit to you in fulfilling the duties of this position?
4. Do you have any plans for personal development that will benefit you in this position?
5. Throughout the course of the year, members of the department may need motivation, direction, and guidance regarding professional training and education needs. Do you see this as part of your role as training officer? Why or why not? If so, briefly describe your thoughts on how you can best provide this need.
6. What is your top priority or priorities that would have to be accomplished in the first 3 months?
7. Describe specifically how you will gain the support, backing, and assistance of those company officers who do not consider training to be a high priority.
8. One of the responsibilities of this position will be to function as the on-scene safety officer at

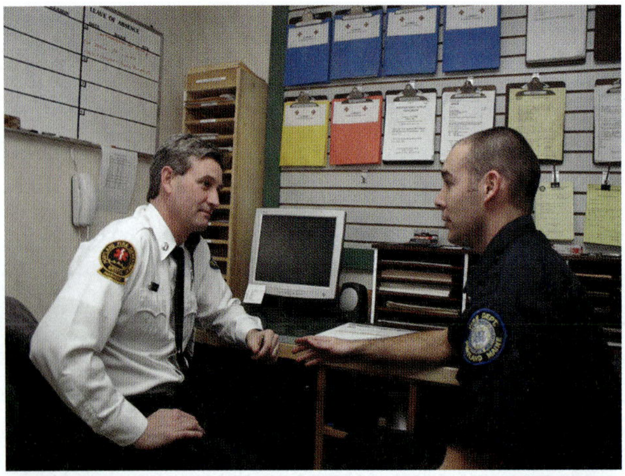

FIGURE 1-13 Succession planning ensures that the goals and objectives for the department or organization continue.

incidents. Have you had prior experience in this type of position? Also, explain your philosophy and approach to the position of scene safety officer.

9. How would you structure, document, and provide follow-up to ensure that all personnel complete required training?
10. How would you structure training sessions to accomplish training and maintain district coverage?
11. Assuming this department is a combination department of full-time and part-time personnel, which additional challenges do you anticipate in developing and conducting training for this type of structure?
12. What is your philosophy regarding the role of the company officer in training?

Written/practical evaluation questions may include the following items:

1. Prepare a written plan (not to exceed three pages—single-sided) describing how you will structure, conduct, and document the self-contained breathing apparatus (SCBA) training program.
2. Full-time personnel hired by the department are required to have prior certification as a Fire Fighter II. These individuals, once hired, are placed directly on shift. A current training issue is to develop a 40-hour program to provide an orientation to the department and complete a basic assessment of skill levels. Prepare a written plan (not to exceed three pages—single-sided) of how you would structure, conduct, and document a new fire fighter orientation/assessment program.
3. An important aspect of department training programs will be the addition of certification courses that are in compliance with the state's certification or training requirements. Prepare a written plan (not to exceed three pages—single-sided) detailing the steps that will be needed to implement an in-house fire apparatus engineer program.

Mentoring

Mentoring is a tool you can use to nurture and develop a fire fighter who has the basic skills and abilities to become a great instructor. As a mentor, you select an individual to begin the process as either a formal or an informal protégé. Your role as a mentor is to demonstrate how to perform functions or skills and to explain and answer questions. Most importantly, you act as a sounding board if your protégé has a problem. The following ideas form the foundation for a solid mentoring program:

- The mentor's job is to promote intentional learning and to provide opportunities for the protégé to learn and grow. This does not mean that you throw your protégé to the wolves and walk away; rather, it means that you give your protégé opportunities to teach or demonstrate a skill while you watch.
- As a mentor, you need to share your experiences, both good and bad. Learning comes from both positive and negative experiences.
- The mentoring process takes time, and patience needs to be shown on the part of both the mentor and the protégé.
- Mentoring is a joint venture and requires both parties to be actively involved in the process.

Sometimes the identification and selection process does not work as anticipated. For example, you might select a person whom you feel is ready for mentoring, but he or she does not respond to the process or fails to perform as desired due to lack of skill or ability. In this scenario, there is still an opportunity to learn and grow from the experience by understanding why the process failed and then learning from it. This allows everyone to part on good terms and leaves the door open to future contact.

Coaching

Coaching is a process usually associated with sports. The coach is a person who has experience and assists players in developing and improving their skills. Coaching is most often tied to manipulative skills development and physical training. The difference between mentoring and coaching is subtle. Coaching is the process of helping an individual see his or her abilities and come up with solutions independently. A coach encourages through words but allows the player to develop his or her own skills. A good coach helps a player see his or her potential and then gives the player the freedom and support to achieve it.

As an instructor, you must have expertise in numerous skills, such as firefighting skills for all levels you could be expected to teach. In addition to your technical skills, you have another set of skills at your disposal—namely, the skills used in the presentation of lessons, lesson and curriculum development, and use and development of evaluation tools. Part of the coaching process consists of allowing the fire fighter you are mentoring the opportunity to develop these skills as well.

Coaching also requires that you evaluate those persons whom you are grooming to replace you. These evaluations may take the form of either formal or informal evaluations or critiques. Just as when teaching a child to ride a bike, you must help your protégé up to a point, and then allow him or her to go on alone. You might run alongside the bike for a while, but as the child gets the hang of it, you back off. The same process applies when coaching a new instructor: You teach your protégé how to do a presentation during training, and then the fire fighter gets to do it for real in a recruit class while you stand in the back of the room and watch. Afterward, you give some advice, highlighting good points and offering suggestions for rough areas. This feedback helps your protégé grow and improve. Coaching involves taking a "big brother" or "big sister" approach toward helping a person use the skills that he or she has and then coaching/teaching the person to do even better.

Sharing

The last skill in succession planning focuses on the basic concept of **sharing**. Sharing is a key part of mentoring and coaching. To be successful in succession planning, you must mentor and coach with a giving attitude. Not only do you need to take your protégé under your wing, you also need to do so with a sharing attitude. You must be willing to share everything that has made you such a successful instructor. This arsenal of experiences includes your skills and knowledge, as well as all the little nuances that have made your job easier and fun. All too often, those persons charged with the task of training their replacements hold back the little tricks of the trade. Some have the attitude, "I had to learn it myself; so can you!" This attitude hurts both the department and your reputation. Share your knowledge and insight with your protégé as he or she takes on the responsibilities of training others. Give your protégé the extra step up rather than making him or her repeat all of your mistakes and waste all of that extra time and effort. When you share what you know with others and help others excel, you benefit both personally and professionally.

When you approach succession planning with this positive attitude and mentor the next generation of instructors by teaching and coaching with a caring and sharing attitude, both you and your department move forward. Leave a legacy of professionalism that will outlive your time on the job.

Summary of Instructor I Duties

At the Instructor I level, the instructor is beginning to develop the basic skills to present a lesson plan to a room of students or a crew of fire fighters sitting around a break room table. Even at this basic level, the instructor must have the basic skills to be effective in delivering the assigned material. The instructor at this level exercises leadership in presenting the material in a way that instills confidence in students and helps build the team. In the process of presenting lesson material, the instructor uses mentoring and coaching skills that will help students obtain new knowledge and build the necessary skills to perform their jobs as part of the organization. As part of the teaching role, the Instructor I evaluates student performance to ensure competency in learning and demonstrating the new knowledge and skill sets.

A critical aspect of the Instructor I role is accurate and thorough recordkeeping, along with reporting and recording test scores and other evaluative information from the course. This type of documentation might not seem important at the time, but future events might require documentation of course material presented, students' scores and evaluation sheets, and the instructor who presented the material.

Training BULLETIN

JBFD Fire Academy

JONES & BARTLETT FIRE DISTRICT
TRAINING DIVISION
5 Wall Street, Burlington, MA, 01803
Phone 978-443-5000 Fax 978-443-8000

Instant Applications: Today's Emergency Services Instructor

Drill Assignment

Apply the chapter content to your department's operation, training division, and your personal experiences to complete the following questions and activities.

Objective

Upon completion of the instant applications, fire and emergency services instructor students will exhibit decision making and application of job performance requirements of the instructor using the text, class discussion, and their own personal experiences.

Suggested Drill Applications

1. Identify the changes in training you have seen or experienced since you began your career in the fire service.
2. Check industry websites and reference materials to identify at least three hot topics facing instructors today.
3. Identify a new piece of equipment purchased by your department. Discuss how the initial training was accomplished on that equipment before it was placed in service. How will your department ensure that the members remain proficient in the equipment's operation after the initial training?
4. Ask the newest or youngest member of your organization about his or her training. Identify similarities and differences between current fire service training and the traditional education of a fire fighter.
5. Review the Incident Report in this chapter and be prepared to discuss your analysis of the incident from a training perspective and as an instructor who wishes to use the report as a training tool.

Incident Report: NIOSH Report F2000-27

Drill Assignment

Review the information in this incident report and prepare a practice presentation for class delivery at the direction of your instructor. Your presentation should include a summary of the incident facts and a review of the NFPA 1403 compliance and noncompliance findings. Use an outline to organize your thoughts. You may be evaluated on your communication skills during your presentation.

Greenwood, Delaware—2000

A volunteer fire department was conducting a live fire training exercise in a 100+-year-old house (**FIGURE 1-A**). Upon completing interior operations, personnel were preparing for the "final burn down" of the 2½-story house.

Three officers were in the attic. One officer was in full protective clothing and SCBA. He was using a sprayer can of diesel fuel to spray fuel. Two other officers, without SCBA, lit multiple fires. The fire spread rapidly and as conditions worsened, the two ignition officers exited to the top of the staircase and told the remaining officer to follow. He agreed to follow, but heat and fire conditions in the attic became untenable very rapidly. The others escaped down the stairs, but fire blocked their colleague's escape.

Multiple rescue attempts were unsuccessful, and the roof quickly collapsed into the attic.

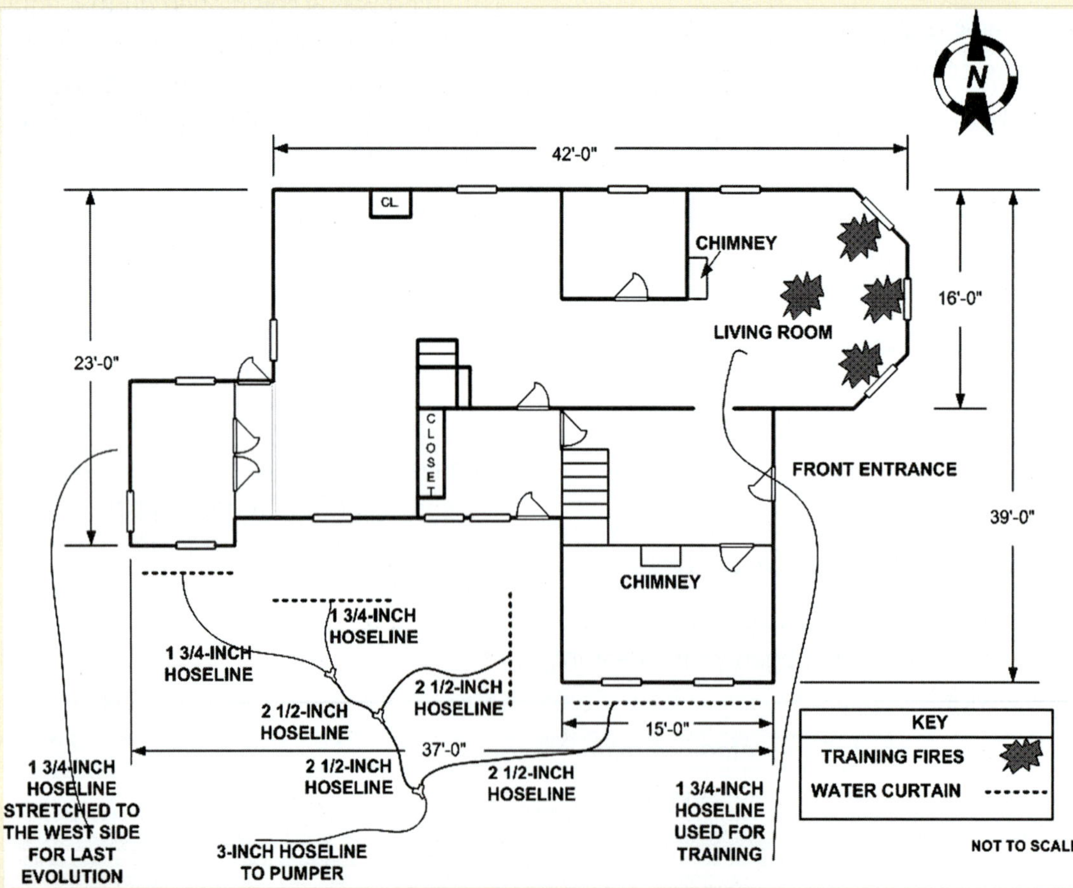

FIGURE 1-A Floor plan of Greenwood, Delaware.

From the NIOSH Fire Fighter Fatality Investigation and Prevention Program, Investigation Report F2000-27.

Postincident Analysis Greenwood, Delaware

NFPA 1403 Noncompliant

- Interior personnel without hose line
- Flashover and fire spread unexpected
- Flammable/combustible liquids used in large quantities
- Multiple fire sets
- Interior stairs only exit other than windows without ladders in place
- Participants not wearing PPE or SCBA

After-Action REVIEW

IN SUMMARY

- NFPA 1041 categorizes instructor duties into three classifications:
  - The Fire and Emergency Services Instructor I is able to deliver presentations from a prepared lesson plan, adapt lesson plans to meet the needs of a jurisdiction, organize the learning environment, and provide appropriate recordkeeping.
  - The Fire and Emergency Services Instructor II meets the requirements of Instructor I and is able to develop lesson plans, schedule training sessions, and supervise other instructors.
  - The Fire and Emergency Services Instructor III meets the requirements of Instructor II and is able to develop training curricula for single or multiple organizations, conduct needs analysis, develop training goals and implement strategies, and develop a comprehensive program and instructor evaluation plan.
- Instructors can have a wide range of ranks, ranging from fire fighter to chief of department.
- Instructors will act in a variety of roles, including leader, mentor, coach, evaluator, and teacher.
- Both physical considerations and emotional issues influence the learning environment.
- Instructors have a responsibility to stay current on topics and aid in succession planning.
- Instructors regularly face ethical dilemmas that require them to make value-based judgments.
- Learning is a lifelong process. An important part of becoming a quality instructor is having the basic desire to always improve and to become a better fire service professional.
- Professional development can take the form of training, certifications, and formal education.
- Professional development can be achieved by participating in local, state, and national organizations and by attending training conferences.
- Networking is a powerful tool that can open the door to sharing or collaborating on an idea and developing a new methodology or course.
- It is important to keep your teaching skills sharp and current. As you grow in your knowledge, stay current with the types of students entering the fire service. Test yourself by teaching a class and be honest with yourself about how effective you were.
- Succession planning is the process of developing individuals who can be mentored and coached to take the lead in the future of the fire department.
- One benefit of training your replacement is that you can select someone who shares your own ideals and goals, thereby ensuring that your training program will continue after you leave. Through this legacy, your influence could be felt for many decades in the department.

KEY TERMS

Access Navigate for flashcards to test your key term knowledge.

Certificate Document given for the completion of a training course or event.

Certification Document awarded for the successful completion of a testing process based on a standard.

Coaching The process of helping individuals develop skills and talents.

Confidentiality The requirement that, with very limited exceptions, employers must keep medical and other personal information about employees and applicants private.

Continuing education Education or training obtained to maintain skills, proficiency, or certification in a specific position.

Degree Document awarded by an institution for the completion of required coursework.

Delegation Transfer of authority and responsibility to another person for the purpose of teaching new job skills or as a means of time management. You can delegate authority but never responsibility.

Direct threat A situation in which an individual's disability presents a serious risk to his or her own safety or the safety of his or her co-workers.

Disability A physical or mental condition that interferes with a major life activity.

Ethics Principles used to define behavior that is not specifically governed by rules of law but rather in many cases by public perceptions of right and wrong. They are often defined on a regional or local level within the community.

Identifying The process of selecting those persons whom the instructor would like to mentor, coach, and develop.

Learning environment A combination of a physical location (classroom or training ground) and the proper emotional elements of both an instructor and a student.

Major life activity Basic functions of an individual's daily life, including, but not limited to, caring for oneself, performing manual tasks, breathing, walking, learning, seeing, working, and hearing.

Mentoring A relationship of trust between an experienced person and a person with less experience for the purpose of growth and career development.

Networking An activity or process of like-minded individuals meeting and developing relationships for professional and personal growth through sharing of ideas and beliefs.

Organizational chart A graphic display of the fire department's chain of command and operational functions.

Reasonable accommodation An employer's attempt to make its facilities, programs, policies, and other aspects of the work environment more accessible and usable for a person with a disability.

Sharing The basic concept of giving to others with nothing expected in return.

Standards A set of guidelines outlining behaviors or qualifications of positions or specifications for equipment or processes. Often developed by individuals within the regulated profession, they may be applied voluntarily or referenced within a rule or law.

Succession planning The act of ensuring the continuity of the organization by preparing its future leaders.

REFERENCES

Austin, Nancy, and Tom Peters. 1989. *A Passion for Excellence: The Leadership Difference*. New York: Grand Central Publishing.

National Fire Protection Association. 2019. *NFPA 1041: Standard for Fire and Emergency Services Instructor Professional Qualifications*. Quincy, MA: National Fire Protection Association.

National Fire Protection Association. 2018. *NFPA 1403: Standard on Live Fire Training Evolutions*. Quincy, MA: National Fire Protection Association.

CHAPTER PRESENTATION EXERCISE

Instructions: Your course instructor will assign individual or group discussions on the key points and teaching tips of this chapter. You or your group will review the chapter teachings and identify the major learning points from the chapter. You should be able to discuss the points, why they are important, and how/where they apply to your responsibilities at your level of instructor training.

REVIEW QUESTIONS

1. Describe some of the main distinctions among the three levels of Fire and Emergency Services Instructors.
2. What are several important factors that create a good learning environment?
3. List some of the initiatives created by the National Fire Academy and explain how they support instructors.

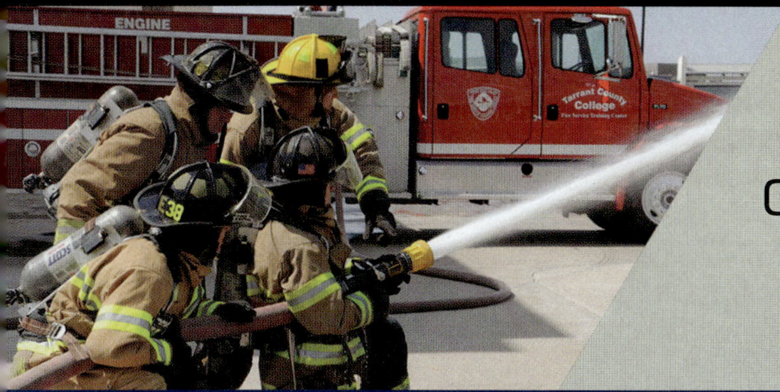

CHAPTER 2

The Learning Process

NFPA 1041 JOB PERFORMANCE REQUIREMENTS

Note: An asterisk denotes that the 1041 standard contains further information in its annex section.

4.3.2 Review instructional materials, given the materials for a specific topic, target audience, learner characteristics, and learning environment, so that elements of the lesson plan, learning environment, and resources that need adaptation are identified.

(A) Requisite Knowledge.

Recognition of student learner characteristics and diversity, methods of instruction, types of resource materials, organization of the learning environment, and policies and procedures.

(B) Requisite Skills.

Analysis of resources, facilities, and materials.

4.4.3 Present and adjust prepared lessons, given a prepared lesson plan that specifies the presentation method(s), so that the method(s) indicated in the plan are used and the stated objectives or learning outcomes are achieved, applicable safety standards and practices are followed, and risks are addressed.

(A)* Requisite Knowledge.

The laws and principles of learning, methods and techniques of instruction, lesson plan components and elements of the communication process, and lesson plan terminology and definitions; learner characteristics; student-centered learning principles; instructional technology tools; the impact of cultural differences on instructional delivery; safety rules, regulations, and practices; identification of training hazards; elements and limitations of distance learning; distance learning delivery methods; and the instructor's role in distance learning.

(B) Requisite Skills.

Oral communication techniques, methods and techniques of instruction, ability to adapt to changing circumstances, and utilization of lesson plans in an instructional setting.

4.4.4* Adjust to differences in learner characteristics, abilities, cultures, and behaviors, given the instructional environment, so that lesson objectives are accomplished, disruptive behavior is addressed, and a safe and positive learning environment is maintained.

(A)* Requisite Knowledge.

Motivation techniques, learner characteristics, types of learning disabilities and methods for dealing with them, and methods of dealing with disruptive and unsafe behavior.

(B) Requisite Skills.

Basic coaching and motivational techniques, correction of disruptive behaviors, and adaptation of lesson plans or materials to specific instructional situations.

KNOWLEDGE OBJECTIVES

After studying this chapter, participating in a structured learning environment, and completing assigned assessments, you will be able to:

- Define learner characteristics and explain their significance for instructors. (**NFPA 1041: 4.3.2**, p 37)
- Identity generational groups and explain general characteristics of each group. (**NFPA 1041: 4.4.3**, pp 39–43)
- Describe the six basic principles or "laws" of learning. (**NFPA 1041: 4.4.3**, p 43)

- Identify methods individuals can use for classroom learning, personal study, and test preparation. (pp 45–46)
- Relate human needs to the instructional environment and process. (pp 46–48)
- Identify the three domains of learning. (p 37; 48–49)
- Define student-centered learning. (p 51)
- Describe common categories of learning disabilities and methods to enhance and adapt instructional techniques to meet the needs of individuals with learning disabilities. (**NFPA 1041: 4.4.4**, pp 60–61)

SKILLS OBJECTIVES

After studying this chapter, participating in a structured learning environment, and completing assigned assessments, you will be able to:

- Perform an audience analysis to determine learner characteristics. (**NFPA 1041: 4.3.2**, pp 39–40)

You Are the Fire and Emergency Services Instructor

Recently, several members of your shift returned from a joint, countywide training program that involved instructors from outside your area, as well as members of neighboring departments who serve as their own department training officers. When asked how the training went, several of those who attended immediately started to remark on how the instructors spent too much time in the classroom telling "war stories" instead of letting those in attendance "get their hands on the equipment on the training grounds." They further criticized the instructors for not understanding that fire fighters are "hands-on" people, contending that the training session was destined to fail because there wasn't enough practical, hands-on involvement. In an effort to learn from this lesson, do the following:

1. Identify the three types of learning domains, and provide examples of different fire service topics that would be appropriate for each.
2. Define the different learner characteristics, and discuss the effects they would have on the success or failure of a specific training session.
3. Compare and contrast the similarities and differences among adult learners.

Introduction

Learning is a change in a person's ability to behave in certain ways. This change can be traced to two key factors—experience with the subject (e.g., in the field) and practice (e.g., in the classroom). Learning can occur both formally (inside the classroom) and informally (around the dinner table) (Connick, 1997). Formal learning does not occur by accident—it is the direct result of a program designed by an instructor (Butler and McManus, 1998). An adult learner may intentionally set out to learn by taking classes or by reading about a subject. He or she may also gather information through the experience of living that changes the learner's behavior. Informal learning occurs spontaneously and continually changes the adult learner's behavior. Ideally, learning is created through the blending of individual curiosity, reflection, and adaptation (Stewart, 2003).

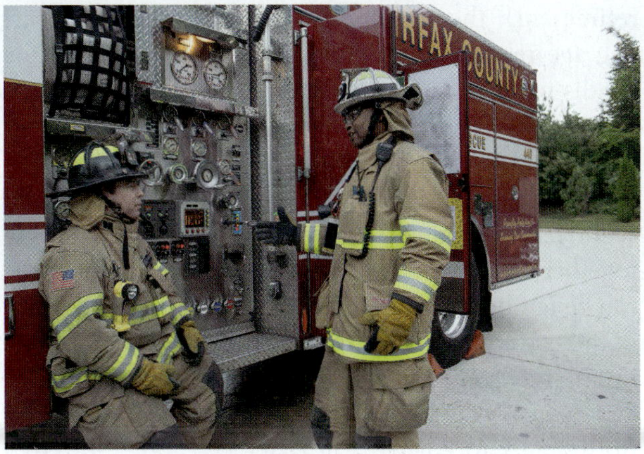

FIGURE 2-1 As a fire and emergency services instructor, you have the opportunity to positively influence fire fighters at all levels of the fire department.

Learning takes time and patience. As a fire and emergency services instructor, you have the opportunity to influence fire fighters positively at all levels of the fire department (**FIGURE 2-1**). As a leader in the fire department, you have a responsibility to teach information, to hone skills, and to promote positive values and **motivation** in your students. A wise fire service leader once said, "Classroom learning plus street experience equals wisdom." As an instructor, you have a major impact on the first part of this equation.

All levels of instructors will learn that each student in your class has different ways that they understand information. As you participate in this course, you are experiencing this phenomenon by reading text and reviewing charts, graphs, photographs, and different text fonts, sizes, and colors. Each of these elements allows different learner characteristics to be experienced. Other characteristics are demonstrated as your instructor presents course materials.

The Interactive Process of Learning

Learning is an interactive process in which the adult learner encounters and reacts to a specific learning environment. That learning environment encompasses all aspects of the adult learner's surroundings—sights, sounds, temperature, other students, and so on. In addition, each adult learner has personal, academic, social, or cognitive attributes that may influence how they learn—that is, **learner characteristics**. Some adults learn by listening to and sharing ideas with others, others by thinking through ideas themselves, and still others by testing theories or synthesizing content and context.

Learning takes place in three domains: cognitive (knowledge), psychomotor (physical use of knowledge), and affective (attitudes, emotions, or values). These domains are discussed later in this chapter.

Effective learning follows a natural process:

1. Adult learners begin with what they already know, feel, or need, based on the groundwork that was laid prior to what is currently taking place. In other words, learning does not take place in a vacuum.
2. Seeing that "newly" learned information has real-life connections prepares the adult learner for the next step—learning something new.
3. Adult learners use the new content, practicing how it can be applied to real life.
4. Adult learners take the material learned in the classroom and apply it to the real world, including in situations that were not always covered in the original lesson.

What Is Adult Learning?

Fire service training and educational programs are designed with the adult learner in mind. An adult learner is defined as someone who has passed adolescence and is out of secondary school. Self-motivation is rarely a problem for these individuals, who typically see the courses as a way both to advance their careers and to better themselves as people (**FIGURE 2-2**).

According to Bender (1999), adult learning is the integration of new information into existing values, beliefs, and behaviors. New information is learned and synthesized so that students will be able to consider alternative answers to never-before-asked questions,

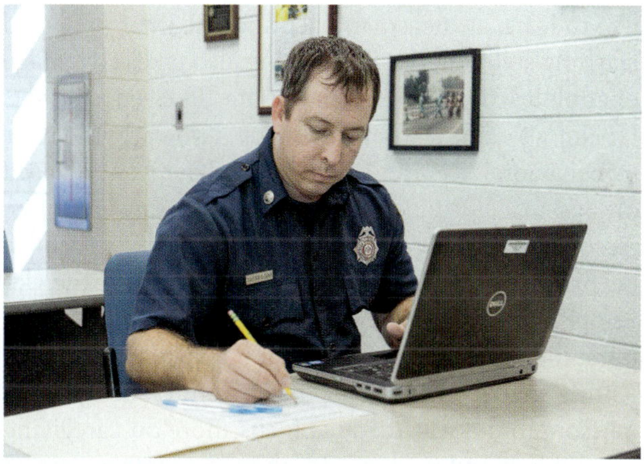

FIGURE 2-2 Fire service training and educational programs are designed with the adult learner in mind.

new applications of knowledge, and creative ways of thinking. Adult students need realistic, practical, and knowledgeable lessons that deliver information in a variety of ways to accommodate their differing learner characteristics. In particular, adult learners may have difficulty imagining a piece of equipment, responding to a written scenario, or performing a skill if they do not have a realistic application for the learning. The more realistic the lesson, the more likely the adult learner will generalize the information and be able to apply it in the field.

Similarities and Differences Among Adult Learners

There are two general lines of thought in the realm of the learning process: pedagogy and andragogy. **Pedagogy** has been defined as the art and science of teaching children. In the pedagogical model, the teacher has full responsibility for making decisions about what will be learned, how it will be learned, when it will be learned, and whether the material has been learned. Pedagogy—or teacher-directed instruction, as it is commonly known—places the student in a submissive role requiring obedience to the teacher's instructions (Knowles, 1984). This process may occur in young adults who are members of an entry-level fire academy or young volunteer fire fighters who have not entered the workforce or higher learning environments. **Andragogy** (adult learning), in contrast, attempts to identify the way in which adults learn and help them in the process of learning. According to this theory's originator—professor Malcolm Knowles—although adult learners differ, some commonalities can be found (Knowles, 1990). For example, adults typically need to know why they need to know something and how they can use it. Adult learners also tend to focus on life-centered (practical) tasks and activities. They like to learn at their own pace and use their preferred learning style. Successful learning also takes advantage of adult learners' rich history of life experiences.

Not all adult learners are alike. Two early theorists in behavioral science, Erikson and Levinson, focused on age to help understand how adult learners differ. According to these researchers, young adults seem to be primarily focused on issues surrounding the development of a sense of identity, establishing a career, pursuing a life dream, having an intimate relationship, getting married, and achieving parenthood. By comparison, middle-aged adults focus more on caregiving for children and perhaps older family members, career changes, physical and mental changes, role changes, and planning for retirement. Older adults, by contrast, often face a series of upheavals—loss of their jobs (via retirement); the transition from parent to grandparent; age-related physical and mental changes; and the deaths of friends, spouses, and eventually themselves. Stage of life, in turn, directly affects the adult learner in the classroom. Many training sessions in the fire station will involve experienced (older) and less experienced (younger) fire fighters sitting side-by-side or working together on the same hose line. Youthful enthusiasm can be tempered by wisdom and naturalization of skills in this setting; when the two are combined, an effective firefighting team will emerge. A young fire fighter in an experienced company may be a motivation for the older fire fighters to engage at a faster and more educated pace than before the young member was introduced.

Houle (1961) identified three types of adult learners:

1. For learner-oriented adults, the content is less important than the act of being involved in learning.
2. Goal-oriented learners acquire knowledge with the intention of improving their job prospects or learning a new skill. Members of this group view the instructor as being responsible for disseminating knowledge that they need.
3. Activity-oriented learners learn by doing. To succeed in learning, they require personal productive time, with control over content and learning style, with the goal of improving social contact rather than the acquisition of knowledge.

With all of these orientations, the adult learners set goals, identify objectives, select relevant resources, and use the instructor as a facilitator for learning.

Influences on Adult Learners

Adult learning theories are based on the premise that adults have had different experiences than children and adolescents, and that these differences are relevant to learning. Although age is certainly a factor that can affect learning, other factors—such as motivation, prior knowledge, the learning context, and influences exerted by situational and social conditions—are influential as well. For example, in the classroom an adult learner might not pay close attention to the topic because a previous experience left the impression that the subject is not important. This view is merely reinforced for the adult learner when others in the class share the same feelings about the subject.

Adult learners are more apt to learn and retain information when it is meaningful to their lives. For instance, information directly related to a new piece of equipment will capture the interest of fire fighters working on that apparatus. In contrast, material that is outside the realm of the adult learner's experience and knowledge is viewed as less meaningful. The prior knowledge and experiences of the adult learner are often more diverse than those of a child or adolescent, yet you must always be aware that some adult learners may lack the expected prerequisite knowledge needed to learn new information.

What influences adult learning? Here is one answer to that question (Merriam & Caffarela, 1999, 107):

> Adults often engage in learning as one way to cope with the life events they encounter, whether that learning is related to or just precipitated by a life event. Learning within these times of transition is most often linked to work and family.

Fire fighters work in a very intense environment. What is learned during times of intense stress inevitably influences learning in the classroom. If a fire fighter was just on an intense call, he or she may have trouble concentrating or sitting still in the classroom. Coping mechanisms (e.g., deflection of emotions, exaggeration of dark humor, being talkative or withdrawn) may affect behavior in the classroom. Always be on alert for signs of critical incident stress. Fire fighters need to discuss incident events in a proper environment.

Other influences on adult learners include social and cultural perspectives, such as social roles, race, and gender. Some adult learners, for example, may feel uncomfortable with classmates who are more educated or who hold a higher rank. You must ensure that in the classroom everyone is equal.

A unique feature of adult learning is that adults often desire to be self-directed learners—that is, they want to take their own direction within the learning process. Self-directed learning is related to humanism, the concept that the adult learner can make "significant personal choices within the constraints imposed by heredity, personal history, and environment" (Elias & Merriam, 1980). Although adults may have the desire to be self-directed in their learning, their prior experience with didactic classroom-based instruction may not have prepared them sufficiently for self-management in the learning environment. As the instructor, it is your responsibility to provide the necessary guidance that keeps your students on track.

Critical reflection—that is, the ability to reflect back on prior learning to determine whether what has been learned is justified under present circumstances—is often a unique advantage attributed to adult learners, and a key asset that you should utilize when teaching. This kind of reflection involves "meta-thinking" about the strategies required to achieve a goal. Such reflection often occurs when adult learners compare their ideas to those of their mentors or those of their classmates. Over time, an adult acquires basic cultural beliefs and ways of interpreting the world. Often such learning and beliefs are assimilated uncritically. In the classroom, however, adult learners may reflect critically on the assumptions and attitudes that underlie their knowledge. Such reflection helps them become deeper thinkers and can enhance their processes of thinking.

The benefits of this evolution in thinking are readily evident in the fire service. How many times have fire fighters gone to training with an attitude of "I really don't want to be here"? These students would rather be doing something else, but they go because the education is mandated. This disdain for training may represent an assimilated attitude—perhaps others in the station feel the same way. It may not indicate the way that a particular fire fighter truly feels about training or education; fire fighters naturally want to fit in socially, so they tend to adopt the attitudes that others around them have. As the instructor, part of your job is to help all students become motivated to learn the information presented.

Factors such as participation in formal educational programs or training programs since high school will also affect the adult learner's ability to learn. For many adult learners, traditional learning skills (e.g., reading and understanding textbook material, taking notes during lectures, and studying for tests) may have been forgotten or, in some cases, were never developed properly. Many adult learners have developed a learning preference that is limited to "doing" (McClincy, 1995). Adult learners with this learning characteristic learn best when they can perform the skill. Difficulty with developing study skills, and problems with unlearning and relearning, present challenges to both the adult learner and you, as the instructor.

Today's Adult Learners: Generational Characteristics

Many types of learners exist, and many groups of students emerge with similar traits and skill sets that the instructor must take into account when developing or presenting a lesson plan. This type of assessment, known as an **audience analysis**, is part of all levels of instructor responsibility when planning instruction. Audience analysis is the determination of characteristics common to a group of people—in this case, students. An audience analysis can be used to choose the best instructional approach. Factors considered in an audience analysis include the following:

- Age of the students and their experience in the subject matter
- Who the lesson is intended for and how students will use the material

- Number of students in the class
- Level of previous knowledge of the class material

Public speaking expert Lenny Laskowski devised the following use of the term *audience* as an acronym to help identify this essential element in presentation preparation and delivery:

- Analysis: Who is the audience?
- Understanding: What is the audience's knowledge of the subject?
- Demographics: What are the ages, genders, educational backgrounds, and other distinguishing characteristics?
- Interest: Why are the students attending your class?
- Environment: Where will this presentation be delivered, and which possible barriers to effective learning will exist?
- Needs: What are the audience's needs associated with your presentation, and how will they use the material in the future or as part of their job?
- Customization: Which specific needs and interests should you, as the instructor, address relating to the specific audience? Are appropriate department SOPs and terminology being used?
- Expectations: What does the audience expect to learn from your presentation? The audience members should walk away having their initial questions answered and explained, or they should be able to perform a task.

The following are some generalized categories of learners divided by the generation in which they were born. Most share common characteristics of behavior, knowledge, and skills. Again, understanding your students is a key behavior for any instructor.

Baby Boomers

The **baby boomers** were born between 1946 and 1964. At the end of World War II, soldiers returned home, married, and began families in the midst of an economic boom. The baby boom ended when the increased use of birth control caused a sharp decline in the birth rate in 1964.

The baby-boomer generation was raised on television, which had a tremendous impact on them and caused many of them to see world events from a single source (**FIGURE 2-3**). The following statements tend to apply to this generation:

- Rock and roll strongly influenced their formative years.
- They have high standards concerning work and place great value on education, and they expect the same of others.

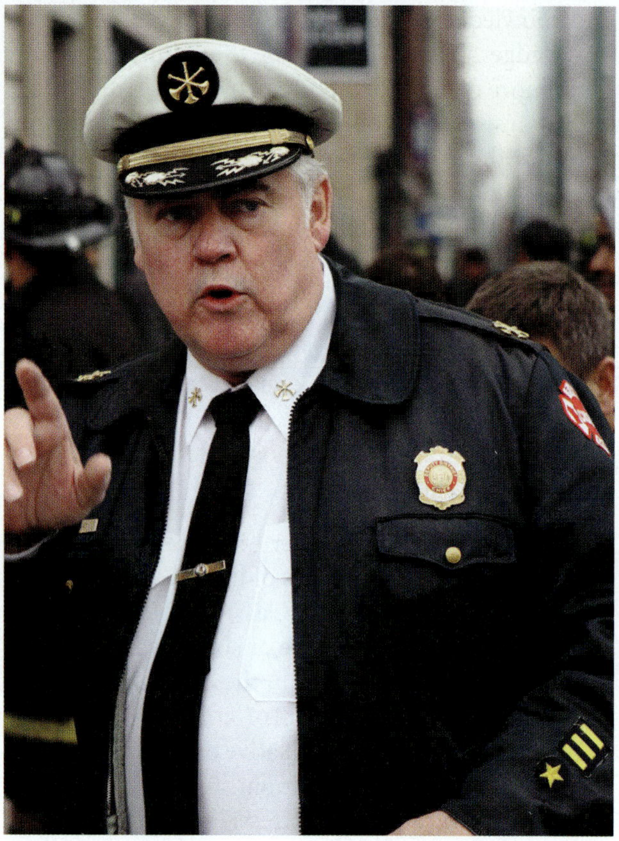

FIGURE 2-3 The baby boomer generation of fire fighters are the backbone of many departments, and their trust must be earned by new instructors.
Courtesy of Fire Chief Gordon J. Nord Jr.

- They are independent, confident, and self-reliant.
- Speaking out against social injustice was a milestone period in their lives.

How do you teach to baby boomers? Today, this generation of individuals may largely compose the upper level management of the department or training division. Look at the senior members of your fire department and observe how you interact with them. As with all students, you must first gain baby boomers' trust and show them respect. Draw on their experience to assist you in teaching your course. Baby boomers will want to share their experiences and knowledge. This generation is known for both accepting change and resisting it because it pushes them out of their comfort zones. An effective method for teaching baby boomers is using group activities that will allow them to take a lead role and share their knowledge.

Generation X

As B. L. Brown points out in *New Learning Strategies for Generation X* the "gap between Generation X and earlier generations represents much more than age and technological differences. It reflects the effect of a changing society on a generation" (Brown, 1997). The term

Generation X has been used to describe the generation consisting of those people whose teenaged years were touched by the 1980s, although this definition excludes the oldest and youngest Gen Xers. In broad terms, members of Generation X are those persons born in the late 1960s to late 1970s. This was the first generation for whom it was common for both parents to work outside the home. Their parents' absence required children to learn to take care of themselves and their siblings until Mom and Dad returned home. While their physical development was the same as earlier generations, the psychological and learning development of Generation X was not. This generation was the first to abandon the traditional family models, to consider divorce to be the norm, and to promote single-parent families. Many Gen Xers prefer to stay childless (**FIGURE 2-4**).

Many members of this generation were raised in single-parent homes, growing up with "fast food, remote controls, entertainment and quick response devices such as automatic teller machines and microwave ovens, all of which provide instant gratification" (Brown, 1997). These life experiences shaped the way they learned and resulted in certain learning characteristics that require some modifications of traditional classroom tactics and new teaching strategies. Members of Generation X are typically familiar with being educated and trained by people from earlier generations. The cultural gap between the generations reflects the diverse life experiences of the individuals in each generation. One of the major challenges facing instructors is the need to bridge the generation gap.

The following statements tend to define the majority of Generation X learners:

- They are independent problem solvers and self-starters. These individuals want support and feedback, but they do not want to be controlled.
- They are technologically literate. Gen Xers are familiar and comfortable with computer technology and using the internet for sourcing information.
- They are conditioned to expect immediate gratification. Gen Xers crave stimulation and expect immediate answers and feedback.
- Members of this generation want their work to be meaningful to them. They want to know why they must learn something before they will take the time to learn the subject.
- They do not expect to grow old working for the same company, so they view their job environments as places to grow. They seek continuing education and training opportunities; if they do not find them, they will look for new jobs where they can get what they want.
- Members of Generation X often seek employment at technology start-ups, start their own small businesses, and even adopt worthy causes.
- Adversity—far from discouraging members of this generation—has given them a harder, even ruthless edge. Many believe, "I have to take what I can get in this world because no one is going to give me anything" (Brown, 1997).

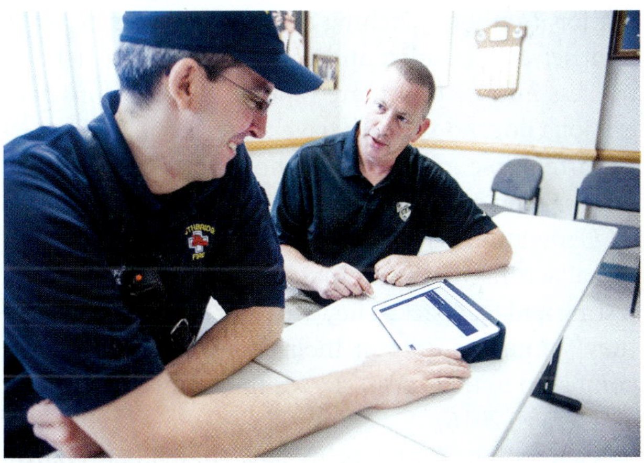

FIGURE 2-4 Instructors must learn techniques to bridge the generation gaps between their students. Generation X firefighters were the first generation of technology literate students to enter the classroom.

In the classroom as well as in the workplace, Gen Xers often clash with baby boomer or traditionalist instructors. As an instructor, you may be the baby boomer trying to teach the Gen Xer. The common value that both generations share is the high priority placed on learning and developing new skills. This point poses a challenge to instructors, who must continually raise the bar in the classroom and perhaps adapt to cross-generational training. To accommodate the unique characteristics of Generation X learners, instructors need to step outside the box and promote learning that has applications in the school, work, and community settings that are part of the Gen Xers' experience.

Generation Y

Generation Y (also known as Millennials) is the name given to those people who were born immediately after Generation X. There is no consensus as to the exact range of birth years that are included in Generation Y or whether this term is geographically specific. The only consensus appears to be that Generation Y includes those individuals born after Generation X.

The "Y" in Generation Y refers to the namelessness of a generation that has only recently come into an awareness of its existence as a separate group. Members of this generation typically feel dwarfed and overshadowed by the baby boomers and Generation X. Nevertheless, members of Generation Y are known for holding wide-ranging opinions on political and social issues, religion, marriage, gay rights, and behavior (**FIGURE 2-5**). This lack of a common perspective may have occurred because these individuals have not encountered a personal situation where their actions or reactions have forced them to consciously choose sides on issues and maintain consistent positions. Most Gen Yers are more tolerant of alternative lifestyles and unconventional gender roles than are previous generations. At the same time, Generation Y tends to be more spiritual than the generation that includes their parents, and disagreement on social issues between the more liberal and more conservative members of this generation is commonplace.

The following statements tend to apply to Generation Y learners:

- They are confident, quick to learn, and sometimes brash.
- They want to work; they tend to have a strong drive to find a career that is fulfilling and satisfying.
- The members of Generation Y have been nurtured and programmed with a slew of activities since they were toddlers, meaning they are both high performers and sometimes considered high maintenance (Armour, 2005).
- They tend to do well at multi-tasking.
- Adapting to and applying ever-evolving technology comes easily to them.

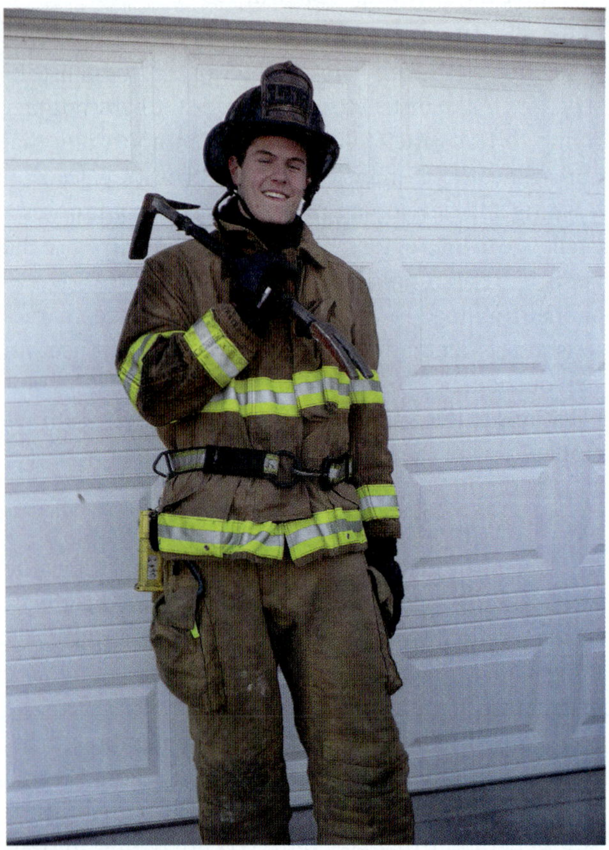

FIGURE 2-5 Many members of Generation Y have been nurtured with a constant flow of activities since they were toddlers, resulting in high-performance and high-maintenance multi-taskers.

Courtesy of Forest Reeder.

Learning in virtual classrooms and virtual labs is ideally suited to Generation Y, as is teaching by technical professionals, because these adult learners can interact with others and get hands-on experience. Virtual labs suit the "click on it and see what happens" experiential approach to learning and have the added benefit that the learner remains in a safe environment.

The Gen Yers in the classroom present a challenge to the instructor who is either a baby boomer or a Gen Xer. The instructor needs to have a general understanding of members of this generation and support their learner characteristics and needs. Instructors need to understand that success in teaching this generation requires gaining their trust by being a good example and "walking the walk" in what instructors say and do.

Generation Z

Generation Z (also called Generation Next, Post-Millennials, or iGen) refers to those born in 1995 and later. They were born into a world where computer use was commonplace, and as a result, have a unique style of learning. Many Generation Z students have had constant computer access from the start of their education, and their learning is based on quick and very visually oriented interaction. Perhaps because of the availability of online videos and the prevalence of instructional videos, this generation prefers to see a skill demonstrated and then try it. This group has grown up teaching themselves how to do things by searching for it online, watching a video, and then trying it themselves (Seemiller and Grace, 2017). They tend to process information more rapidly than previous generations do, and seem to have a greater ability to perform multiple tasks at once; however, they may also have shorter attention spans.

Generation Z learners have grown up in an educational setting that has provided regular standardized testing and feedback. They are used to knowing where they stand, not only in their own classroom, but as compared to their peers across the country (Seemiller and Grace, 2016).

Generation Z prefers to have individual control over their learning with the option to collaborate. They expect active participatory learning environments and student-centered learning environments. (Seemiller and Grace, 2016).

The Laws and Principles of Learning

Numerous theorists, including Edward L. Thorndike and his contemporaries Edwin R. Gutherie, Clark L. Hull, and Neal E. Miller, have studied learning and developed ideas that have become recognized as the basic laws or principles of learning. According to Thorndike, there are six laws of learning: readiness, exercise, effect, primacy, recency, and intensity. They are described here:

1. **The law of readiness:** A person can learn when he or she is physically, mentally, and emotionally ready to respond to instruction.
2. **The law of exercise:** Learning is an active process that exercises both the mind and the body. Through this process, the learner develops an adequate response to instruction and is able to master the learning through repetition. For example, a fire fighter can master ropes by practicing tying knots every night for a month. The opposite is also true: A skill that is not exercised after it is developed will be lost. In some areas, this concept is referred to as the principle of disuse.
3. **The law of effect:** Learning is most effective when it is accompanied by or results in a feeling of satisfaction, pleasantness, or reward (internal or external) for the student—for example, when the student receives an A on a pop quiz.
4. **The law of primacy:** This principle states that the first method or way a concept is taught will be the way the student learns and remembers it. As the saying goes, "First impressions are lasting impressions"—and when it comes to learning, this holds true. The concern here is that if a student learns a new skill incorrectly, then the instructor has to help the student "unlearn" and correct the knowledge.
5. **The law of recency:** Practice makes perfect, and the more recent the practice, the more effective the performance of the new skill or behavior. Running drills on new skills will reinforce and perfect training in fire fighters. This law is why we retrain fire fighters and review information that is not used on a daily basis. If a skill is not used, it goes away, just as a muscle that is not exercised loses its strength over time.
6. **The law of intensity:** This principle states that the more of the senses that are stimulated, the more likely the student will be to change his or her behavior—which is what learning is all about. A lesson that moves from lecture to real-world videos to hands-on application of the skill will increase the student's ability to learn. The more the material is presented in a real-world manner, the stronger the learning effect (Thorndike, 1932).

Use of Senses

Adult learners use the five senses—hearing, seeing, touching, smelling, and tasting—to obtain information (**FIGURE 2-6**). The type and number of senses used to learn determines how learning occurs and what is remembered. Of the five senses, seeing (e.g., a visual demonstration of a skill) is generally the most effective means of learning, followed by hearing (e.g., listening to a lecture), smelling (e.g., smelling smoke), touching (e.g., handling fire equipment), and tasting (rarely used in training fire fighters, especially due to hazardous materials and other safety concerns). As an instructor, the more senses you can engage during the learning process, the greater the students' ability to retain the information that was presented. Effective lesson plans will address this issue by allowing time for questions, hands-on training, and other methods that bring all of the senses together.

The Behaviorist and Cognitive Perspectives

Two schools of thought have developed to explain how behavior evolves: behaviorist and cognitive. According to the **behaviorist perspective**, learning is a relatively permanent change in behavior that arises from experience. Not all changes in behavior reflect classroom learning. Many changes in behavior take place owing to a person's maturation and physical changes as he or she ages (Rathus, 1999).

According to the **cognitive perspective** (mental), learning is an intellectual process in which experience

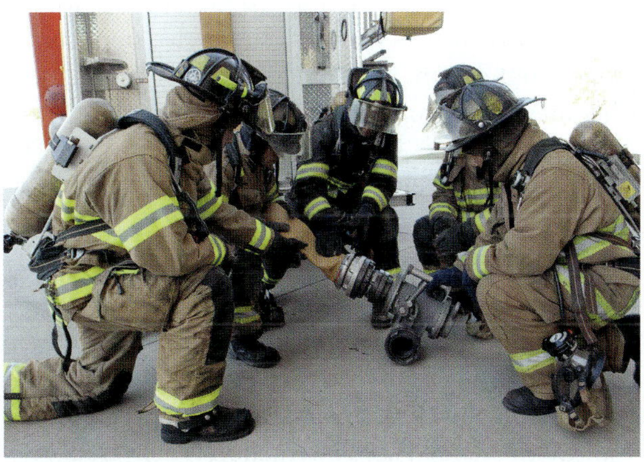

FIGURE 2-6 Adult learners use their senses to obtain information.

contributes to relatively permanent changes in the way individuals mentally represent their environment. Cognitive theories stress the use of mental capabilities to change behavior. Cognition is defined as the acquisition of knowledge through the use of perception, encounters with ideas, and obtaining of experiences (Lefrancois, 1996). Thus, cognitive learning is demonstrated by recall of knowledge and use of intellectual skills. It entails the comprehension of information, organization of ideas, analysis and synthesis of data, application of knowledge, choice of alternatives in problem solving, and evaluation of ideas or actions. According to this perspective, learning is an internal process that is demonstrated externally by behavioral changes.

Competency-Based Learning Principles

Learning that is intended to create or improve professional behavior is based on performance, rather than on content. Such **competency-based learning** is usually tied to skills or hands-on training. Not surprisingly, much of what is accomplished on the fire ground occurs through hands-on activities that require proficiency with skills—for example, the ability to force entry on a door. Competency-based learning is based on what the adult learner will do or perform.

Competency-based learning originates with the identification and verification of the needed competencies to perform particular skills. These competencies are actually job requirements, and ideally, they will have been identified through a job task analysis. For the fire service, this job task analysis has been done by the National Fire Protection Association (NFPA) via its professional qualification standards, which are all written in job performance requirement (JPR) format.

To ensure the success of a competency-based course, it is essential to follow a standardized process. This process ensures that each successive step has the proper foundation. Without the proper foundation, what may look like an excellent course might not address the real skills issues of the fire department. The design of a competency-based course includes the following requirements:

- Competencies exist.
- Job task analysis is performed.
- Standards are identified and set.
- Course goals are identified and written.
- Lesson objectives are identified and written.
- Competency-based instruction is delivered.

The most critical facet of competency-based learning is the notion that the skills must be mastered by the adult learners for each of the competencies. To ensure that this requirement is met, students must be given enough time and appropriate instruction to both learn and master the skill. Both the instructor and the students must understand that with mastery comes the responsibility of maintaining a particular performance level. Thus, learning objectives, instruction, and the evaluation of the skills must be tailored to performance in the field, not just to the acquisition of abstract knowledge that is out of context.

A competency-based learning process must be flexible enough to be adapted to the needs of all students. Each student inevitably learns at his or her own pace and in his or her own individual fashion. Some students may take longer than others to learn the skill, so you must take each individual's abilities into account when teaching skills. Also, appropriate and immediate feedback needs to be provided to students to allow them to achieve mastery of the skill, thereby applying the principles of primacy, recency, and intensity (**FIGURE 2-7**).

Forced Learning

There is an important fact of which you need to be aware: Adult learners cannot be forced to learn. Unfortunately, too many adult learners attend training programs or engage in educational situations only because they are required to do so or because they are motivated by the wrong reason. Understanding the dynamics of the fire service, there always seem to be new continuing education credits to be accumulated for recertification or some new required certification to be obtained. Mandating learning often results in a lack of motivation related to classroom activities and a poor attitude toward the learning process in general,

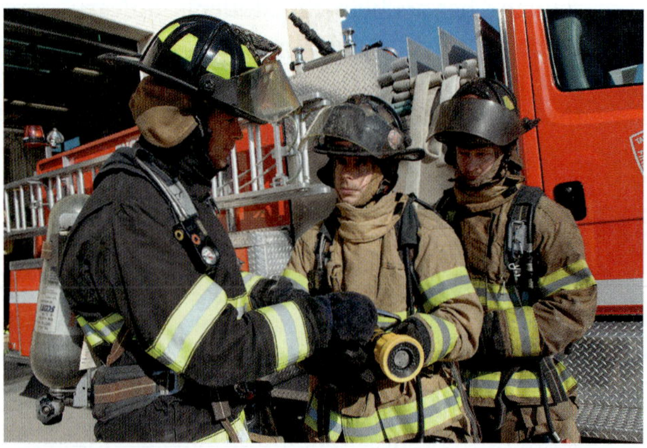

FIGURE 2-7 Immediate feedback needs to be given on the training ground to ensure that each student masters the skill.

both of which present quite a challenge to the instructor who is tasked with teaching the course.

The presence of students who are mandated to attend a class or training session should alert you to the possibility that the lesson plans might need to be altered. For example, if you are assigned to teach a cardiopulmonary resuscitation (CPR) recertification course to paramedic students, then you might look for ways to involve students in both the teaching process and the learning process. The creation of such dual roles will help capture their attention and enhance the learning process.

Areas of Interest

All adults have certain areas of interest. Tapping into these areas may help reinforce the desire to learn. The source of this interest is less important than its mere presence, because all students need to have encouragement if learning is to take place. Such positive reinforcement can serve to increase the motivation of students who are forced into your classroom. You may need to acknowledge the areas of special interest of reluctant students to guide them through the learning process and to keep them engaged in your class. Knowing your students and their areas of interest allows you to capitalize on their knowledge base and become a more effective instructor.

When teaching adults, you are really more of a facilitator than a traditional teacher. Here are some core qualities that will help you become a good facilitator:

- **Be genuine in your relationships with adult learners, rather than consistently adhering to the traditional role as "teacher."** Show that you really care about the students and their success in the classroom.
- **Accept and trust in the adult learner as a person of worth.** Provide positive reinforcement and engage the learner with respect and value. Remember—people learn more from individuals whom they trust than from individuals whom they mistrust. Establishing a mutual climate of trust is important in fostering learning.
- **Provide nonjudgmental understanding of adult learners' perspectives.** Respond with empathy to both their intellectual and emotional perspectives. Remember that people are more open to learning when they are respected and feel supported than when they feel judged or threatened.
- **Establish a climate for learning.** Openness and authenticity are essential for maintaining this supportive atmosphere. People will be more likely to examine and embrace new ideas in an open and authentic environment.

Learning Skills for Adult Learners

As an instructor, you may find yourself teaching adult learners who have not been in a classroom setting since high school or college or rookie school. Study habits that these students developed while in primary school, secondary school, or college could have become rusty over time. Perhaps the most important study skill to develop as a student (and instructor) is to have the right attitude toward learning and studying. A positive attitude toward learning will help you learn new material and enjoy the classroom environment.

To assist your students in becoming effective learners, you can share study skills that enhance what they learn during classroom and personal study time. Study tips can be viewed as belonging to one of three categories: classroom, personal study, and test preparation.

Classroom Study Tips

In the classroom environment, students can learn to develop the following skills to help them in the learning process:

- **Ask questions.** If students do not understand the material being presented by the instructor, they should be encouraged to ask questions. Students should not wait for someone else to ask a question or feel that they are the only student who does not understand. In most situations, other students have the same question.
- **Take notes.** A good study technique is to develop an outline format for notes that follows the syllabus or outline given by the instructor.
- **Participate in class.** Participate in classroom activities and discussions and group activities.
- **Turn off your phone.** If students want to get the most out of classroom instruction, they should turn off their cell phones and other technological distractions and listen to the instructor.
- **Connect with peers.** As appropriate, students should get the names and phone numbers of other students in the class to contact for notes or information in case of a missed class.

Personal Study Time

Outside the classroom, students will need to study on their own. This is the time when most adult learners really learn the new material and develop effective learning skills and habits, including the following:

- **Time management.** Adult learners must learn to budget their time. This can be done by setting

aside a predetermined period of time each day to study and sticking with that schedule.
- **Study location.** If studying in the fire house after hours, the student should find a location to study that is free of distractions and will allow him or her to focus on the material to be learned.
- **Material prioritization.** A student should review what needs to be studied and determine what is the highest priority and what needs to be covered first.
- **Class notes review.** To aid the student in focusing personal study time, he or she should review notes from class.
- **Reading skills.** One technique that will help students retain what they have read is to take brief notes of the material read. These notes can be used later to help in test preparation.
- **Study groups.** Depending on the class format and the material being learned, study groups can be an effective method for learning new material. These groups can be formal groups assigned by the instructor or informal groups that are organized by students who desire to study together.

Test Preparation Skills

Testing and course evaluation during instruction are commonly used methods for instructors to determine whether students have learned the material presented in class. Testing can take the form of quizzes or questioning by the instructor. Many courses require a comprehensive test to be administered at the end of the course to assess the students' learning. The following techniques can be used to help students prepare for a test:

- **Participate in study groups.** Study groups are effective methods for students to quiz one another and help one another in test preparation.
- **Do not cram.** Preparing for a course exam should begin on the first day of class, not hours before the test by cramming. Students should not wait until the last hours before a test to study; this method does not work.
- **Use mnemonic devices.** Fire service members and paramedics have long used mnemonic tools to help them remember information, such as RECEO-VS or SAMPLE. (RECEO-VS: Rescue, Exposure, Confinement, Extinguishment, Overhaul-Ventilation, Salvage; SAMPLE: Signs/symptoms, Allergies, Medications, Past illnesses, Last oral intake, Events leading up to present illness)
- **Take a break.** One skill that students need to learn is knowing when to take a 10-minute break from studying and refresh yourself—let your mind stop thinking, get some fresh air, and then go back to work.

To be a successful instructor, you must truly know yourself. Some of us are excellent speakers, whereas others are effective writers. What are your strengths? What do you need to work on? Taking a personal inventory assessment such as the Myers–Briggs Type Indicator can clue you in to behaviors that you may need to improve. Sometimes you will find that the fire fighters in your department are ready and willing to learn and experience training as a group. When it comes down to individual fire fighters, however, blocks to learning may spring up. For example, a fire fighter may be tired and unable to concentrate because he worked an incident all night. When basic needs are not met, learning becomes a second priority, which can in turn create a safety issue. A student may perform an unsafe act due to his or her less-than-optimal physical or mental state, or a student may miss information (because of inattention) that he or she must know to be able to perform at actual incidents.

COMPANY-LEVEL INSTRUCTOR TIP

Think back to a dynamic and unique instructor you encountered during school. Which characteristics or approaches did that instructor use to motivate you to learn the material? Then recall an instructor who did not motivate you, and identify the characteristics that may have played into that. Pinpointing the instructor traits or techniques that you found positive or negative can help you determine the style you want to incorporate in your own approach.

Maslow's Hierarchy of Needs

Abraham H. Maslow was a psychologist who researched mental health and human potential. He is most often associated with the concepts of a hierarchy of needs, self-actualization, and peak experiences. Maslow's initial work in 1943 was followed up in 1954 by his development of what is commonly referred to today as the "hierarchy of needs." Maslow took a unique approach in conducting his research, called "biographical analysis," wherein he reviewed the biographies and writings of 21 people he identified as being "self-actualized." His subjects included such major figures as Albert Einstein, Jane Addams, Eleanor Roosevelt, and Frederick Douglass. Based on his research, Maslow determined that certain needs should be satisfied to enable a person to move forward toward self-actualization. He perceived human needs as being arranged like a ladder or a pyramid (**FIGURE 2-8**). According

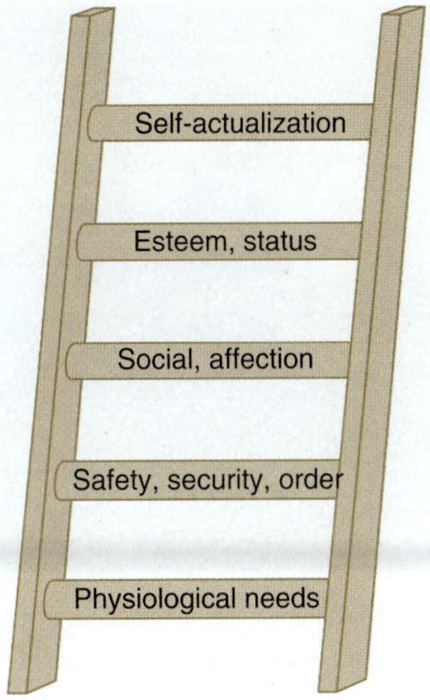

FIGURE 2-8 Maslow's hierarchy of needs.

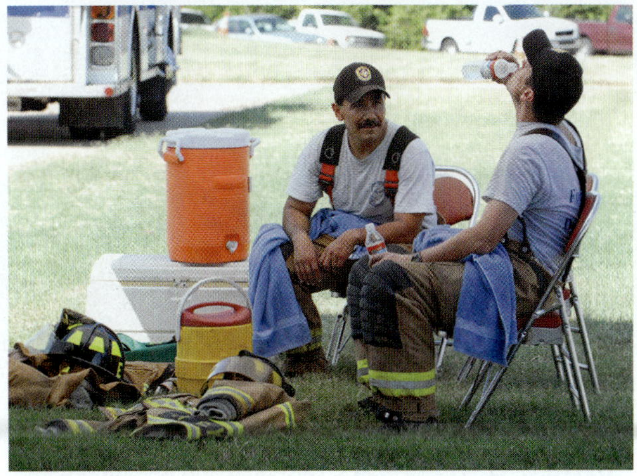

FIGURE 2-9 Fire fighters need periods of rest and rehydration to meet their most basic physiological needs.

to Maslow, unfulfilled needs at the lower levels on the ladder will inhibit a person from climbing to the next step. As he pointed out, a person who is dying of thirst quickly forgets the thirst when deprived of oxygen.

Understanding the basic needs of people can facilitate an appreciation of which basic needs your students have. An instructor should keep these needs in mind when creating, adapting, or modifying lessons and the classroom dynamic.

Level One: Physiological Needs

The most basic human needs, at the bottom of the ladder, are physical—air, water, food, and shelter. It is hard to be creative or productive when you are exhausted and hungry. For the instructor, this means staying alert for conditions where the students are hungry, exhausted, dehydrated, too hot, or too cold. Although some of these conditions may arise in a long classroom session, they are more likely to occur in off-site training, during which reasonable breaks must be given for food, water, and rest. An example of a basic need that is too often overlooked is restroom facilities at a remote training site.

Sometimes fire fighters have to work at the extremes of discomfort and personal inconvenience during emergency activities, but these situations should be the exceptions and not a normal way of getting the job done. Making a fire company train or work without a rest and rehydration period will fail to meet their most basic needs (**FIGURE 2-9**).

Level Two: Safety, Security, and Order

Safety, security, and order are next on the ladder of needs. Safety is obviously a primary concern in the fire service, although a fire fighter's perceptions of safety are probably quite different from those of a typical office or factory worker. If students feel that their instructor is leading them in an unsafe manner or that a particular policy or practice in the fire department is exposing them to an avoidable risk, safety is likely to become a very significant issue.

The concept of security is more closely associated with maintaining employment or status within the organization. This need could be as subtle as a fear that a personality clash with a particular instructor will impede a fire fighter's professional development. An individual who feels threatened may do what is necessary to survive, but will not feel highly motivated to advance the fire department's objectives.

The need for security and order could become a factor when a fire department is undergoing a significant reorganization, such as a change in a standard procedure that the fire fighter was accustomed to over a long period of time. If a department adopts a new procedure or operational structure, the fire fighter may feel apprehension over new training responsibilities, evaluations, and scrutiny by upper levels of management. Any type of change in the established order is likely to arouse insecurities. The anticipation of significant changes in the organization can easily impede the fire fighter's creativity and motivation.

Level Three: Social Needs and Affection

Social requirements and affection, as identified by Maslow, are the psychological or social needs that are related to belonging to a group and feeling acceptance by the group (**FIGURE 2-10**). Group acceptance and belonging are particularly strong forces within the fire service. The majority of fire fighters have some

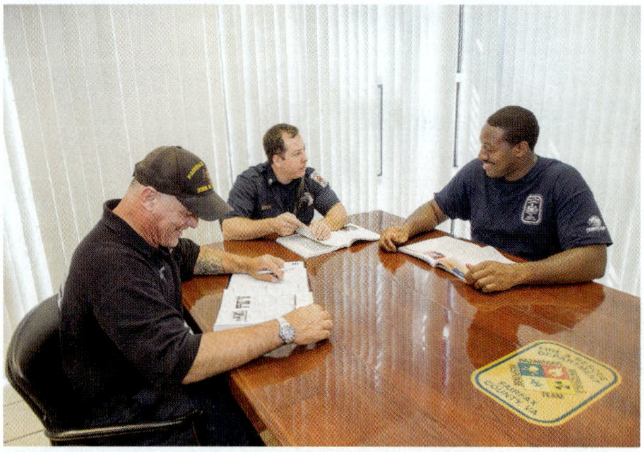

FIGURE 2-10 Group acceptance and belonging are particularly strong forces within the fire service.

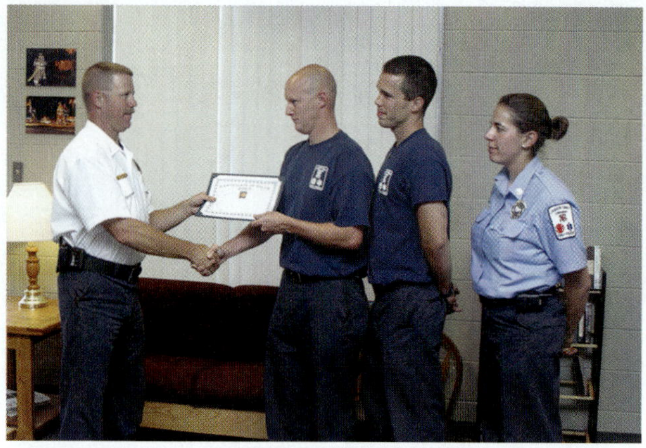

FIGURE 2-11 An instructor can positively affect a fire fighter or company's esteem and status by making efforts to recognize new certifications or training milestones.

type of identification on their personal vehicles that visibly declares their local fire department affiliation and membership in the fire service at large. Transferring a fire fighter away from a "good" assignment can be a strong demotivator, just as suspending a volunteer from responding to calls can have a significant impact on him or her at the social and affection levels. Fire fighters who are temporarily or permanently assigned to a company other than the one they have worked with and for over a long period of time will feel the same impact. For example, they must learn how they will fit into the formal and informal rank structures and work groups in the new station. In fact, many newly placed but experienced members feel like they do not fit into the company until they can begin to socialize with the new crew members.

Make your class its own community of social acceptance by acknowledging that all students present are to become the future of the fire service. This group acceptance leads the class to a greater cohesion even when many of its members come from differing backgrounds and departments.

Level Four: Esteem and Status

Promotions, certifications, and special awards are all symbols that relate to the student's esteem and status level (**FIGURE 2-11**). For example, membership in an elite fire department technical unit is often an indicator of advanced qualifications or achievements. Many fire fighters are willing to invest money and off-duty time to compete for a high-esteem or high-status position. For example, fire fighters may spend months preparing for a fire officer promotional exam or taking courses to qualify for a rescue company. Most elite fire units have more applicants than available positions. As an instructor, keep these motivational factors in mind. Every student is in your class for a reason, and it is your responsibility to guide them toward meeting the course objectives, and in doing so getting another step closer to their own goals.

As an instructor you need to be aware of how self-esteem plays out in the classroom environment and the importance of protecting your students from negative comments both from you as the instructor and from their fellow students. The fire service is known for joking in a "brotherly" fashion to foster camaraderie, but as the instructor you need to be careful not to allow this type of joking to cross the line where it affects a student's self-esteem.

Level Five: Self-Actualization

Peak experiences are profound moments of love, understanding, happiness, or rapture, when a person feels more whole, alive, self-sufficient, and yet a part of the world—more aware of truth, justice, harmony, and goodness. Self-actualizing people have many such peak experiences. These individuals tend to focus on problems outside of themselves and have a clear sense of what is true. Self-actualization in the learning environment is seen when students finally complete a skill or task they have been struggling with and can turn their attention to the next challenge. Graduation day at a recruit academy is an ultimate moment and point of self-actualization for those students, when they have completed a hard training process and receive their badges as fire fighters.

Learning Domains

In 1956, Benjamin Bloom and his research team identified three types of **learning domains**—that is, categories in which learning takes place (**FIGURE 2-12**).

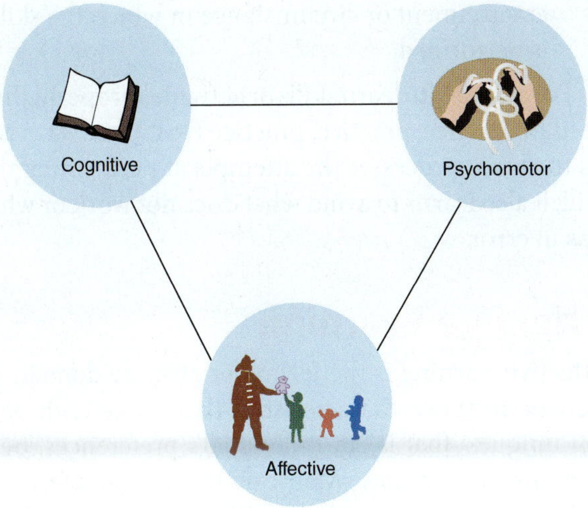

FIGURE 2-12 The three types of learning domains are cognitive, psychomotor, and affective.

- **Cognitive domain**: knowledge
- **Psychomotor domain**: physical use of knowledge
- **Affective domain**: attitudes, emotions, or values

Today, this classification system is widely known as Bloom's Taxonomy of the Domains of Learning (Bloom, 1984). **Bloom's Taxonomy** has had a widespread influence in the field of learning research. Researchers have since developed new strategies of classifications and identified additional learning domains to build upon Bloom's original taxonomy.

Although Bloom identified three general learning domains, the learning process seldom takes place solely in one domain. Additionally, within each of the domains, the levels of learning build one upon the other. These levels, which have been expanded and refined by subsequent researchers, serve as the building blocks of the learning process. Within each level are found three basic sublevels: knowledge, application, and problem solving. Being aware of these levels and Bloom's three original learning domains will assist you in developing lesson objectives and course material to address a specific level of learning.

Cognitive Learning

The most commonly understood of the learning domains is cognitive learning, which results from instruction. Bloom's Taxonomy distinguishes six levels of cognitive learning:

- Knowledge: remembering knowledge acquired in the past
- Comprehension: understanding the meaning of the information
- Application: using the information
- Analysis: breaking the information into parts to help understand all of the information
- Synthesis: integrating the information as a whole
- Evaluation: using standards and criteria to judge the value of the information

Each of these levels builds on the previous one. The most basic is the knowledge level; the highest is the evaluation level. By understanding the cognitive domain of learning, you will be able to build more effective lesson plans and use students' thinking processes to encourage them to learn the information and apply that new knowledge. Adult learners should be able to fit the abstract thinking, facts, and information you present into the context of their jobs.

Consider these examples of cognitive learning and their application for fire fighters:

- Learning terms, facts, procedures, or principles: The fire fighter uses cognitive learning to learn the standard operating procedures (SOPs) of the fire department.
- The ability to translate and explain facts and principles: The fire fighter is taught the basic principles of fire and then asked to identify types of fuels.
- The ability to apply facts and principles to a new situation: The fire fighter is able to size up the scene, formulate a plan based on that analysis, and evaluate all possible outcomes.

Psychomotor Learning

For fire fighters, psychomotor learning is the most common learning domain. The term *psychomotor* refers to the use of the brain and senses (psycho) to tell the body what to do, and the use of the muscles (motor) to tell the body how to move. The psychomotor learning domain involves the ability to physically manipulate an object or move the body to accomplish a task or perform a skill. This kind of learning is also referred to as **kinesthetic learning**.

As in the cognitive domain, the learning phases in the psychomotor domain build progressively one upon the other. Building on Bloom's work, Ravindra Dave (1970) added the following six levels to the psychomotor domain model:

- Observation: watching the skill or activity being performed
- Imitation: copying the skill or activity in a step-by-step manner
- Manipulation: performing the skill based on instruction
- Precision: performing the skill or activity until it becomes habit
- Articulation: combining multiple skills together

- Naturalization: performing multiple skills correctly all the time

Each level of learning in Dave's psychomotor domain model builds upon the previous level: observation → imitation → manipulation → precision → articulation → naturalization. By understanding that the physical use of knowledge is the basis for students learning to perform the skill, you will be able to develop a lesson plan that involves demonstrating the skill to students, who then practice until they are able to perform that skill flawlessly. As students progress from one level to the next within the psychomotor domain, they may experiment with new ways to perform the skill. This trial-and-error process is completely natural as students learn how to adapt the skill and become more familiar with the activity.

Awareness of the following aspects of human behavior will assist you in teaching the psychomotor skill and developing an effective lesson plan:

- Gross body movement: the ability to move the arms, legs, and shoulders in a coordinated, controlled manner
- Fine motor control: the ability to use hands, fingers, hand–eye coordination, and hearing
- Verbal behaviors: the use of sound to communicate
- Nonverbal behaviors: the use of facial expressions and body gestures to communicate

In your delivery of lesson plans, ideally you will identify how a student should perform a skill or activity by carrying out a task analysis and identifying the steps involved in performing the activity. Here are some examples of psychomotor learning and its application:

- Comprehensive skill approach: The skill is demonstrated by the instructor and the fire fighter watches.
- Step-by-step approach: The fire fighter performs the skill in a precise step 1, step 2 manner until the entire skill activity is accomplished.
- Repetition of the skill or activity until it becomes habitual and is correct: The fire fighter performs the skill until it becomes second nature and he or she executes the skill flawlessly. The instructor then presents "what if" questions to help the student determine when to perform the skill.
- Combination of multiple skills: The fire fighter is able to adapt to changing situations and defend his or her choice of skills for the activity.
- Performing multiple skills correctly all the time: The fire fighter can perform the skill, and it is truly a natural activity regardless of the environment or circumstance in which the skill is performed.

For students to learn skills or activities properly, they need to practice, practice, practice (**FIGURE 2-13**). As the brain processes the attempts at performing the skill, it also learns to avoid what does not work or what was in error.

Affective Learning

Affective learning is the feeling or attitude domain. It focuses on those characteristics that make each person unique—that is, an individual's preferences, perceptions, and values. Many of these characteristics will have evolved in individual fire fighters over long periods of time, so attitudes may not change immediately after the introduction of a new concept. Instead, learning within this domain progresses from simple awareness, to acceptance, to internalization, and finally to acting out the attitude. Bloom's work with Masia and Krathwohl (1965) led to the development of the affective domain and identified the following five learning levels:

- **Receiving:** becoming aware of the skill or concept
- **Responding:** acknowledging the implications of the skill or concept and altering behavior accordingly
- **Valuing:** internalizing the skill or concept and having it become part of everyday life
- **Organizing:** comparing and contrasting skills or concepts
- **Characterizing:** adopting and personalizing skills or concepts

Each level of affective learning in Bloom's *Taxonomy of Educational Objectives: Book 2* builds on the previous level: receiving → responding → valuing →

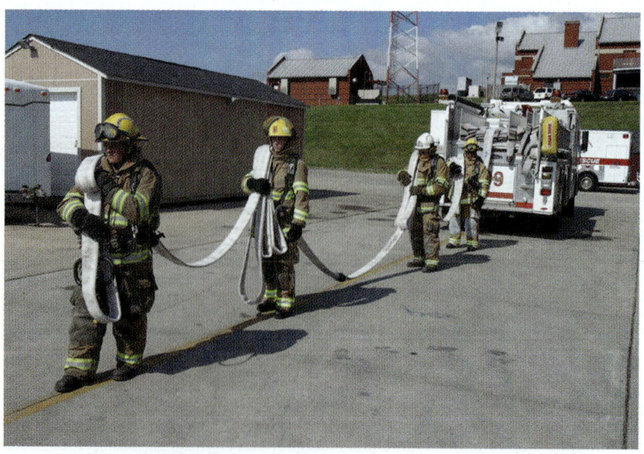

FIGURE 2-13 For students to learn skills or activities properly, they need to practice.

organizing → characterizing. Because much of this learning takes place inside the mind, it is important to look for subtle changes in students to confirm that affective learning is occurring. Here are some examples of affective learning:

- **Acquisition of new values:** The fire fighter is willing to learn the information and attends class regularly.
- **Acknowledgment of the concept:** The fire fighter studies for tests and participates in class activities.
- **Internalization of values:** The fire fighter volunteers to participate in an extra-credit activity.
- **Internalization of the organization of information:** The fire fighter decides to pursue continuing education because the additional training can keep him or her abreast of new developments and technologies.
- **Full adoption of the new values:** The fire fighter decides to pursue a degree in fire service management.

The affective domain is difficult to measure, but it should not be overlooked. The instructor must be observant to identify a student's reaction to the learning situation and changes in his or her value system. Another way of looking at the affective domain is as the marriage of cognitive knowledge with the psychomotor skills and their application in the real world by the student.

Learner Characteristics

How Does an Individual Learn?

When preparing for a class, you must ask, "What is learning?" as well as "How does a particular individual learn?" To answer these questions, you need to recognize that each student has different learner characteristics—that is, a way in which he or she prefers study and consider information and the ways he or she views the world around them. To use the terminology introduced by Bloom's Taxonomy, learning styles comprise characteristic cognitive, psychomotor, and affective behaviors.

Additional information on how students learn and retain new information and knowledge was provided by Jean Piaget, a biologist from Switzerland who developed his learning theory based on his observations of children and how they learn. Piaget's theory (Piaget and Inhelder, 1958) states that children learn "through motor actions, develop intelligence by using their natural intuition, develop cognitively through the use of logic and finally develop the ability to think abstractly." While Piaget's theories apply to adult learners in many ways, most of all they help us see how to help a student learn by going back to basics.

Although learning is an invisible mental and emotional process, the results of the learning process are frequently visible in that they may be traced back to certain experiences (e.g., a training session) and are evident in behaviors (e.g., performance of a skill).

Every individual has different characteristics and abilities as a learner. A successful instructor must take into account individual learner characteristics and abilities to ensure that all students' needs are met. This concept of considering learner characteristics and abilities is part of **student-centered learning**. Student-centered learning shifts the focus of teaching from the student as a passive observer watching a teacher to the student as an individual with an active role in the learning process (Student-Centered Learning Definition, 2014).

While learners have individual characteristics, groups of students may share common characteristics. Discovering these characteristics in the preparation phase of planning a lesson might involve contacting the organizer ahead of time and gathering specific information about the audience's demographics, their learning backgrounds, and their experience levels.

Of course, it is inappropriate to make assumptions about a group based on a single group identifier. For example, if you were assigned to teach a group of senior citizens in an assisted living center and assumed that all of them would be sitting in chairs all day, you would be very surprised to learn that most of them cook, play golf, and lead very active lives.

Groups of learners may have subsets within the larger group. To see how this works in practice, consider a group of fire fighters in a class on fire-ground support operations. Although the majority of the class wants to start placing ladders immediately and practicing ventilation, a minority prefer to watch a video and discuss the skills before actually practicing the operations (**FIGURE 2-14**). Both groups want to learn, but the preferred method is different for each.

Your students may have different ways they prefer to study or review information and different ways they think about concepts. In learning environments, using varying modes of instruction benefits all students. Using a variety of means and methods allows individual students to better grasp ideas by presenting the same ideas in different ways. Multimedia is the most common way of incorporating multiple modes of presentation. The availability of computer programs and educational websites has significantly expanded the ease of incorporating multimodal learning options.

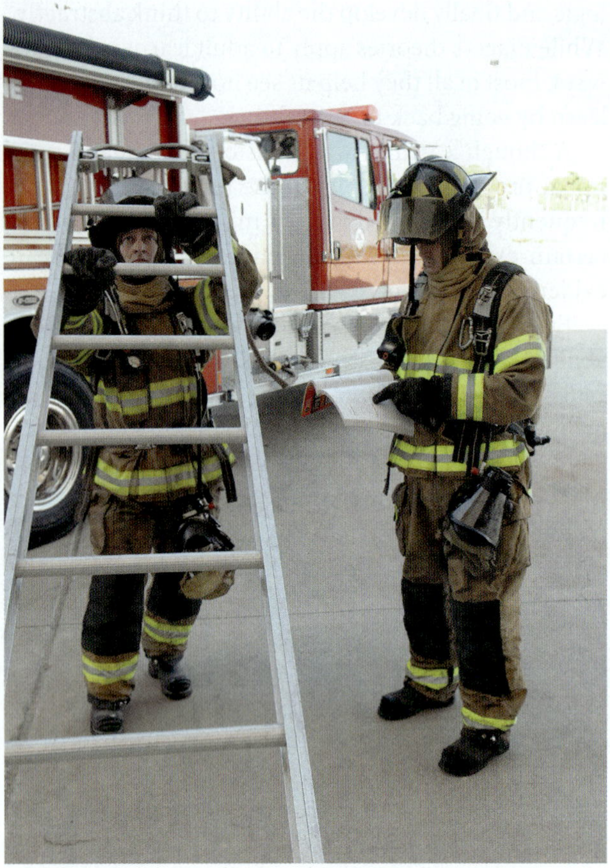

FIGURE 2-14 Both fire fighters want to learn how to raise the ladder; they simply have different learner characteristics.

Effective Teaching and Learning for All Students

Fortunately, despite the differences in learners, there are some common features to learning and effective learning experiences that inform teaching practice. Many fields of study contribute to the body of knowledge known as *learning science*. Our understanding of how people learn is incomplete and evolving, but more than a hundred years of research has led to a strong base of knowledge in the discipline. Being aware of some key concepts of learning science is useful in developing your skills as an instructor and in meeting the needs of all students. The following five learning science concepts are particularly useful for the fire and emergency services instructor:

1. **Starting points are important.** The process of learning involves connecting the new ideas and concepts to existing ones (National Research Council, 2000). Every student you will encounter brings with them preexisting ideas and perspectives. It is not uncommon for students to have an incomplete or even erroneous understanding of concepts that can interfere with their ability to add and integrate the knowledge you are presenting. As an example, students who have seen fire sprinklers go off on television may believe that a typical sprinkler activation includes multiple heads all over a building going off simultaneously. It may be harder for that student to comprehend a lesson on sprinklers because their existing knowledge will not fit with the new information. Likewise, students who have watched fire fighters work in a burning structure on television may have an unrealistic expectation of visibility in a fire setting that impedes their attention to the importance of specific communication details of a search and rescue lesson. An important step in making sure the lesson will be effective for all is assessing the base knowledge of your students and clearing up any misconceptions that may exist.
2. **Real learning is an active process.** Adults and children learn when they are involved in **active learning**. Active learning can be defined as "anything that involves students in doing things and thinking about the things they are doing" (Bonwell and Eison, 1991). "Doing things" does not mean just performing physical tasks such as raising a ladder. Doing things can include having a discussion, drawing a diagram, or working in a group. Students are doing things when they are using the information to construct their understanding of a concept. Listening and reading are passive and do not require the student to make any use of the information. To deliver effective instruction, you must do more than stand in front of the class, show a slide presentation, and talk. Learning environments that provide opportunities for students to use and integrate knowledge have more successful outcomes.

   The second aspect of this definition is *metacognition*, meaning "thinking about thinking." Students need to think about what they are doing and consider how they learn as individuals. Good instruction helps learners to be aware of their thought processes. Recall from earlier in this chapter the idea of critical reflection. This is a form of metacognition. Providing learners opportunities to develop awareness of how they learn, what helps them learn, and ways to meet their needs is part of a successful learning environment (Hacker, Dunlosky, and Graesser, 2009).
3. **Organization of knowledge is a critical part of learning.** To gain mastery in an area, students must not only know facts and concepts, but must be able to organize them into a conceptual

framework and retrieve it as usable knowledge (National Research Council, 2000).

Good teaching provides students with guidance in developing conceptual frameworks. It is important to make sure you are presenting the big picture and emphasizing the important overall concepts. Visually organizing the lesson can help students to see the connections between concepts. Pay attention to how students are thinking about the concepts being presented. Ask students to explain their thinking or "think out loud" and give feedback and guidance. Provide a model of what more advanced thinking about the topic looks like. For example, explain how an experienced fire fighter would think about conditions present on arrival at a fire. Scaffolding, which is discussed in more detail later in this chapter, is an effective way to provide frameworks for students.

4. **Practice matters.** Deliberate, goal-directed practice with feedback, is necessary for learning. This is intuitive to many fire instructors when thinking about practical skills. We have all experienced a situation in which we were shown a skill, practiced it with guidance to correct our mistakes, and finally mastered it. What is less intuitive is that this is true for not only physical skills but mental skills as well. Students need to practice using and applying knowledge (National Research Council, 2000). Again, this is easy to see when we think about specific instances. If you are teaching students a formula for determining friction loss, it is important to provide the opportunity for them to practice not only using the formula with guidance, but also determining when to apply the formula. It is less apparent, but equally as necessary, when presenting a complex idea. For example, in a lesson about combustion, students need to have opportunities to practice retrieving and applying the concept. In the classroom, this may involve asking students studying combustion to predict what would happen if they tried to light a match on the moon. After letting them apply their knowledge to make a prediction, discuss the correct answer and why it is correct. This allows them to practice applying the concepts and get feedback on how well they did.

   Part of being able to provide students with the feedback they need to learn is assessment. Assessment can be informal, like asking a question, or more formal, like testing. Often, students and teachers see testing and assessment as a required behavior at the end of a session that is unrelated to the classroom. In reality, assessment is fundamental to helping students determine what they know and what they have not yet mastered. Assessment is not just performed by the instructor for the students. Encouraging students to do continual self-assessment is part of metacognition and helps them develop their learning skills (Ambrose, Bridges, DiPietro, Lovett, and Norman 2010).

5. **Learning is social.** The majority of our learning takes place with the input of others. Consider the exchange of information and skill that occurs when you are engaged in an activity with friends. Golfing, fishing, a school organization, a sports team, an office group: whether working or playing, we transfer knowledge and skills within groups. Humans use peers to clarify their understanding and learn new things on a regular basis. You have probably used this technique yourself multiple times. Maybe you read the directions to set up something on your phone but do not quite understand, so you ask a friend for help and you walk through it together. Working together helps people to refine concepts.

   Explaining things to others is a prime example of "doing things" with new knowledge that active learning requires. It turns out that explaining a concept to others is a very effective way of developing understanding. Many people have experienced the "a-ha!" moment when something becomes clear as they are explaining it to another person. Given this, it should come as no surprise that research indicates that peer interaction and cooperative learning improve outcomes (Crouch and Mazur, 2001).

Student-Centered Learning

Think about teaching and learning. What comes to mind first? Probably a scene where students are seated in rows, focused on the instructor, occasionally looking at a whiteboard or overhead presentation and exhibiting boredom, fatigue, and apathy. Contrast this picture with a classroom where students and instructor are engaged equally, where the instructor is facilitating the work of the students who are working in groups and practicing a skill, creating energy, synergy, and excitement.

Teacher-centered passive learning requires little involvement on the part of the student. Learners simply receive information by listening, watching, reading, or observing. The instructor disseminates information and is at the center of activity. Passive involvement leads to limited retention of knowledge by students. Unfortunately, this is historically the type of teaching fire fighters have been subject to. Because most fire and emergency services instructors had limited, if any, teaching experience and little exposure to the field of learning science, the fire service developed a pattern of instructor-centered teaching that provided the least effective avenue for retention.

Over the past 20 years, there have been significant advances in the field of teaching and learning. As learning science has provided more insight into what works, educational practices have moved from this older instructor-centered learning model to a more effective student-centered learning model. Teaching in a student-centered learning setting is called *learner-centered* or *student-centered teaching*.

In a student-centered learning model, the focus is on the students and their learning rather than the instructor and teaching. Responsibility for learning is a shared responsibility of both the instructor and the student.

Student-centered learning is active learning. Active learning is anything students do more than simply receiving instruction and passively listening to a lecture or watching a movie. Students are required to participate by reading, writing, discussing, solving problems, and engaging in higher-level thinking. Activities may include group discussion, questioning, brainstorming, problem solving, participation in demonstrations, or a variety of other hands-on techniques for involvement. Frequent assessment opportunities are provided to assist the student in understanding how well they have mastered skills and concepts.

In a student-centered learning environment, the role of the instructor is that of a facilitator. The instructor's job is to work with the students to facilitate their learning by providing guidance and feedback to enable students to develop skills and knowledge. This should not be interpreted as a philosophy that removes all responsibility for the educational process or outcomes from the instructor or as a system that lets students "do whatever they want," because this is not the case at all. Learner-centeredness is a partnership model where the instructor and the students work together to achieve the course goals.

One of the keys to student-centered learning is providing frequent feedback so students know how they are doing. Assessment is one of the main ways instructors and students get feedback. Assessment does not mean testing; while testing is one method of assessment, there are a wide variety of other ways that learner progress can be measured. Assessment can be as simple as watching a student do a task and providing feedback on his or her performance. In addition to being useful to students, assessments are helpful to instructors in knowing where to focus their attention. Providing frequent low-stakes assessments can ensure that assessment is viewed as a positive experience by both the learner and the instructor.

Lessons involving active, student-centered learning take more planning and organization but are always worth the effort in the end. An Instructor I must be prepared to use a wide range of student-centered teaching methods and strategies that are called for in lesson plans.

Student-Centered Teaching Methods and Strategies

The best teaching includes a variety of methods, often referred to as strategies, used to meet the diverse needs of the learners. The decision to use one strategy over another will depend on the time available, number of students, objectives of the lesson, type of information to be presented, availability of materials and resources, domains and levels of learning, and personal preferences of the instructor. Most instructors tend to teach in the ways that they themselves learn best. It takes a knack to select an instructional method that best fits both the instructor's teaching style and the lesson situation. Often, one teaching method will naturally flow into another, all within the same lesson. Experienced instructors have the skills to make this process seamless and productive for students without overloading their ability to process information. There is no one "right" method for teaching, but certain criteria specific to each style help the instructor make the best choice possible for the learners. We will discuss some of the more common teaching strategies in this chapter in terms of their advantages and disadvantages as well as some tips for implementing each.

Discussion

A discussion format is different from a lecture-and-discussion format in that learners are as much a part of the presentation as the instructor. In fact, the instructor's role shifts to that of facilitator. Traditional discussion can tend to be instructor centered. A true discussion creates an exchange of ideas to provide two-way communication throughout the session, allowing everyone to participate. The educator speaks directly to the learners, asking questions or making comments and waiting for a response, or groups of learners can discuss views with each other. This method is very useful when trying to engage the affective domain and when working with concepts, ideas, and feelings. The participants can express themselves and learn from each other. This method deals less with facts, although the facts may be presented in the beginning as a reference for discussion. Discussion groups are effective in combination with or after a demonstration or film presentation.

This method, although very productive, is not recommended for groups larger than 20. Even in smaller groups, some participants may withdraw, not feeling comfortable enough to participate. Other group members may dominate discussions or become overbearing when voicing their opinions. It takes careful planning on the part of the facilitator to prevent these bumps in the road. When planning to use this method, be sure to design questions that evoke critical thinking and a sense of cooperation. Be clear that all ideas will be considered and that no idea or suggestion will be considered incorrect. The facilitator should allow time for a well-constructed summary that includes information gathered during the session. Another technique that can foster more engaged discussion is called think-pair-share, wherein the question is directed to the class, students formulate responses, share with another student, then share with the class.

COMPANY-LEVEL INSTRUCTOR TIP

An effective way to reinforce learning with a group that meets for more than one session is to use a sum-up. Sum-ups are short paragraphs or fill-in-the-blanks that capture the main ideas of a presentation. At the beginning of the next session, review the sum-ups from the last class. These can serve as an evaluation tool to discover whether the main points made their way to the learners.

Small Discussion Groups

Small discussion groups offer some of the same advantages as the larger group discussion, but they may even provide for more engagement and interaction. Some people feel more comfortable in smaller groups and will become more verbal. Each member will have more opportunities to participate, which will generate more viewpoints. To ensure that each person is engaged and contributing, assign roles such as reporter, scribe, timekeeper, and organizer. Sometimes these roles will be taken by participants and need not be assigned; other times, the instructor will need to be aware of the group dynamics and assign the roles. When handled correctly, the small-group discussion method facilitates active learning and can create energy conducive to learning in the room. Groups that develop their own synergy are capable of a heightened level of problem solving and creativity. Small-group discussions lend themselves well to the method of guided discovery, wherein participants are coached as they work to come up with solutions to problems on their own. Problem solving is an important element of learning; participants in the experience are more likely to remember the solutions when they were involved in the process of discovery. However, it takes a skilled facilitator to keep several small groups focused and on task. There is a tendency for the groups to get side tracked and run out of time before the objectives are met. Planning a session with small-group discussions requires preparing specific, well-crafted tasks or questions for the groups to address. The makeup of the groups must be considered. Will the instructor assign groups or allow members to form their own groups? It will also be important to build in time during and after the group time for reporting and summarizing. The facilitator should stroll around the room to make sure groups are focusing on the problems, while still allowing for an atmosphere of fun and creativity. The clock will be ticking, so occasional reminders to the groups will keep them cognizant of the amount of time they have left to finish their work.

Demonstrations

The purpose of a demonstration is to transmit the big picture to a group in a short period of time. This method is more instructor centered than student centered, but it is useful for teaching skills or situations that are difficult to fully explain through a verbal description alone. By seeing a task performed, learners become more aware of what materials are needed, better remember the steps in the process, and are able to observe the final outcome. Demonstrations generally take more preparation and usually need to be supported by audiovisual materials or other equipment, but the benefits will be well worth the effort for the

COMPANY-LEVEL INSTRUCTOR TIP

When teaching a group that meets more than once you can 'flip" the classroom. Instead of showing your students a video or giving a lecture during class time, assign those as pre-class work to the students. Have them watch the video or lecture or read the information before the class. Then when they come to class, use the class time to check for understanding and practice the skills. This is flipping the classroom. Think about people learning to play a musical instrument. They practice on their own and then see the instructor to get feedback on how well they are doing and correct mistakes. The instructor's time is not used to watch the student practice but rather to check progress, clarify questions, set goals, and evaluate mastery.

A critical part of this is that the students must know that completion of the pre-class work is required and essential for their learning. Instructors can help bring that point home by holding students accountable for being prepared by checking for the preparation and for understanding in class and attaching value such as points or grades to the preparation.

participants. Field trips, tours, and simulations are all variations of the demonstration method.

Instructors using demonstrations should make sure all students are in a position where they can see and hear. Decide how many students and how much room and equipment will be needed. To hold the audience's attention, demonstrations should not exceed 20 minutes. It is important to practice and time the demonstration before presenting it to an audience. Without an actual run-through, presenters are often surprised that their planned demonstration takes far less or much longer than they anticipated. Either situation can be perceived as unprofessional, especially if the instructor does not have backup materials to fill the gap. Handouts with pictures or written instructions and information serve to support and clarify the demonstration for the audience.

Fire instruction has many opportunities to present demonstrations of interest to students. Personnel need to remember that although students are intrigued by what they see, educational objectives should be at the core of the presentations. The objectives will provide the reasons for giving the presentation in the first place and dictate the arrangement of the information from beginning to end.

COMPANY-LEVEL INSTRUCTOR TIP

Give students a short pre-lesson quiz. This can be informal through a show of hands at a station training session, it can be done on paper with partners correcting it, or software or web-based applications can be used. Doing this will not only improve the students' learning but it will also help you assess what level the students are starting at and what you might need to focus more attention on in class.

Questioning

One of the best ways to evoke a response from an audience is by asking good questions. Socrates knew that he was able to get students to think more critically by challenging them with questions rather than relying solely on a direct lecture approach. Generally, questioning is used in conjunction with other methods. The learner becomes more actively involved and begins to think at higher levels. Questions and their responses also allow an instructor to evaluate the learners' level of understanding and make adjustments immediately. Instructors should be aware that there is an art to using questions to produce the greatest learning. Poorly crafted questions limit the success of using this method. The give and take of a questioning session will also take more time than straight lecture (**TABLE 2-1**). You also can pose a question or topic for the class, and then allow them the opportunity to research and develop responses, instead of simply asking the question.

Following are several tips to keep in mind when using questioning as a method of instruction:

- Ask challenging, open questions. This means avoid phrasing questions that are closed or require straightforward factual answers unless you are only checking for retention. Questions that begin with who, when, or where and yes-or-no questions do not require learners to think as critically as when they are asked questions that begin with why, how, and what if. For example, you might ask a group of students if they should perform ventilation at a fire. The answer is simply "yes" and could be answered with almost no thought at all. It would be better to ask "What could happen if a fire fighter started ventilation before a water supply was established?" More than one answer exists, and the feedback will generate further discussion.
- Closed questions, or those requiring a specific answer, will work best in the classroom with students who cannot focus well.
- Ask uncluttered questions. Questions with many sub-questions or interspersed with background information can confuse students because it becomes unclear as to what is being asked of them.
- Make sure the questions are crafted at a level the students are prepared to understand. Ask if the question is clear and write questions down where they can be seen by everyone, if possible.

Role Playing

Role playing brings students into a lesson and encourages them to become part of the learning and teaching. The instructor and the student take on roles to act out situations, providing for more active learning than direct teaching methods and a more interesting way to present material. For a brief time, the classroom becomes a stage where an audience member is given an opportunity to practice newly introduced knowledge or skills. As the instructor, you are able to introduce problem situations more dramatically and observe students' reactions. The students can explore alternative solutions, and you can see how the material plays out in a fairly realistic scenario. This method is particularly effective with skills that involve an interaction between people, such as taking an emergency call or interviewing a witness. The experience can be rewarding because learners retain more by observing members of their

TABLE 2-1 Questioning Techniques

Type of Question	Purpose and Strength
Factual	Soliciting simple, straightforward answers based on facts, observation, or awareness. Answers are usually right or wrong. Example: How often should hose be tested?
Convergent	Looking for answers that fall within a very finite range of acceptable accuracy. The student can make some inferences based on personal awareness or other forms of information. Utilizes organizing, planning, sequencing, and structuring skills. Example: If you were sitting in front of the fire station and a person ran up and reported a fire, how would you handle the situation? What would you do first?
Divergent	Requiring students to explore different avenues and create many different variations, alternatives, and scenarios based on existing knowledge as a springboard. Students may arrive at answers through intuition, imagination, inference, projection, or conjecture. May not be a right or wrong answer. Higher-level cognitive thinking is necessary than for factual or convergent questions. Divergent questioning lends itself to better discussions and engagement. Hypothetical questions provide interesting discussions. May become essential questions for a lesson. Example: You are applying high volumes of water to a warehouse fire through an open loading dock door, but it does not appear to be having the expected effect. Why do you think the suppression efforts are not working?
Evaluative	Asking for more sophisticated levels of cognitive and/or emotional judgment. Students will combine multiple logical and/or affective thinking processes, or comparative perspectives, to synthesize information for conclusions. Example: What are reasons that fire fighters might fail to follow safety procedures like wearing seatbelts?
Combination	A blend of any of the types of questions in this table. Example: If you were asked to prepare a list of objectives for a community class about fire safety, what five messages would you consider, in order of importance, and why?

own groups; however, be aware of some of the pitfalls of using this approach. It is difficult to use in large groups. Some students may be too self-conscious to fully engage in the activity. Not everyone wants to be the center of attention. To prepare for successful role play experiences, define the problem situation and roles clearly, give clear instructions, watch the time, and plan for correcting incorrect responses as they occur.

Peer Tutoring

Peer tutoring occurs when a student with adequate or excellent mastery of an idea helps another student while a lesser degree of mastery. Peer tutoring works because the students are likely to more readily express opinions, ask questions, and risk untested solutions. They also may speak a more similar language with each other than in an instructor–student relationship. This approach provides many positive benefits for both the tutor and the tutee in all three domains of learning. Fire and emergency services instructors can easily make use of this teaching method when the student group has a mixed level of experience or when some of the group is mastering skills or knowledge faster than the rest. For example, if an instructor presents a lesson on knot tying to a group of fire fighters, members new to knot tying can be paired up with members with knot tying experience to practice with feedback.

Storytelling

Everyone loves a good story—especially fire fighters. Stories do have a place in the learning environment. Told correctly, they can be an effective hook, reeling in the audience to the world of the speaker. The storyteller must ensure the tale is relevant to the lesson content and interesting to the audience. Tell a story in which all audience members are in the story. Using imagery, walk them through to generate a mental picture. For example, begin with, "Imagine you are on the second floor of a home with a fire in the attic. You are about to open the door to the attic stairs. Picture the hallway and your crew. How is everyone positioned?" If you are animated and believable, the method is sure to set the stage for learning. But if the story is too long or irrelevant or if stories are overused during a presentation, this method will fail. Keep the lesson objectives in mind when choosing and preparing a story for presentation. Instructors should avoid telling too many stories during one presentation, especially about themselves; use these stories sparingly to maintain interest! Effective storytelling is an art and should be practiced before using it in a presentation.

Brainstorming

Brainstorming is a fast-paced activity in which group members arrive at answers or solutions by bringing ideas to the table for discussion and resolution. Learning flourishes when the audience members are active learners sharing in a spirit of cooperation. Full participation is encouraged because all ideas are welcomed and recorded. One idea often sparks a series of questions, new ideas, and dynamic creativity. The activity draws on the entire group's knowledge and experience. Again, the instructor becomes a facilitator or coach, and learning is student centered.

Instructors new to this technique may find that participants have difficulty getting "off the ground" or that the activity can easily become unfocused and chaotic; therefore, actual brainstorming sessions should be around 5 to 7 minutes long.

Sessions must be well facilitated to avoid criticism and discussions going off on tangents. Facilitators need to carefully select and focus the issues and prepare ideas for stimulating the groups that are slow to get the main idea. Most importantly, brainstorming sessions require the instructors to prepare guidelines and objectives and make them clear to the participants. Instructors must also be ready to intervene if the groups get bogged down. It will always help the "brainstormers" to have guidelines posted on an easel or a whiteboard as a reference to center their thinking. Flip charts for each group are also helpful for groups to record their ideas as they evolve. Following are some rules for brainstorming:

1. Define the problem and set directions.
2. Encourage participation from everyone. All ideas are valuable. All ideas become the property of the group rather than of a particular individual.
3. Build on the ideas put forth by others. Use the word "yes" instead of "but" when responding to another idea. Piggyback on ideas rather than discounting them.
4. Suspend judgment. Not everyone is comfortable with brainstorming. Aim to minimize barriers and inhibitions.
5. Encourage outside-the-box thinking. Be creative. No idea is too absurd. Wild and exaggerated ideas can lead to other possibilities.
6. Go for *quantity*, not quality. Reality checks and fine tuning will come later.
7. Record and display ideas. Be complete in writing down ideas; use more than one word so the intent is not forgotten. Sticky notes and flip charts work well.
8. When the session is finished, circle 20 percent of the most workable or interesting ideas. Think in terms of the 80/20 rule: look for 20 percent of the ideas that will accomplish 80 percent of the desired results.
9. Watch the clock. Start and finish on time. Encourage a brisk pace to maximize investment in the process.
10. Have fun! Keep the atmosphere light; it increases creativity.

COMPANY-LEVEL INSTRUCTOR TIP

The K-W-L (what I *know*, what I *want to know*, and what I *learned*) is a predictive approach to learning, but it can easily be incorporated into a strategy for discussion formats. Create a simple form with three columns, titling them "What I Know," "What I Want to Know," and "What I Learned" and provide the form to each member of the group. Lead students through brainstorming on the topic. You can participate as a contributor of relevant questions. Ask each participant to fill in the "K" and "W" columns with what they already know or believe about the topic and what more they would like to know about it. Show a video or give a brief presentation. After the presentation, have group members go back to check which questions were answered by the information provided; these can be written in the last column.

Motivation and Learning

Motivational factors make students feel enthusiastic and eager to learn. Motivation affects how students practice, what they observe, and what they do—all of which are critical to learning. As an instructor, you need to understand how learning and motivation work together to make a great fire fighter. Instructors will face various motivations themselves that will require them to become more vocal, animated, or intense to emphasize why information is important to the student.

Learning is the potential behavior, whereas motivation is the behavior activator. Learning and motivation combine to determine performance in training. Without a motivated student and an expert instructor, learning will not take place. If the student's motivation is poor, then his or her performance in training will be sloppy and inaccurate. If the student's performance in training is sloppy and inaccurate, then the fire fighter's response at an incident will be sloppy and incorrect. This sort of shortcoming is not acceptable on the fire ground.

Motivation of Adult Learners

Cyril Houle (1961) identified three types of adult learners: goal oriented, activity oriented, and learning oriented. Each type is associated with different motivational issues, which in turn affects how learning takes place (Draper, 1993).

Goal-oriented learners are the most common type of adult learner. Their learning decisions are guided by clear-cut goals, as the learner takes a "utilitarian" or "pure" stance toward education. An example of a goal-oriented learner is a fire instructor attending a workshop on using distance learning to enhance a department's training program.

The second type of adult learner is the activity-oriented learner. For these individuals, participation is based on reasons other than the stated purpose of the learning activity. Examples of activity-oriented learners include a full-time worker who attends evening noncredit courses with a friend or a fire fighter attending a conference with other department members just to attend social events after the conference.

The third type of adult learner, the learning-oriented learner, seeks knowledge for the purpose of learning something new. For this learner, education is a way of life and, as such, is an intrinsically valued activity. Because this type of learner focuses on the content of a learning activity, he or she can participate either within a group or individually (Houle, 1961).

Consider the example of two fire fighters who are attending a CPR training class. A fire fighter who is a goal-oriented learner might attend the class in an effort to improve her job skills, whereas the fire fighter who is an activity-oriented learner might take the class to spend time with his friends and possibly learn CPR at the same time. Although the learning agendas and goals of these fire fighters are quite different, both are in the same class. Learner-oriented adults focus on the act of being involved in learning.

Another factor that greatly influences success in the classroom is whether the adult learners grasp how the material relates to the real world and how this learning can be beneficial to job performance. This factor is well documented as affecting the learning outcome (Wlodkowski, 1999). Experienced instructors use real-world applications and can point directly to how information translates to use in the workplace. Theory into practice is a concept that can work to an instructor's advantage in this sense. For example, as part of their training, recruits learn that a gallon of water weighs a little more than 8 pounds. That statistical information is fairly simple to recall, but if you show recruits that a master stream flows 500 gallons per minute × 8 pounds per gallon, the students can quickly see that when they use a master stream in the real world, they are putting 4000 pounds of live load per minute into a structure, which may cause collapse.

Yet another key factor is the adult learner's psychological state. Mild anxiety can help the adult learner to focus on a particular task. Conversely, intense negative emotions (e.g., anxiety, panic, rage, insecurity) may detract from motivation, ultimately either interfering with learning or contributing to a low performance. To counteract this possibility, make your students feel welcome in the class session or at the drill ground by explaining the context and content of the training and allowing for a positive-outcome-based environment.

The current position of adult learners in the life cycle also influences the quality and quantity of learning. Research suggests that each phase of life is characterized by the need for learning certain behaviors and skills. Because they are adults, adult learners invariably want to be treated as autonomous, independent learners.

Geographical changes (moving from one location to another), physical changes (reaction times), visual and auditory acuity, and intellectual functioning influence the adult learner's performance as well. The adult learner's internal world of ideas, beliefs, goals, and expectations for success or failure can either enhance or interfere with the quality and quantity of thinking and information processing. In addition, the adult's attitudes about his or her ability to learn and judgment as to whether learning is an important life goal affect motivation. Moreover, motivational and emotional factors influence the quality of thinking and the processing of information.

No matter where the adult learner is and what he or she believes about his or her abilities, the adult learner continues to acquire knowledge both intentionally and unintentionally (Butler and McManus, 1998). The effectiveness of the learning process relates directly to the learning environment and the adult learner's interactions with that environment. In short, the adult learner's mental and emotional processes for learning can either help or hinder the fire fighter during training.

Motivation as a Factor in Class Design

Motivation is the primary learning component for adult learning. It generates the question "Why?" Why is the adult learner in the class? Why does the adult learner want to take (or not want to take) this class? When you can identify the why, it will allow you to tap into the how—the precise motivation and techniques that will help the adult learner achieve the goal of learning.

For example, knowing that attendance at a training class is mandatory allows you to design the lesson plan for the captive audience to maximize motivation. Unfortunately, most adult learners who are mandated to attend a class do poorly during such training, simply because they are unmotivated. Some adult learners may not know why they must learn the information or what is expected from the training or educational program, whereas other adult learners may have high expectations of the class. The unmotivated adult learners, the questioning adult learners, and the adult learners with high expectations all share the same classroom.

Find out from your students why they are in your class and what they expect. This information will enable you to design the lesson plans to meet every student's needs and sow the seeds of self-motivation in every student. You will inevitably need to employ a variety of motivational techniques to stimulate students. To learn, a student must be stimulated by the subject (McClincy, 2002).

If you are motivated, your enthusiasm may prove contagious in the classroom. When you are dynamic, outgoing, charismatic, and generally interested in the topic, your lessons will be taught with energy. Your personality will shine through in the classroom and will serve as a motivational factor for your students.

The use of audiovisual aids, teaching strategies, teaching methods, and even the classroom itself may serve as motivational factors. How you incorporate any or all of these motivational factors into the classroom will be reflected in the success of the learning process. For example, live-action video used to highlight a key point or term will motivate and engage the learner to observe the action much more than a still photo will, and even more than text on a slide will. Nevertheless, you must ensure that your video enhances your presentation but does not become the presentation. The next two chapters will expand on this topic.

Motivational factors are part of each level of instruction, from design to delivery to evaluation. The best courses you have attended motivated you to learn and provided you with the topic's relevance and application. Take time to consider ways to engage your learners throughout the presentation. Students are motivated to learn when they can understand how the material applies to them and how they will use it. An adult learner's motivation may change throughout a session. The number of factors that can affect motivation is limitless. You need to be able to recognize the changing motivational needs of adult learners. Frequently cited course improvement suggestions include more periodic input on student grades, ongoing monitoring of progress in a course, and the ability to provide more feedback between the instructor and the student.

Learning Disabilities

As an instructor, you may encounter students with a wide variety of learning disabilities. The Americans with Disabilities Act (ADA—federal legislation that was originally passed in 1990) classifies learning disabilities into these major categories:

- Reading disabilities range from the inability to understand the meaning of words, to the inability to read or comprehend, to **dyslexia**. This disability could become apparent in class if a student is asked to read a section of course material aloud or to summarize a paragraph from a textbook.
- Some students lack the ability to write, to spell, or to place words together to complete a sentence. This type of disability, known as **dysphasia**, might present itself when a student submits work for a course and the work is poorly written.
- Other students might suffer from **dyscalculia**, or difficulty with math and related subjects. Students with this disability might struggle on a hydraulics course or test.
- **Dyspraxia** is the inability to display physical coordination of motor skills. This condition could be observed on the training ground as a student's inability to complete a task such as climbing a ladder.
- A disorder that affects children but can be carried into adulthood is known as **attention-deficit/hyperactivity disorder (ADHD)**.

A person with ADHD has a chronic level of inattention and an impulsive hyperactivity that affects his or her ability to function on a daily basis. This disorder is a documented condition identified by the Centers for Disease Control and Prevention (CDC). Although it can be treated, there is no known cure for ADHD.
- Other types of disabilities that could affect the learning process include color blindness and poor vision, even if it is just difficulty in seeing the screen in a classroom.
- Some adult learners may have poor hearing and cannot properly hear material presented in the classroom. Hearing loss is a common problem that occurs with aging, so instructors may often teach older fire fighters who are dealing with being unable to hear.
- English as a second language (ESL) is a factor that some organizations are facing that can affect the learning environment and create a challenge to the instructor.

Knowing and understanding each of these learning disabilities will help you teach. Unfortunately, in most cases you will not know that students have these problems until a class has already begun. If you are a guest lecturer, you will not get the opportunity to know your students until after the first few hours of instruction. Once you have identified students with some type of learning disability, you need to adjust your teaching as necessary. There are many ways to help students in your class who are struggling to learn. For example, a few positive words in private or suggestions on a written assignment might help a struggling student understand a concept that is just beyond his or her reach. Students who have learning disabilities are not unintelligent or unable to learn; they simply learn in different ways. They usually have average to high intelligence, but may perform poorly on tests because of their disabilities if accommodations are not made for their special needs.

A student who is a hesitator may be suffering from a learning disability. Such a student is often shy, reluctant, at a loss for words, and quiet. Although he or she may know the material and have much to offer, the individual's shyness, fear, or lack of confidence may keep him or her from participating in class activities or answering questions. You can engage this student by asking nonthreatening questions and offering encouragement. You need to let a hesitator know that his or her contributions are worthwhile and important. Every student's participation in the classroom is important, so provide reassurance to this type of student as necessary.

Making accommodations for students with learning disabilities is largely a fact-based situation. Under the ADA, reasonable accommodations must be made for students with disabilities; however, accommodations are not necessary if they create an undue hardship to the employer or agency or pose a direct threat to the safety and security of others.

Instructing Students with Disabilities

Instructors can employ a variety of strategies to assist students with learning disabilities. For example, breaking the material into smaller steps or components will allow a student to comprehend the material more easily. Supplying regular, positive feedback in a manner that does not single out the individual is very effective in encouraging a student with a disability to learn. Use of diagrams, graphics, and pictures to support a lecture is effective in tying learning material together.

A new teaching technique that has been developed over the past few years is called scaffolding. Scaffolding is intended to assist students with learning disabilities, but could be used with any student. Think of metal scaffolding that surrounds a building as it is constructed, serving as a support system. As the structure takes shape and is able to stand on its own, the scaffolding is removed until we see the final building. When working with a student who has a learning disability, the instructor who is using scaffolding establishes a support system when presenting the new material. The instructor gives the student the content, motivation, and foundation of the new material. In building and establishing the scaffolding, the instructor can use some of the following strategies:

- Activate the student's prior knowledge with questions or ask for others' experiences.
- Offer the student a situation, involving the subject being taught, that gives the student a chance to think and give a response from his or her own experiences.
- Break complex course material into easier pieces that will allow a student learning "successes" in understanding the new material.
- Show a student an example of the desired outcome before he or she completes the task.
- Allow a student to "brainstorm" or think out loud while seeking a solution to questions or problems.
- Teach the student mnemonic techniques to help in memorizing material or procedures.
- Teach key vocabulary terms before reading to help improve what is learned while reading.

When using this technique, you offer students support to learn the new material and then slowly or strategically remove the scaffolding to allow the students to stand on their own. For learning to progress, scaffolds should be removed gradually as instruction continues, so that students will eventually be able to demonstrate comprehension independently.

Disruptive Students

Other types of students may pose challenges as well. For example, some students, for one reason or another, feel the need to establish their presence in the class by acting out in other ways (also discussed in Chapter 3, *Methods of Instruction*).

- The class clown feels the need to make comments or jokes about the course material or perhaps others in the classroom.
- The class know-it-all has been there and done that already, regardless of the topic.
- The gifted learner is very familiar with the course material or has the ability to read quickly. This individual becomes bored because he or she is so far ahead of the rest of the class.

Most often, these types of students have other underlying issues that cause them to seek out attention in a negative way. A variety of methods may be used to deal with these types of students, but in general the most effective method is to minimize their impact on the class by not giving into the same type of behavior. Most often a stern look is enough to get a class clown to stop cracking jokes (**FIGURE 2-15**). If this measure fails to quell the disruptive behavior, then engage the student with a question that is meant to bring him or her into the class discussion. If this technique does not work, then at the next break a one-on-one discussion might be appropriate. The last step in dealing with a student who continues to disrupt the learning environment would be to ask him or her to leave the class. In using this form of progressive discipline, the goal is to bring the student back into the classroom in a positive way that does not embarrass either the student or you as the instructor.

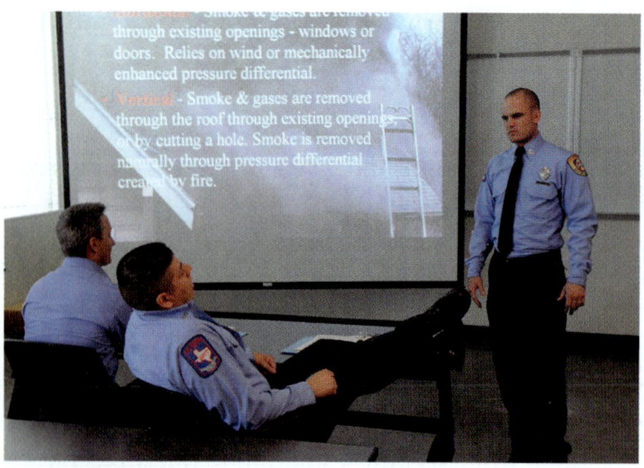

FIGURE 2-15 Occasionally, an instructor will have to deal with inappropriate behavior. How might you deal with this situation?

The student who is bored or quiet may be displaying that behavior because of a particular circumstance. Sources of this problem may include a lack of interest in the subject, an objection to being forced to take the class, unfamiliarity with the terminology in the class, boredom, and long and technical lectures. This student may just drift off mentally and refuse to participate in the classroom or become disruptive in other ways. As the instructor, you need to keep all students interested and focused on the material. Make your lectures interactive and concise. See Chapter 3, *Methods of Instruction*, for more on this topic.

Other students may not be interested in the topic. They may be in the class simply because they have to be. These students lack energy and attention, and you should try to determine whether this is a regular problem. If so, these students may have a disability or other problem that you may need to discover and address through counseling, tutoring, or other means.

A student who is a slow learner may be the most difficult for you to deal with. Such an individual has trouble keeping up and may not understand some or all of the material. One technique for handling this situation is to encourage input from other students—hearing the information differently may help. During a break, have a respectful one-on-one talk with the student to ensure understanding and comprehension.

Many students have some kind of impediment to learning, and most of those students have found unique ways to compensate for these obstacles. We all have times when our attention drifts or our energy is low, but if this failure to engage in the learning process is a recurring event it needs to be addressed because it will interfere with long-term learning. Some students may need help in the form of tutoring or individualized instruction, for example. These options should be discussed with students who have learning disabilities, and together you and the student should design a learning plan.

Training BULLETIN

JONES & BARTLETT FIRE DISTRICT
TRAINING DIVISION
5 Wall Street, Burlington, MA, 01803
Phone 978-443-5000 Fax 978-443-8000

Instant Applications: Lesson Plans

Drill Assignment

Apply the chapter content to your department's operation, training division, and your personal experiences to complete the following questions and activities.

Objective

Upon completion of the instant applications, fire and emergency services instructor students will exhibit decision making and application of job performance requirements of the instructor using the text, class discussion, and their own personal experiences.

Suggested Drill Applications

1. During several upcoming company training sessions, evaluate your shift members and identify their learner characteristics.
2. Identify and demonstrate different methods of dealing with learning disabilities.
3. Prior to participating in a company-level training session, identify several of the influences that may affect the ability of your shift members to learn during the session.
4. Review the laws and principles of learning from the text, and identify which of those appear to have the greatest impact on your shift-level training.

Incident Report: NIOSH Report F2007-09

Drill Assignment

Review the information in this incident report and prepare a practice presentation for class delivery at the direction of your instructor. Your presentation should include a summary of the incident facts and a review of the NFPA 1403 compliance and noncompliance findings. Use an outline to organize your thoughts. You may be evaluated on your communication skills during your presentation.

Baltimore, Maryland—2007

The Baltimore City Fire Department was conducting a live fire training exercise in a row house following the department's Fire Fighter I program. The program had not been successfully completed by all participants, and some of the recruits did not successfully complete the physical performance requirements during training. Some of the recruits had also never participated in interior live fire training evolutions.

The involved building was a three-story row house, and was one of a series of very narrow row houses, only 11 ft 4 in. (3.5 m) wide. It was a 1200 ft^2 (111.5 m^2) unit, built as a single-family home. It had been vacant for almost 7 years, and condemned for 3 years. Each unit had separate exterior walls and the side walls touched on one or two sides of the adjacent unit(s). The units were trapezoidal in shape, and this was an end unit (**FIGURE 2-A**).

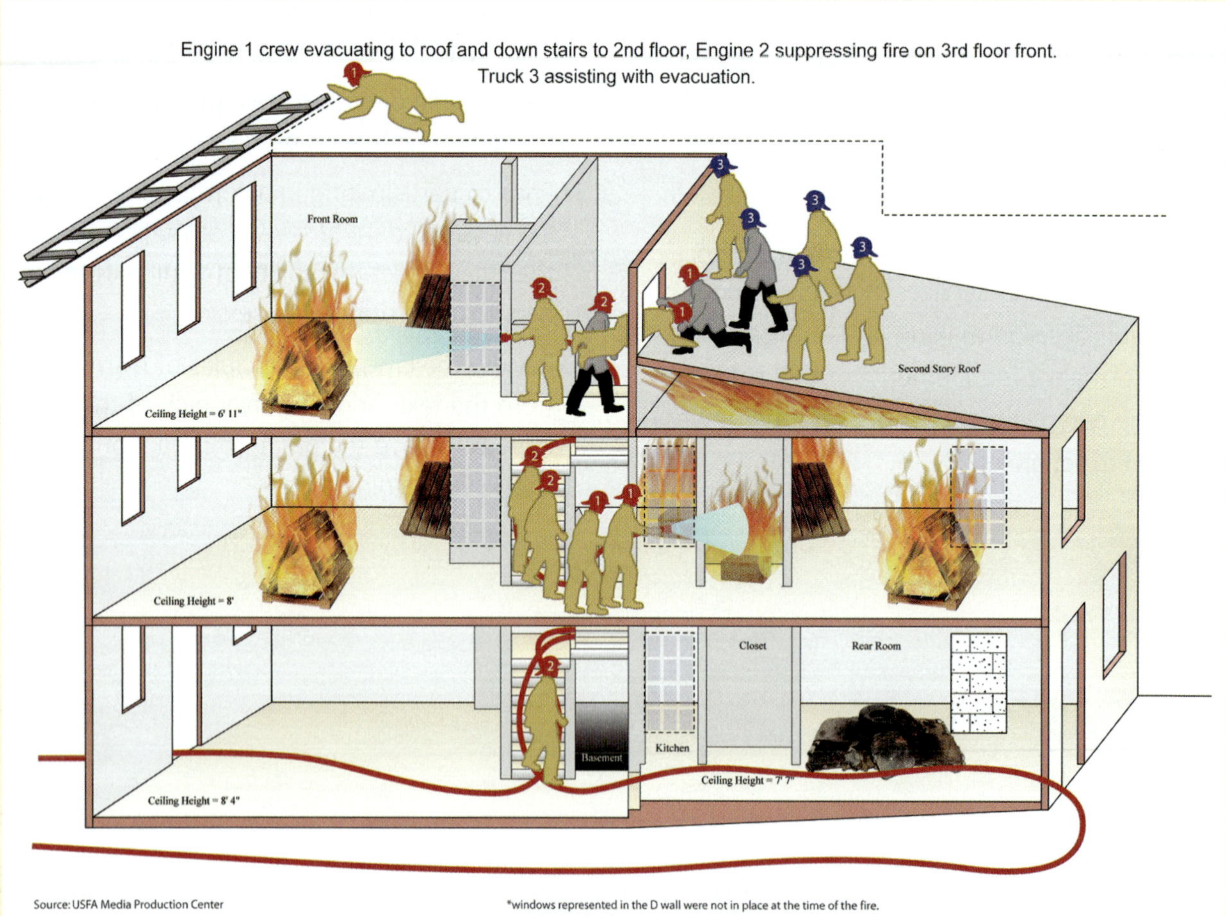

FIGURE 2-A Baltimore floor plan. Note fire locations.
Courtesy of the USFA Media Production Center.

The live fire exercise consisted of multiple fires on all floors. The investigation indicates that approximately 11 bales of excelsior and at least 10 wooden pallets were used for the fires. Pallets were propped against the walls in several locations, with excelsior underneath. Excelsior was also placed in openings in the ceilings and in walls. In the backroom on the first floor, an automotive tire, two full-size mattresses, one twin-size mattress, one foam rubber chair, tree branches, and other debris were piled up and burned. The exact number of fires set could not be definitely determined, but there were at least nine separate fires.

It appears that the ignition of the fires was not coordinated with the preparation of students entering. Several students were not ready when the fires were ignited, and that delay allowed the fires to burn unimpeded while crews made final preparations to enter.

Five separate crews were expected to operate simultaneously as engine and truck companies. A sixth crew was designated as the rapid intervention crew (RIC), but they were not briefed and did not have a hose line.

An adjunct instructor and four students of the first crew, designated as Engine 1, entered through the front door. All of the students had personal alert safety system (PASS) devices, but the adjunct instructor did not, nor did he have a portable radio. Per the direction of the instructor-in-charge, Engine 1 began making their way to the third floor and expected a second hose line to follow. They advanced an initially uncharged 1¾-in. (44-mm) hose line to the centrally located stairs on the first floor. There is disagreement as to when the line was actually charged.

Another crew of recruits was to advance a hose line to the second floor from the rear door. When they entered the rear of the house, they encountered the large pile of debris burning, which inhibited their ingress and egress. The fire was spreading across the ceiling, and they extinguished the fire before making a delayed advance to the second floor. As with the first crew, the four students had PASS devices, but the adjunct instructor did not, nor did he have a portable radio.

The Engine 1 crew advanced to the second floor and encountered heavy fire conditions. Although directed to go to the third floor, the instructor determined it was necessary to knock down the fire before proceeding upstairs to the third floor. Two of the crew's members stayed on the landing between the second and third floors to pull hose, while the remainder of the crew advanced upstairs. Conditions on the third floor became too hot, and the instructor did not have a radio to advise command of their situation or of the interior conditions. The instructor lifted himself up and climbed out of a high window onto the back roof of the second floor. The first student was able to lift her upper body out of the window. The instructor then grabbed her self-contained breathing apparatus (SCBA) straps to pull her out the rest of the way onto the second floor roof. She was then hoisted to the third floor roof by Truck 3, where she told them that her crew needed help.

The other student was now at the window as the instructor attempted to pull her through, using her SCBA harness as he had done with the other fire fighter. She was initially able to talk to the instructor to tell him that she could not help, and that she was burning up. It appears that she still had her SCBA face mask on at this time. The instructor lost his grip, and the student fell back into the room, landing on her feet. When he was able to get hold of her again, she was still conscious, but her mask was partially dislodged or removed. Her face had visibly started to blister. The instructor did not have a radio, but yelled for help. He lost his grip on her a second time, and the student fell back into the room. Shortly after regaining his grip on her for the third time, she became unresponsive. At this point, the crew jumped about 6 ft down from the third floor roof to help pull the student out, but they were unable to do so. With additional assistance, they were eventually able to help lift her onto the roof, where a student used a portable radio to advise of the fire fighter down.

Assistance was requested from the on-duty battalion, engine, and truck units that had come by to watch. The engine company engaged the fire, while the truck company entered the structure to ensure that the students were all out.

Two members of the on-duty truck company climbed the aerial ladder to the roof; they assisted in placing the victim in a Stokes basket and carried her down the ladder. An advanced life support ambulance initiated advanced life support and transported her to a shock trauma center, where her care continued until she was pronounced dead.

Incident Report continued

Postincident Analysis Baltimore, Maryland

NFPA 1403 Noncompliant

NOTE: Near-total lack of compliance with NFPA 1403. 50 issues considered to be violations of NFPA 1403 by investigative team.

- Flashover and fire spread unexpected
- Walk-through was not performed
- Multiple fires on different floors
- Excessive fuel loading
- Fire was beyond the training and experience of the students to participate in live burn exercises in an acquired structure
- No incident safety officer
- Noncompliant gear on victim
- Instructors without PASS
- Instructors not equipped with portable radios
- Adjunct instructors had little to no prior instructional experience

NFPA 1403 Compliant

- 22 students, 11 instructors
- EMS (ALS transport) on standby on scene

Other Contributing Factors

- Students not informed of emergency plans/procedures
- Rapid intervention crew staffed by students and unequipped or unprepared

After-Action REVIEW

IN SUMMARY

- As an instructor, you are a leader and have a responsibility to teach information, to hone skills, and to promote positive values and motivation in your students.
- According to Edward L. Thorndike, there are six laws of learning: readiness, exercise, effect, primacy, recency, and intensity.
- Of the five senses, seeing (e.g., a visual demonstration of a skill) is generally the most effective means of learning, followed by hearing (e.g., listening to a lecture), smelling (e.g., smelling smoke), touching (e.g., handling fire equipment), and tasting (rarely used in training fire fighters).
- Two schools of thought have developed to explain how behavior evolves: behaviorist and cognitive.
  - According to the behaviorist perspective, learning is a relatively permanent change in behavior that arises from experience.
  - According to the cognitive perspective, learning is an intellectual process in which experience contributes to relatively permanent changes in the way individuals mentally represent their environment.
- Learning that is intended to create or improve professional behavior is based on performance, rather than on content. Such competency-based learning is usually tied to skills or hands-on training.
- Mandating learning often results in a lack of motivation in classroom activities and a poor attitude toward the learning process in general, which present quite a challenge to the instructor who is tasked with teaching the course.
- To assist your students in becoming effective learners, you can share study skills that enhance what they learn during classroom and personal study time. Study tips can be viewed in three categories: classroom, personal study, and test preparation.
- Abraham Maslow determined that certain needs should be satisfied to enable a person to move forward toward self-actualization:
  - Physiological needs
  - Safety, security, and order
  - Social needs and affection
  - Esteem and status
  - Self-actualization
- Benjamin Bloom and his research team identified three types of learning domains:
  - Cognitive domain (knowledge)
  - Psychomotor domain (physical use of knowledge)
  - Affective domain (attitudes, emotions, or values)
- Adult learners can be divided into three types: learner oriented, goal oriented, and activity oriented. Each type is associated with different motivational issues, which in turn affects how learning takes place.
- Researchers focused on learner characteristics are divided into two distinct camps: those emphasizing the cognitive learning domain and those highlighting other learning-related factors, such as motivation and personal preferences.
- Once you have identified students with some type of learning disability, then you need to adjust your teaching as necessary to ensure their learning. There are many ways to help students in your class who are struggling to learn.
- Most often, disruptive students have other underlying issues that cause them to seek out attention in a negative way.

KEY TERMS

Access Navigate for flashcards to test your key term knowledge.

Active learning Anything students do beyond simply receiving instruction and passively listening to a lecture or watching a video.

Affective domain The domain of learning that affects attitudes, emotions, or values. It may be associated with a student's perspective or belief being changed as a result of training in this domain.

Andragogy The art and science of teaching adults.

Attention-deficit/hyperactivity disorder (ADHD) A disorder in which a person has a chronic level of inattention and an impulsive hyperactivity that affects daily functions.

Audience analysis The determination of characteristics common to a group of people; it can be used to choose the best instructional approach.

Baby boomers The generation born after World War II (i.e., 1946–1964).

Behaviorist perspective The theory that learning is a relatively permanent change in behavior that arises from experience.

Bloom's Taxonomy A classification of the different objectives and skills that educators set for students (learning objectives).

Cognitive domain The domain of learning that effects a change in knowledge. It is most often associated with learning new information.

Cognitive perspective An intellectual process by which experience contributes to relatively permanent changes (learning). It may be associated by learning by experience.

Competency-based learning Learning that is intended to create or improve professional competencies.

Dyscalculia A learning disability in which students have difficulty with math and related subjects.

Dyslexia A learning disability in which students have difficulty reading due to an inability to interpret spatial relationships and integrate visual information.

Dysphasia A learning disability in which students lack the ability to write, spell, or place words together to complete a sentence.

Dyspraxia A lack of physical coordination with motor skills.

Generation X People born after the baby boomers.

Generation Y People born immediately after Generation X.

Generation Z People born immediately after Generation Y, starting in the late 1990s.

Kinesthetic learning Learning that is based on doing or experiencing the information that is being taught.

Learner characteristics Designating a target group of learners and defining those aspects of their personal, academic, social, or cognitive self that may influence how and what they learn. (NFPA 1041)

Learning A relatively permanent change in behavior potential that is traceable to experience and practice.

Learning domains Categories that describe how learning takes place—specifically, the cognitive, psychomotor, and affective domains.

Motivation The activator or energizer for an activity or behavior.

Motivational factors States of the person that are relatively temporary and reversible and that tend to energize or activate the behavior of the individual.

Pedagogy The art and science of teaching children.

Psychomotor domain The domain of learning that requires the physical use of knowledge. It represents the ability to physically manipulate an object or move the body to accomplish a task or use a skill.

Student-centered learning Educational methodologies that focus on student engagement and require students to be active, responsible participants in the learning experience. (NFPA 1041)

REFERENCES

Ambrose, S. A., M. W. Bridges, M. DiPietro, M. C. Lovett, and M. K. Norman (Eds.). 2010. *How Learning Works: Seven Research-Based Principles for Smart Teaching*. San Francisco: Jossey-Bass.

Armour, Stephanie. 2005. "Generation Y: They've Arrived at Work with a New Attitude." USA Today, November 6, 2005. http://www.usatoday.com/money/workplace/2005-11-06-gen-y_x.htm.

Bender, D. 1999. *Unique characteristics of adult learning*. www2.bw.wdu/~dbender/csu/adultlearn.html. Accessed August 10, 2018.

Bloom, Benjamin S. 1984. *Taxonomy of Educational Objectives*. Boston: Allyn and Bacon/Pearson Education.

Bloom, Benjamin S., David R. Krathwohl, and Bertram B. Masia. 1965. *Taxonomy of Educational Objectives: Book 2*. London: Longman.

Bonwell, C. C., and J. A. Eison. 1991. Active learning: Creating excitement in the classroom (ASHE–ERIC Higher Education Rep. No. 1). Washington, DC: The George Washington University, School of Education and Human Development.

Brown, B. L. 1997. *New learning strategies for Generation X*. ERIC Clearinghouse. http://www.ed.gov/databases/ERIC.

Butler, Gillian, and Frida McManus. 1998. *Psychology*. Oxford: Oxford University Press.

Connick, G. 1997. "Beyond a Place Called School." *NLII Viewpoint* (Fall/Winter).

Crouch, C. H., and E. Mazur. 2001. "Peer Instruction: Ten years of experience and results." *American Journal of Physics, 69* (9): 970. doi:10.1119/1.1374249

Dave, R. H. 1970. *Developing and Writing Behavioral Objectives*. Tucson: Educational Innovators Press.

Draper, J. 1993. *The Craft of Teaching Adults*. Toronto: Culture Concepts.

Elias, J. L., and S. Merriam. 1980. *Philosophical Foundations of Adult Education*. Malabar, FL: Krieger.

Erikson, E.H., 1959. Identify and the life cycle: Selected papers. *Psychological Issues*, 1: 1–171.

Hacker, Douglas J., John Dunlosky, and Arthur C. Graesser (Eds.). 2009. *Handbook of Metacognition in Education*. London: Routledge.

Houle, C. 1961. *The Inquiring Mind*. Madison, WI: University of Wisconsin Press.

Knowles, M. 1984. *The Adult Learner: A Neglected Species*. 3rd ed. Houston, TX: Gulf Publishing.

Knowles, M. 1990. *The Adult Learner: A Neglected Species*. Revised ed. Houston, TX: Gulf Publishing.

Laskowski, Lenny. A.U.D.I.E.N.C.E. Analysis—It's Your Key to Success. Presentation-Pointers website, copyright 2000-2010. http://www.presentation-pointers.com/showarticle/articleid/248/. Accessed August 17, 1018.

Lefrancois, Guy R. 1996. *The Lifespan*. 5th ed. Belmont, CA: Wadsworth.

Levinson, Daniel J. 1977. The Mid-LIfe Transition: A Period in Adult Psychosocial Development. *Psychiatry*, 40: 99–112.

McClincy, W. D. 1995. *Instructional Methods in Emergency Services*. Englewood Cliffs, NJ: Brady Prentice Hall.

McClincy, W. D. 2002. *Instructional Methods in Emergency Services*. 2nd ed. Englewood Cliffs, NJ: Brady Prentice Hall.

Merriam, Sharan B., and Rosemary S. Caffarella. 1999. *Learning in Adulthood*. San Francisco, CA: Jossey-Bass.

National Fire Protection Association. 2019. *NFPA 1041: Standard for Fire Service Instructor Professional Qualifications*. Quincy, MA: National Fire Protection Association.

National Fire Protection Association. 2018. *NFPA 1403: Standard on Live Fire Training Evolutions*. Quincy, MA: National Fire Protection Association.

National Research Council. 2000. *How People Learn: Brain, Mind, Experience, and School: Expanded Edition*. Washington, DC: The National Academies Press.

Piaget, Jean, and Barbel Inhelder. 1958. *The Growth of Logical Thinking from Childhood to Adolescence*. London: Routledge.

Rathus, Spencer A. 1999. *Psychology in the New Millennium*. 7th ed. Fort Worth, TX: Harcourt Brace College.

Seemiller, Corey, and Meghan Grace. 2017. "Generation Z: Educating and Engaging the Next Generation of Students." *About Campus* 22 (3), 21–26.

Seemiller, Corey, and Meghan Grace. 2016. *Generation Z Goes to College*. New York: San Francisco: Jossey-Bass.

Stewart, D. 2003. "Computer and Technology Skills." http://www.ncwiseowl.org/Kscope/techknowpark/Kiosk/index.html.

"Student-Centered Learning Definition." *The Glossary of Education Reform*, Great Schools, 7 May 2014, www.edglossary.org/student-centered-learning/.

Thorndike, Edward L. 1932. *The Fundamentals of Learning*. New York: Teachers College Press.

Wlodkowski, Raymond J. 1999. *Enhancing Adult Motivation to Learn: A Comprehensive Guide for Teaching All Adults*. Revised ed. San Francisco, CA: Jossey-Bass/Pfeiffer.

CHAPTER PRESENTATION EXERCISE

Instructions: Your course instructor will assign individual or group discussions on the key points and teaching tips of this chapter. You or your group will review the chapter teachings and identify the major learning points from the chapter. You should be able to discuss the points, why they are important, and how/where they apply to your responsibilities at your level of instructor training.

REVIEW QUESTIONS

1. Two schools of thought have developed to explain how behavior evolves: behaviorist and cognitive. Describe each of these.
2. Learning takes place in three domains. List and explain them.
3. Provide examples of *convergent* and *divergent* questioning techniques.

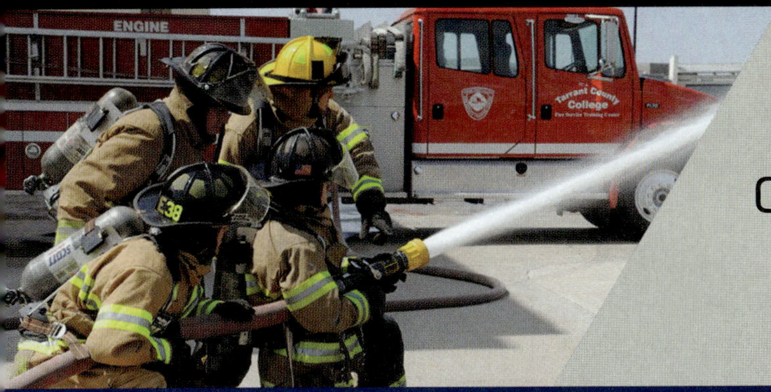

CHAPTER 3

Methods of Instruction

NFPA 1041 JOB PERFORMANCE REQUIREMENTS

Note: An asterisk denotes that the 1041 standard contains further information in its annex section.

4.3.2 Review instructional materials, given the materials for a specific topic, target audience, learner characteristics, and learning environment, so that elements of the lesson plan, learning environment, and resources that need adaptation are identified.

(A) Requisite Knowledge.

Recognition of student learner characteristics and diversity, methods of instruction, types of resource materials, organization of the learning environment, and policies and procedures.

(B) Requisite Skills.

Analysis of resources, facilities, and materials.

4.3.3* Adapt a prepared lesson plan, given course materials and an assignment, so that the needs of the student and the objectives of the lesson plan are achieved.

(A)* Requisite Knowledge.

Elements of a lesson plan, selection of instructional aids and methods, and organization of the learning environment.

(B) Requisite Skills.

Instructor preparation and organization techniques.

4.4.2 Organize the learning environment, given a facility and an assignment, so that lighting, distractions, climate control or weather, noise control, seating, audiovisual equipment, teaching aids, and safety are addressed.

(A) Requisite Knowledge.

Learning environment management and safety, advantages and limitations of audiovisual equipment and teaching aids, classroom arrangement, and methods and techniques of instruction.

(B) Requisite Skills.

Use of instructional media and teaching aids.

4.4.3 Present and adjust prepared lessons, given a prepared lesson plan that specifies the presentation method(s), so that the method(s) indicated in the plan are used and the stated objectives or learning outcomes are achieved, applicable safety standards and practices are followed, and risks are addressed.

(A)* Requisite Knowledge.

The laws and principles of learning, methods and techniques of instruction, lesson plan components and elements of the communication process, and lesson plan terminology and definitions; learner characteristics; student-centered learning principles; instructional technology tools; the impact of cultural differences on instructional delivery; safety rules, regulations, and practices; identification of training hazards; elements and limitations of distance learning; distance learning delivery methods; and the instructor's role in distance learning.

(B) Requisite Skills.

Oral communication techniques, methods and techniques of instruction, ability to adapt to changing circumstances, and utilization of lesson plans in an instructional setting.

4.4.4* Adjust to differences in learner characteristics, abilities, cultures, and behaviors, given the instructional environment, so that lesson

objectives are accomplished, disruptive behavior is addressed, and a safe and positive learning environment is maintained.

(A)* Requisite Knowledge.

Motivation techniques, learner characteristics, types of learning disabilities and methods for dealing with them, and methods of dealing with disruptive and unsafe behavior.

(B) Requisite Skills.

Basic coaching and motivational techniques, correction of disruptive behaviors, and adaptation of lesson plans or materials to specific instructional situations.

KNOWLEDGE OBJECTIVES

After studying this chapter, participating in a structured learning environment, and completing assigned assessments, you will be able to:

- Describe methods of instruction typically used in adult and fire service education. (**NFPA 1041: 4.4.3**, pp 73–75)
- Describe the four-step method of instruction. (pp 75–76)
- Explain how distance learning can enhance instruction. (**NFPA 1041: 4.4.3**, pp 76–77)
- Describe communication techniques that will improve your presentation. (**NFPA 1041: 4.4.3**, pp 77–80)
- Explain methods for controlling the physical learning environment. (**NFPA 1041: 4.3.2**, pp 80–82)
- Describe how to create a learning environment that facilitates the learning process. (**NFPA 1041: 4.4.2**, pp 83–90)
- Identify issues unique to outdoor learning environments and explain how to address them. (**NFPA 1041: 4.3.2**, pp 87–90)
- Identify considerations when arranging learning environments for testing functions. (**NFPA 1041: 4.3.2**, p 87)
- Describe the effect of demographics on the learning environment. (**NFPA 1041: 4.4.3**, pp 91–92)

SKILLS OBJECTIVES

After studying this chapter, participating in a structured learning environment, and completing assigned assessments, you will be able to:

- Deliver an instructional session using prepared course material. (**NFPA 1041: 4.4.1; 4.4.3**, pp 73–80)
- Manage disruptive and unsafe behaviors in the classroom. (**NFPA 1041: 4.4.4**, pp 80–82)
- Organize the learning environment to meet the requirements of the students and the material to be presented. (**NFPA 1041: 4.3.2; 4.4.2**, pp 83–90)
- Present material to a diverse audience following acceptable presentation methods and techniques. (**NFPA 1041: 4.3.3**, pp 83; 91–92)

You Are the Fire and Emergency Services Instructor

As the newest member assigned to your shift, your shift officer has asked you to conduct a training session about the department's fire fighter safety and survival program. Prior to the session, however, he warns you that several of the more veteran fire fighters on your shift have no interest or buy-in to the topic as your department has never experienced a fire fighter line-of-duty death or even a close call. Knowing that you are going to be evaluated on how well you present this topic, address the following:

1. Identify several motivational techniques or methods you can use to promote interest and buy-in among your audience, especially the more veteran fire fighters.
2. List the steps of the four-step method of instruction and how you can use these steps to deliver a successful training session.
3. Consider different evaluation and questioning techniques you can use to assess the learning process during your training session.

JONES & BARTLETT LEARNING NAVIGATE 2 *Access Navigate for more practice activities.*

Introduction

As a fire and emergency services instructor, you must constantly ask, "How can I best help my students to learn?" It is your responsibility to present information and have a clear understanding of the course objectives. Instruction is the single most important factor in students' success: Teaching has a greater impact on achievement than all other factors combined.

Whether the class is a large introductory course for recruits or an advanced course for fire officers, it makes good sense to start off well. Students decide very early—maybe even within the first class—whether they will like the course, its contents, the instructor, and their fellow students.

Fire fighters are adults. This point may seem obvious, but sometimes instructors can lose sight of that fact. Some of the strategies that work with second graders also work well with adults, but there are important differences in the way adults and children learn. Never treat your fire service students like children—you are teaching adults. Remember, too, that although you are teaching to a class, the individual may require a particular learning strategy.

Methods of Instruction

The **method of instruction** is the process of teaching material to students. You can also identify it as how your lesson plan will be given to your students. Many different and diverse methods of instruction exist, and each applies to different types of materials as well as different types of students. Each of the various student demographics and categories discussed earlier in this chapter will respond differently to the material according to how they are motivated and the method(s) of instruction used. If you are an Instructor I, the method of instruction will be identified on your lesson plan by the lesson plan developer. Chapter 5, *Using Lesson Plans*, discusses formatting of and placeholders in the lesson plan that developers can use to identify the methods of instruction they have determined to be most appropriate for the material. The same chapter also discusses the parts of a lesson plan and provides guidance on how lessons are constructed, considering the method of instruction to be used.

Determining which method of instruction should be used to deliver information is accomplished based on several factors:

- The experience and educational level of the students
- The classroom setting or training environment
- The objectives of the material to be taught
- The number of students to be taught

As an instructor at the Instructor I level, you should understand the different methods of instruction and master those methods. Based on this fundamental knowledge, when a lesson plan states that Instructor I personnel are to deliver a "lecture," they understand the method of instruction to be used. For Instructor II personnel, as they develop a lesson plan, they will select the most appropriate and effective method to deliver the material in the lesson plan they have created. Any level of instructor should be able to adapt a lesson plan to the learning environment as well as to the audience who will receive the instruction so as to make it most effective. All instructors will perform an audience analysis by looking at the demographics of the audience, including age, learning level, previous experience, and other factors, and then adapt the lesson plan accordingly.

Ask yourself three basic questions when reviewing and planning for the delivery of a lesson plan:

- What are the goals of the lesson?
- Who is the intended audience?
- What are the resources and learning environment characteristics?

Methods of instruction vary among disciplines, but for the fire service the following techniques are known to be the most effective in teaching new and in-service personnel.

Lecture

The lecture method is used widely in the fire service. It consists of the instructor being the primary source of information and delivering the course material while using various multimedia tools (**FIGURE 3-1**). As part of your Instructor I job duties, you will be required to present an illustrative lecture in a practice teaching environment to a group of fellow students. An illustrative lecture allows the instructor to use a visual aid such as a presentation slide to illustrate key points, which is important to effective communication and is probably the most common and familiar method of fire service instruction.

Demonstration or Skill Drill

This method is used when teaching skills or hands-on learning. This type of learning is used when the instructor demonstrates the use of a new tool or demonstrates how to perform a specific task-oriented skill (**FIGURE 3-2**). Several variations in the sequence of how these types of drills should progress are possible, especially when learning a new skill. You might

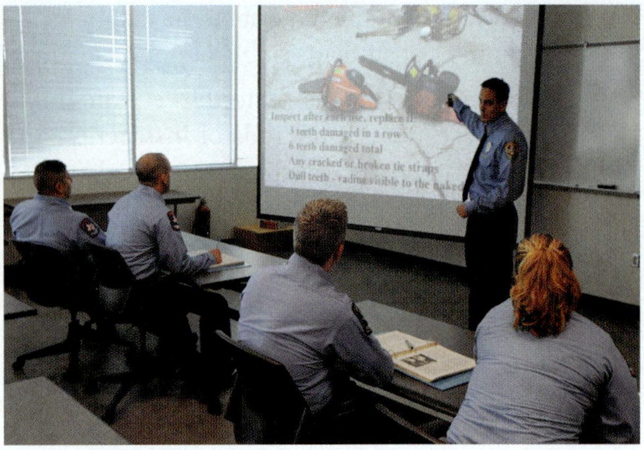

FIGURE 3-1 The lecture method of instruction consists of the instructor being the primary source of information and delivering the course material while using various multimedia tools.

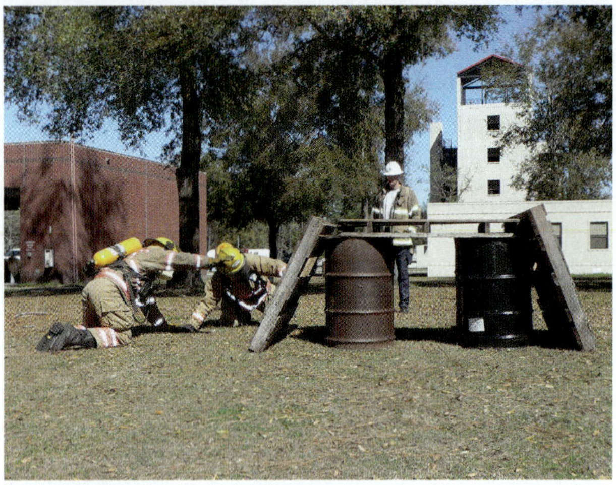

FIGURE 3-2 Skill drills allow the student to learn by actively participating and physically using the new tool or practicing the new skill.

view the training as a crawl–walk–run sequence or engage in an instructor-led demonstration—that is, you might demonstrate the skill at full speed for the students, then slowly explain each step and stop at each step point, then perform it one more time at full speed while explaining the step. This approach is also known as a psychomotor lesson or hands-on method of instruction. As part of the Instructor 1 job duty area, you may be required to present a demonstrative presentation where a student will perform a task from a prepared skill sheet as part of the student instructor's practice presentation.

Most fire fighters and other adult learners respond very well to hands-on training. This method gives each student the opportunity to learn by actively participating and physically using the new tool or practicing the new skill. While the student engages in hands-on application during this method of learning, the instructor needs to monitor student safety. This method of instruction references a skill drill and requires the instructor to ensure that personal protective equipment (PPE) is in use and proper student-to-instructor ratios are maintained to ensure student and instructor safety. Chapter 7, *Training Safety*, discusses appropriate levels of safety considerations that must be applied to this method of instruction.

Discussion

The discussion method is used to facilitate the learning process by having a two-way open forum, from instructor to student and from student to student (**FIGURE 3-3**). This method fosters interaction among the instructor and the students; the instructor's role in this method is more of a facilitator or monitor to ensure the discussion stays on track. Time keeping will be an essential element when this method of instruction is employed. Discussion is typically used as the method of instruction when consensus is needed or when new ideas are necessary to explore higher levels of learning and application. In most cases, this method requires students to have some prerequisite level of topic knowledge.

Based on the material to be covered and the make-up of the class, most instructors use a combination of these methods while delivering course material. For example, instructors might deliver course material via lecture and then engage in a discussion to determine the level of understanding from the students. When teaching a new skill or use of a tool, the instructor might begin with a lecture and then demonstrate

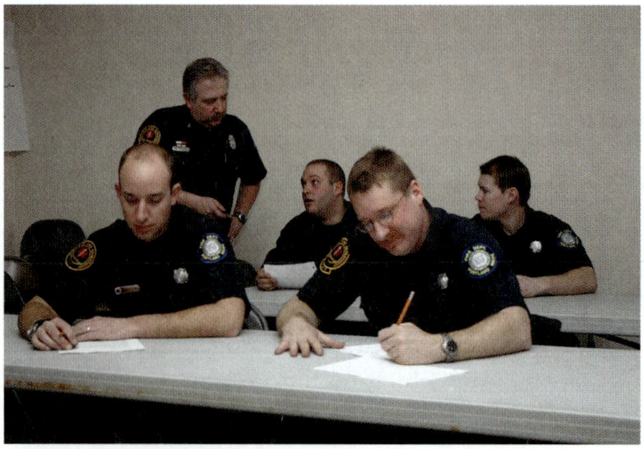

FIGURE 3-3 Discussion is used to facilitate the learning process by having a two-way open forum between instructor and student.

how to use the tool; the class might then move to the training ground to practice using the new tool.

The Four-Step Method of Instruction

While reviewing and preparing for class with your lesson plan, the **four-step method of instruction** is the primary process used to relate the material contained in the lesson plan to the students (**TABLE 3-1**). These four steps are found within the lesson plan. The four-step method of instruction is the most basic method of instruction used in the fire service.

TABLE 3-1 The Four-Step Method of Instruction

Step in the Instructional Process	Instructor Action
1. Preparation	The instructor prepares the students to learn by identifying the importance of the topic, stating the intended outcomes, and noting the relevance of the topic to the student. This should not be confused with the time used by the instructor to prepare course material and review lesson plan content.
2. Presentation	The presentation of content is usually organized in an outline form that supports an understanding of the learning objectives. Varied presentation techniques should be used to keep the students' interest and to maximize learning.
3. Application	The instructor provides opportunities for the students to *apply* what is being presented through questions, exercises, and discussion. Typically, this is not a graded activity, since it is the opportunity to practice under the supervision and support of the instructor.
4. Evaluation	The students' understanding is evaluated through written exams or in a practical skill session.

Step 1: Preparation

The preparation step is the first phase in the four-step method of instruction. The preparation step—also called the motivation step—prepares or motivates students to learn. When beginning instruction, you should provide information to students that explains why they will benefit from the class. Adult learners need to understand what they will get out of attending the class, because very few adults have time to waste in sitting through a presentation that will not directly benefit them.

The benefit of a class can be explained in a few ways:

- The class may count toward required hours of training.
- The class may provide a desired certification.
- The class may increase students' knowledge of a subject.

Whatever the benefit may be, you should explain it thoroughly during the preparation step. In a lesson plan, the preparation section usually consists of a paragraph or a bulleted list describing the rationale for the class. During the preparation step, the Instructor I needs to grab students' attention and prepare them to learn when he or she begins presenting the prepared lesson plan. Adult learners like to learn quickly how the class material will affect them: Will it make them safer or more knowledgeable about their job? Will it improve their efficiency on the fire ground or make them better leaders? This step in the process is critical as a motivational tool to encourage the students to participate in the learning process, not just sit in on the class as a way to pass the time.

Step 2: Presentation

The presentation step is the second step in the four-step method of instruction; it comprises the actual presentation of the lesson plan. During this step, you lecture, lead discussions, use audiovisual aids, answer student questions, and perform other techniques to present the lesson plan. In a lesson plan, the presentation section normally contains an outline of the information to be presented. It may also contain notes indicating when to use teaching aids, when to take breaks, or where to obtain more information.

Step 3: Application

The application step, which is the third step in the four-step method of instruction, is the most important step because it is during this phase that students apply the knowledge presented in class. The root word *apply* is very important to illustrate what the instructor needs to let the students do: apply what they are learning to examples or actual hands-on practice. Normally, this is where learning occurs, as students practice skills, perhaps make mistakes, and retry skills as necessary. You should provide direction and support as each student performs this step. You must also ensure that all safety rules are followed as students engage in new behaviors.

In a lesson plan, the application section usually lists the activities or assignments that the student will perform. In the fire service, the application section of a psychomotor objective lesson often requires the use of skill sheets for evaluation purposes. The experienced instructor uses the application step to make sure that each student is progressing along with the lesson plan. This step also allows students to participate actively and to remain engaged in the learning process.

Step 4: Evaluation

The evaluation step is the final step of the four-step method of instruction. It ensures that students have correctly acquired the knowledge and skills presented in the lesson plan. The evaluation may, for example, take the form of a written test or a skill performance test. No matter which method of evaluation is used, the student must demonstrate competency without assistance. In a lesson plan, the evaluation section indicates the type of evaluation method and the procedures for performing the evaluation.

Pre-Course Survey and Prerequisites

Some instructors use programs that require students to take a pre-course survey. This survey might try to determine student motivation for taking the class or the students' educational level, work experience, or previous training. Its results can also be used to adapt the lesson plan based on the students' needs.

A tool used in some classes is a pre-course test or quiz, which is used to gauge the students' knowledge of the material. After reviewing the results, you can adjust the course material accordingly to meet the needs of the students better. These tests or quizzes do not count toward the final grade, but they do provide an understanding of how the instructor can best help each student.

Some programs require that students take prerequisite classes before attending certain advanced classes. The fact that students have completed such preliminaries ensures that the students taking your course have a certain base level of training and education. It also ensures that students do not get into a course that is beyond their experience level. Success in a class will be impaired if a student is already behind the knowledge level for the course. You must ensure that your students have the correct competencies before moving to the next level.

Enhanced Instructional Methods

Instructors have other tools at their disposal to enhance the learning process and increase the retention of the material being taught. These tools include the use of role play, labs/simulations, case studies, and assignments to be done after class, such as handouts or assignments in a course workbook:

- **Role play:** Students become part of the lesson by assuming roles and "acting out" a situation or scenario meant to reinforce material from the lesson. Many leadership and management classes feature a senior instructor role-playing a problem employee or angry citizen to allow students to practice handling confrontations.
- **Labs/simulations:** Students are placed in a "real-life" situation, albeit in a controlled environment. A table-top fire-ground lab where the student can run a fire scene is an example of such a tool. Placing students under pressure in a controlled scenario strengthens information learned in the classroom. Many simulation programs that create a very realistic learning environment now exist to simulate actual fires and incidents (**FIGURE 3-4**). A simple online

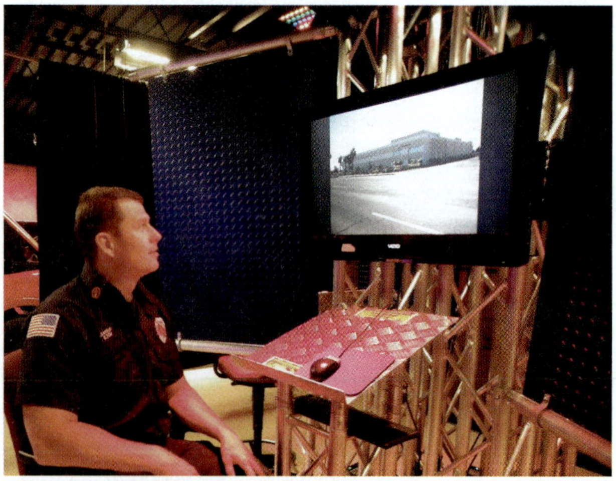

FIGURE 3-4 Many new simulation programs that create a very realistic learning environment now exist to simulate actual fires and incidents. Pictured here is a Command Training Center using the Blue Card Certification program.
Courtesy of Orland Fire Protection District.

search of fire scene simulations will reveal multiple sources of simulation-based programs.

- **Case studies:** Instructors often take advantage of examples from the real world to teach material. Using an incident report that was generated after a line-of-duty death and allowing students to read the report, discuss the material, and then determine ways to apply the knowledge is an effective way to work with a case study. The National Institute for Occupational Safety and Health (NIOSH) fire fighter fatality reports provide tremendous learning opportunities in many types of training sessions. The Charleston, South Carolina, furniture store fire investigation, for example, has become a staple in case study presentations discussing fire behavior, risk assessment, and tactical options. Most fire fighters can recall a presentation that included case studies when such scenarios relate to the lesson being presented, especially if the scenarios are from incidents with which they are familiar. All fire fighters should be aware of the significant fire fighter fatality investigations that have shaped our profession (such as the Hackensack, New Jersey, car dealership fire; the Worcester, Massachusetts, cold storage warehouse fire; and the Phoenix, Arizona, supermarket fire), as they have greatly influenced modern firefighting knowledge.
- **Out-of-class assignments:** Assignments given to students to be completed outside of class are another effective method of helping students learn. Many courses require pre-course work to be completed prior to class; the instructor might then give assignments in a workbook to be completed during the course. If the instructor does use this tool as part of the coursework, the instructor needs to make sure that these assignments are evaluated and that feedback is provided to the students. Failure to follow through with these measures will give the impression that the material was not important to learn.

Three other methods of instruction are becoming prevalent in today's fire service: online learning, independent study, and blended learning. These methods of learning are gaining popularity for many reasons (such as budget constraints or distance to a training location) and are being used in many disciplines for new or continuing education training.

Online learning (or distance learning) is conducted on the internet and takes the form of students entering a "classroom" that is hosted by an organization or campus. Delivery methods for the classroom consist of either a "synchronous" or "asynchronous" delivery method. In **synchronous learning**, the entire class meets at the same time, and the instructor delivers the course material in real time by voice and/or video. Students interact with the instructor and class verbally or with instant messaging. In **asynchronous learning**, in contrast, the course material is provided in the online classroom and students enter and exit it on their own schedule. Classroom discussion in an asynchronous class is facilitated by use of discussion boards where the instructor will post discussion questions or assignments and students are required to post responses to the instructor or to classmates and complete assignments that students then upload to the instructor.

Independent study has been used for many years (primarily in the military) to help students complete course material at distant locations. It entails registering for a course, receiving course material in the mail, completing assignments, and submitting them back to an instructor for evaluation. This method is one example of distance learning for those who might not have access to the internet.

A third method of instruction combines online/independent study with a face-to-face meeting with the instructor. This **blended learning** format allows for students to learn material on their own at remote locations. Then, at certain benchmarks within the curriculum, the class gathers to complete the hands-on portion of the training. Chapter 6, *Technology in Training*, further discusses technological resources, distance delivery, and creative ways for instructors to enhance their presentations.

All of these methods of instruction are dependent on the instructor knowing how to use each method and applying them while delivering the material as outlined on the lesson plan.

Lesson Presentation Skills and Techniques

No matter which methods of instruction you use or which generations you teach, the following communications techniques will help you improve the delivery of your information to your class:

- **Dress professionally.** Students should see you as a professional and recognize you instantly as a subject-matter expert. Even though we like to believe that we don't "judge a book by its cover," you will be sized up by your students. A professional appearance lays the groundwork for making a good first impression.
- **Welcome each student.** Your first impression begins the moment that students enter the

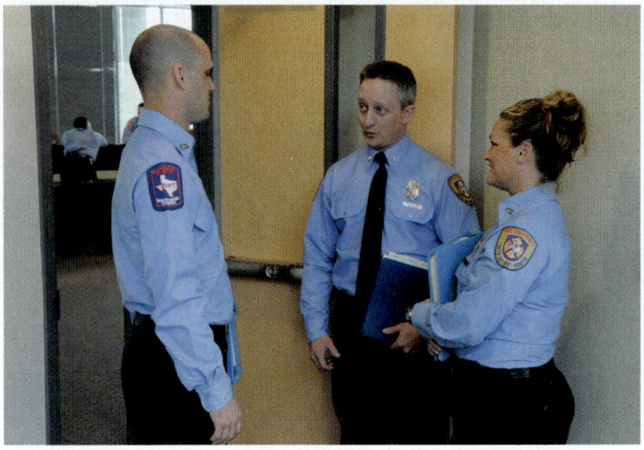

FIGURE 3-5 A good way to make a positive impression is to greet your students as they enter the classroom.

classroom. Shake students' hands as they arrive, introduce yourself, and have a warm smile on your face—this will immediately convey that you are an approachable person who cares about your students (**FIGURE 3-5**).

- **Call students by name.** Making every student feel important is essential in creating motivation and maintaining attention. Calling students by their names is one of the most effective methods of demonstrating to them that they are valued. Although it may not be possible in large, lecture-style courses that meet only once, most fire service courses are small enough to allow you to learn the students' names. Many of us struggle to learn names, but a variety of methods have been developed that can help you with this task. One of the most basic strategies is to use name tents or cards with the students' names. Another technique is to keep a seating chart in front of you. Name association may also work well. Each method has its own advantages and disadvantages, but determining a method that works best for you will go a long way toward helping you manage your class.
- **Use eye contact.** In our culture, it is important to make eye contact with people to whom you are speaking. Making eye contact with each fire fighter for a few moments in the course of your presentation will help students feel that you are communicating directly with them. Resist the temptation to look at the wall, at the clock, or over students' heads. Lack of eye contact makes people think you are not willing to be straight with them or that you are not confident in what you are saying. In fact, a lack of eye contact is probably one of the most disturbing mannerisms you can display.
- **Use your normal speaking voice but instill enthusiasm in your message.** As an instructor, you have a strong motivation to build a positive relationship with your class. If you are committed to the importance of what you are teaching, then that commitment will be revealed in your voice and by the enthusiasm that you display for the topic. Remember that enthusiasm is contagious—let it show!
- **Speak with respect.** You are teaching adults, and it is important that they perceive that they are respected as adults. When you are respectful to them, they will be respectful to you.
- **Use pauses when you speak.** A short pause can be used to signal an important point or a transition in your lecture. A pause can also indicate the conclusion of one topic and the beginning of another. It allows you the opportunity to view your students and visually check for comments, interest levels, or questions.
- **Use information appropriately.** It is important to gauge your students' level of understanding correctly. For example, Fire Fighter I students will have a different understanding of information than seasoned fire officers. Make sure you speak at a knowledge and vocabulary level that students will understand and explain concepts or information on the same level. You may have to spend time ensuring that the level of training or education is appropriate for all participants in the course.
- **Use gestures sparingly, for emphasis.** Avoid meaningless gestures—for example, jingling keys or change in your pocket, playing with a pencil, or tapping mindlessly on a podium or desk. Try to avoid playing with things, chewing on the ends of pencils, or repeatedly tapping your foot. Hide those tempting items if playing with them has become an unconscious habit for you. Eventually, these habits will become intrusive—and distracting to your students—and students will be placing bets on whether you will swallow the pencil or how many times you will tap your foot in a minute.
- **Practice positive mannerisms.** Well-placed mannerisms can increase your effectiveness in presentation of your lectures, and appropriate gestures can add to the verbal messages. Vary your position and movement, because your ability to change the pace of the lesson will increase involvement. Your body language and facial expression can give a fire fighter support and encouragement even when you are not saying anything aloud.

- **Choose your teaching aids appropriately.** The technology that you have at your fingertips in the classroom is simply a way to communicate with students and reinforce information. Eraser boards and paper pads have some unique advantages in communicating, as they can be used to convey a variety of information during a single lesson. If you use these tools, make sure that your writing is legible. These teaching aids also provide a visual reinforcement of your verbal message. Slide presentations, charts, models, and videos are other means of communicating information to students and can reinforce information being presented verbally. Your wise use of technology can enrich your classroom and assist you in teaching. Even so, you should not rely on technology alone to teach: It can malfunction, so always have a backup plan.
- **Know how to use your chosen teaching aids in the classroom.** Your communication with your students is interrupted when you do not handle technology smoothly. Each time you are guilty of mishandling your teaching aids, you will weaken the impact of the lesson by sending an unintended message ("I don't know what I'm doing").
- **Transition techniques during presentations.** While presenting your lesson plan, make sure that you make smooth transitions between your media and verbal communication techniques. Distributing handouts before you want to have the students read them is an example of using media (nonprojected materials/handouts) at the wrong time. If you want to hold students' attention, then use media in the correct manner and use transition techniques that enhance the learning process rather than distract from it.

Transition techniques also are used during a presentation to move from one topic to the next. Many students get lost during a lecture when the instructor moves on and the students do not realize or understand the instructor has changed topics. To help students follow a presentation, instructors need to learn transition techniques. Five effective techniques are delineation, words/phrases, pictures, voice, and body language:

- **Delineation.** This is the simplest way to make a transition. As an instructor, you tell your class that you will be covering four points and then begin by stating "point number one," and then move to point two, point three, and point four, and then summarize the material.
- **Words/phrases.** Use phrases such as "the next point we need to discuss," or summarize the topic and then use a phrase like "the next step in the process . . ."
- **Pictures.** Because so many of today's lessons use PowerPoint presentations, an effective tool to use within such a presentation is the insertion of historic or unique pictures between points or topics. This visual signal will allow you to pause and switch topics, and the students will quickly pick up on the fact that the topic has changed.
- **Voice.** Use your voice by changing your tone or pitch, by using different volumes to emphasize change from one idea to another, or by inserting an effective pause. Pausing will draw students' attention to you and will develop anticipation about what is coming next.
- **Body language.** Effective use of body language will assist you in moving from one topic to the next. Moving from the podium to one side of the classroom with a change in voice will clearly inform students that the topic has changed or is very important. Make your movements conscious and meaningful, and try to avoid nervous pacing.

All of these techniques or methods will allow you to make transitions during a presentation, but they need to be practiced to be used effectively. Some instructors will develop all of these transition techniques; others will not. The goal is to develop transition techniques that work best for you.

Effective Communication

Effective communication is fundamental to ensuring that the students learn—that they receive and remember the information you intended to transmit to them. As a general guideline, consider these findings noted by educator Edgar Dale in 1969:

- We remember 10 percent of what we read.
- We remember 20 percent of what we hear.
- We remember 30 percent of what we see.
- We remember 50 percent of what we see and hear.
- We remember 70 percent of what we say.
- We remember 90 percent of what we say while doing.

It is important to choose the right kind(s) of communication when you are preparing for class. It is also important to use the selected communication methods effectively. Understanding how the communication process works will help you develop lesson plans or adapt lesson plans based on your students' learning characteristics. For example, if your students are visual learners, then you may need to include more visual presentations. See Chapter 4, *Communication Skills*, for a discussion of the elements and role of the communication process.

Questioning Techniques

An important part of the learning process is to assess the learning process during class. One simple method used over and over is to ask students questions from the material that is being taught from the lesson plan. Many lesson plans will build in questions for the instructor to ask the students to determine whether the students are picking up the new information and understanding what is being taught.

When using questions during the teaching process, it is important to ask the correct question at the correct time. Again, many lesson plans will identify the appropriate time to ask questions to support what has just been taught. Another appropriate place to seek student feedback is at the end of a lesson during a summary activity. There are times during a presentation at which an instructor can use a question to stimulate discussion, to bring class focus to a new topic, or to break up side discussions in the classroom. When used correctly, a question can also be used to challenge a disruptive student positively and bring him or her back into the classroom.

Numerous types of questions can be used during the learning process, including the following:

- **Direct questions.** Direct questions are those beginning with *who*, *what*, *where*, *when*, *why*, or *how*. They are meant to elicit specific information and limit discussion. This type of question is used when the instructor is seeking an answer from a specific student and is often effective in dealing with a student who is being disruptive or whose attention seems to be somewhere besides the classroom. It is important to exercise caution with this type of questioning, as it could be perceived as singling out a student.
- **Rhetorical questions.** This type of question is usually asked to stimulate discussion or to prepare the learners' minds for a new topic. Often a rhetorical question does not have an answer, or it may have multiple correct answers.
- **Open-ended questions.** This type of question could be answered with varying correct answers based on the question and the situation presented.
- **Closed-ended questions.** This type of question seeks a specific answer based on the question asked.

Other types of question formats could be added to this list, but these are the most common forms of questions used within a classroom during a presentation. Knowing which question to ask and when to ask the question is very important, but dealing with a student's response to a question is just as important. Instructors are there to teach students and to foster a positive learning environment, so responding to a student's answer is critical to maintaining a good learning environment. If the student gives the correct response, the instructor can build on the response and move on with the lesson. But what happens when a student's response or answer to a question is incorrect? Effective instructors should use the answer that was given and highlight the positive and downplay any negatives. Instructors who make light of a student's incorrect response can destroy a student's desire to learn and dampen the learning environment. Students are in a classroom to learn; if they respond incorrectly, then the instructor has an opportunity to correct the information, reinforce the positive, and help the student learn new material.

COMPANY-LEVEL INSTRUCTOR TIP

One of the instructor's most important responsibilities is to maintain a positive learning environment where students can feel comfortable with the instructor and their peers and feel free of judgment.

Managing Disruptive Behavior

There are many types of disruptive behavior, and your strategy for handling the problematic situation will vary depending on the type of behavior. The most important thing to remember is that you are in charge of the classroom. If you do not control your classroom, you are setting the stage for problems. You may be perceived by your students, peers, and administration as being a less competent instructor. Disruption in the classroom can significantly reduce or limit the amount of learning time for students (**FIGURE 3-6**). It can also lead to unsafe and negative learning that could have serious implications when students apply what they have learned in the field. You are responsible for providing a safe learning environment and proper, safe instruction to all students.

The type of disruptive behavior a student exhibits might fall into one of the general categories described here:

- The *monopolizer* has a tendency to take control of classroom discussions and dominate class time. To deal with this type of student, make certain to call on other students during classroom discussions. You can also call a break or, when a class break occurs, pull the monopolizer aside and discuss your concerns about his or her "over-participation"

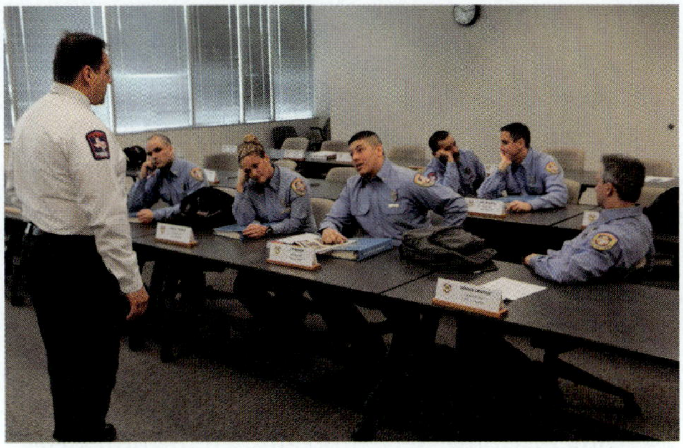

FIGURE 3-6 You are responsible for providing an appropriate learning environment to all of your students, which includes minimizing disruptive behavior.

during the class. Instructors have been successful positioning themselves between the monopolizer and other students as a physical barrier in an effort to engage other students. More direct approaches may be to ask an overhead question: "Anyone other than 'John' have an idea how this term applies to fire department operations?"

- The *historian* has some experience and wants to make sure that everyone is aware of it. Real historians have the benefit of years of experience and share their experiences to help illustrate an instructor's lesson; they focus on helping the instructor and other students. By contrast, artificial historians focus on helping themselves and interject their opinions to show other students how much they know. Real historians can be disruptive if their stories become distracting for the other students, in which case you should carefully guide the discussion back to the main topic. Another way to redirect real historians is by pairing them with struggling students. Artificial historians are almost always distracting. Assertively redirecting the discussion back to the lesson plan generally corrects this issue. If not, take the student aside and discuss the need for the class to stay focused on the lesson plan. Treat your adult students as adults—with respect.
- The *daydreamer* is preoccupied with anything other than the lesson. He or she may have been forced to attend the training class or may be participating as part of a job assignment. Often, this student is focusing on life outside of the classroom. Daydreamers may not directly disrupt other students, but are more of a distraction to you, the instructor. Try to draw such students into the class by using direct questioning techniques and making maximum eye contact.
- The *expert*, or the *know-it-all*, is a student who may become confrontational or monopolize the class in an attempt to show off his or her brain power and perceived expertise, often as a measure of competitiveness. The expert will provide up-to-date information, factoids, applications, and case information about the topic and can easily subvert your position as the classroom authority. You may have to discuss his or her contributions to the class during a private break.
- The *class clown* is the student who seeks attention by acting out or making jokes about course content, the instructor, or other students in the class. Most often the reason for this type of behavior is to draw attention to the individual. Two effective methods for dealing with this type of behavior are to ignore the class clown or to engage him or her with a direct question. Sometimes a stern look will deflate this type of student. Another option is, during a break, to take a moment to engage the student in conversation and to get to know him or her better and seek the individual's help in setting an example for others in the class.
- Another type of student who can be a challenge in the classroom is the *gifted learner*. This type of student is usually not disruptive, but becomes a challenge to the instructor because he or she seems to be disengaged in the learning process. These students might appear to be shy or daydreaming, but in reality, they are usually intelligent and are "bored" with the material being presented because they have read the material already or have good working knowledge of it. An effective method to manage this type of student behavior is to have such students assist you as an instructor during the course.

Some behaviors are clearly inappropriate in the classroom because they are unsafe or illegal. Other worrisome behaviors may include actions or words that are threatening or offensive, or that create risks to students, instructors, or property. These behaviors must be dealt with immediately and without hesitation.

Behavioral problems in the classroom arise for many reasons, ranging from complex to simple. For example, the student who falls asleep in class may have been on a working fire during all or part of the previous night and is just plain tired. This issue is relatively easy to identify and is not a persistent problem. By contrast, the student who falls asleep in class every day may have a medical disorder that causes him or her to be unusually drowsy. Learn more about human behavior, behavioral problems, and their causes to become a more effective instructor.

Behavioral problems displayed by the disruptive student may be rooted in other problems as well. As the instructor, you may be put in the position where you must deal with behaviors that are the result of situations outside the instructional environment. These problems may be as simple as hunger or thirst, illness, or medical needs. On other occasions, disruptive students may be experiencing personal problems. Your first priority is to create a positive learning environment for the whole class so all behavioral expressions can be addressed. Your second priority is to ensure the existence of a positive learning environment for the individual student. If you are able to determine the reason for the behavioral issue, and it is one that you can address, this will allow the individual student to learn as well.

Other behaviors that may prove disruptive to the class include calling out, asking irrelevant questions, and giving excessive examples. In these cases, students may be seeking attention from the class or from you. Some students may seek to gain power by being argumentative, lying, displaying a temper, or not following directions. These students need to be dealt with quickly and directly before their behavior gets out of hand.

Some of these problem behaviors can be easily addressed. The hungry student may need to take a break so he or she can eat. The bored student may need a more stimulating lesson to motivate him or her to learn. No matter what the problematic student behavior is, understanding the sources of some basic behaviors will help you control the classroom environment.

As the instructor, you have the opportunity to make positive behavioral changes possible for your students. Here are some simple ways to do so:

- **Lead by example.** You set the tone for the class through your own behavior; in doing so, you set a standard for the class. Act as a professional.
- **Take steps to prevent undesired behaviors.** By preventing the behavior from occurring, you will have changed it before it happens and disrupts the class. For example, in your opening discussion with the class, you can outline the rules that govern the classroom and tell students which kind of behavior is (and is not) expected of them (Bear, 1990).
- **Know what to expect.** By putting the rules in writing, you will have anticipated what the behaviors may be. When formulating these policies, it is important to include the consequences for their violation and to let the students know what rights they have in the classroom situation.
- **Stick to the rules.** Do not contradict the facility's or administration's rules.
- **Communicate.** Talk to problem-causing students and explain that it is unfair for their behavior to continue to disrupt the class.
- **Reward good and appropriate behavior.** This can be done through special assignments or may be as simple as a pat on the back—in front of the class, of course (Walker and Shea, 1991).
- **Act like a professional.** This includes being prepared, approachable, and good natured.
- **Do not either overreact or underreact.** Some issues may bother some people and not bother others. Conversely, problems left unaddressed seldom resolve themselves.

When all else fails, know when it is "time to clean house." If a student continues to be disruptive after you have attempted to speak with him or her one-on-one and used the chain of command to resolve disruptive behavior, the time might come when the instructor requests that the student leave the class. This is an extreme step and one that should be used only when all other efforts have failed to correct disruptive or inappropriate behavior.

Transitioning Between Methods of Instruction

The Instructor I should acquire skills to effectively apply problem-solving techniques, to facilitate and lead conferences, and to employ discussion methods during presentations. These techniques are frequently used to conduct small-group sessions where participants have advanced knowledge and experience in the subject matter and the goal is to reach a group solution to a problem or issue. When students become engaged in the learning process and actively participate in a class, the instructor can shift from a lecture format to a guided discussion. The same effect can occur when a student has adapted to a basic skill level in a hands-on training session, allowing the student to perform simultaneous actions and progressive skills.

Some disconnects in learning occur when a student who has learned in high-tech environments is suddenly dropped into a fire service classroom that is a traditional lecture-based format. The Generation Z student may easily become bored and not engaged unless the instructor is able to motivate them using many application questions and more hands-on methods. Instructors may use more directed study applications and preload the lesson plan content by providing resources and information ahead of time to the students.

Whereas a chalk board and overhead projector were common to a Generation X student, an interactive board and flat panel would be more recognizable to the Generation Z student. This underlines the importance of knowing your audience characteristics and adapting the learning environment to them to increase retention and understanding of class material. As more and more Generation Z students enter the work force and the fire and emergency medical services field, instructors will have to adapt the learning environment to varied generations of students who will all bring different learning backgrounds and different ways that learning is retained and put to use in the future. Chapter 2, *The Learning Process*, discusses the different generational traits that are important considerations when determining your teaching approach.

Audience and Department Culture

To be effective in teaching, you must know your audience, the message you are trying to convey, your best delivery method, and the ideal atmosphere in which to deliver your message. This information is not always easy to come by. You may not know exactly with whom you are going to speak or even the context in which you will be presenting. You must be able to think on your feet and be prepared to take the presentation in the direction it needs to go so that the learning objectives are met. Remember—a good instructor always has a backup plan.

Audience

Depending on whether you are presenting at a conference with attendees from multiple jurisdictions or presenting locally to your own department, the manner in which you share the material with your audience will change. When presenting to a diverse audience, your presentation may need to be more generic. Avoid using specifics, such as the exact procedures of any one department. Consider speaking in generalities or giving examples instead of describing mandates or specific procedures. Taking this kind of broader perspective will allow each audience member to adapt your message for his or her own department. For example, when speaking about a procedure, give examples of several procedures used in fire departments across the country. Even when you are presenting to one department, be careful not to mistake instruction for department policy.

You may also need to adapt your presentation style to better match the learning environment. As your audience and your space increase in size, your presentation loses its intimacy. If you typically encourage a lot of student interaction, you may have to adapt your style to deliver a more traditional lecture because the larger room may not allow for personal student interaction. Avoid the phrase, "If I were you, I would do it this way." The best instructors help lead students into making the best decisions for their own departments based on the knowledge that the instructors provide.

Department Culture

When making a presentation or teaching a class, you must also be aware of culture. Here we speak not of customs associated with a particular national origin, but rather of departmental culture. Every department has its own culture. It is what makes fire fighters different, yet exactly the same. It is based on the mission of each and every fire department in the world. Departmental culture specifies what we will do, what we can do, and what we will not do. When you instruct students, you must put aside your personal culture. If you are brought in to teach, you must be able to separate facts from opinions.

Your misgivings about a technique do not automatically make that approach a bad idea. For example, some fire fighters might insist that positive-pressure ventilation causes a building to burn down; they may even show examples and argue that this technique introduces air into a hostile environment. These people may have had unpleasant experiences with positive-pressure ventilation, but that does not mean the technique is at fault. The misapplication or misuse of any technique will end poorly. This is the information a student needs—not personal opinions.

You must listen to the culture in which you are instructing and adapt your training accordingly. Every fire department says it is in existence to save lives. Likewise, every department says it is in existence to protect property. But how will the members of that culture save lives and property? To what extent are they willing to risk their own lives? These are the questions a departmental culture must answer.

As fire fighters, a major portion of our job is risk management. Risk management must be viewed within the context of the fire department's culture so that you can place the correct emphasis on the decision-making process. For example, although you may not agree with the decision to go offensive, you must respect and acknowledge the department's decision.

The Learning Environment

There is an old saying: When two people are together, one is always the leader. In training, whenever two fire fighters are together, one is always the instructor. The setting is not important, the time is not important, and the subject is not important—what *is* important is that you use the environment to ensure that learning takes place.

The **learning environment** is not always a classroom, because learning takes place in many different locations. In many company officer training classes, the concept of tailboard chats is encouraged. Many fire officers report that a great deal is learned sitting around the kitchen table in a firehouse or standing around a charred table in a kitchen that has just been overhauled (**FIGURE 3-7**). The place is not as important as recognizing the opportunity to share a message or thought and to deliver a piece of knowledge with others. Training might start in the classroom lecture or a demonstration by the instructor. From the classroom, the demonstration moves to the training ground, where the students get to apply hands-on training to further develop the skill set. Skill sets become building blocks that develop into scenarios, and scenarios move to larger-scale evolutions that are based on training as close to reality as possible. This process encompasses a variety of learning environments that require the instructor to know how to teach in each venue.

Many agencies are now using online training for their personnel for either initial or continuing education needs. As an instructor, the time may come when you will present a lesson in an online environment, which is different than the traditional classroom but is now considered standard for many agencies. The learning environment for an online course is different because you do not have a classroom to prepare or set up. However, depending on the type of online learning platform, you can have a big impact on how your virtual classroom is set up and how the students feel in that environment. Chapter 6, *Technology in Training*, has more information on online courses.

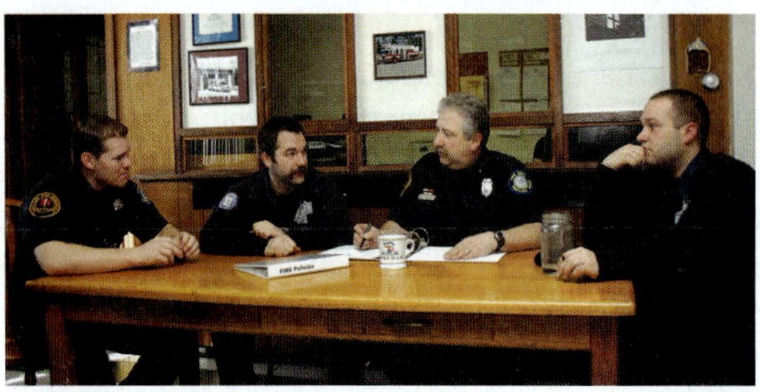

FIGURE 3-7 Learning can take place almost anywhere, and in some cases it can be even more effective in informal settings than in a classroom or on a drill ground.

To be an effective instructor, you need a solid understanding of the benefits and weaknesses of potential learning environments, and you must be able to select the best environment for presenting your message. First and foremost, you need to ensure the safety of your students, yourself, and others involved in the training. Eliminating all safety hazards and concerns should be priority number one. After evaluating the learning environment for safety, you next need to address the environment to ensure that learning can take place.

The Physical Environment

The perfect environment for students is one in which all of their needs are met. In Abraham Maslow's hierarchy of needs, the first need relates to creature comforts and physiological needs. Warmth and shelter make you feel safe in your environment. In the teaching sense, this need would be met when the classroom has enough light, the temperature is comfortable, and the seating and work space are adequate. In the case of an outdoor classroom, it may mean a place of shelter is available where students can warm up in cold weather and cool off in hot weather.

Learning takes place in two general settings: formal and informal. The formal environment consists of a classroom plus learning objectives, lesson plans, lesson outlines, and a final evaluation. By comparison, informal learning takes place every day in every location. Controlling the learning environment is a critical task for instructors. Consider the following factors to ensure you have a positive learning environment that will facilitate the learning process:

- Classroom environment
- Classroom setup
- Safety
- Lighting
- Teamwork and self-actualization
- Minimizing distractions

If you are instructing locally, the venue could be anything from the back of a fire engine to a formal classroom in a training center. Knowing where you will present the information is important so that you can tailor your presentation style to the venue. The size of the room is one factor; the seating in the room is another. The receptivity of students to your message will vary depending on whether the instruction takes place in a formal classroom with tables and chairs or in an apparatus room where students are just standing around. A formal training center with tables and chairs automatically puts students in the learning mind frame; that is, students are more focused in this venue. Because this venue represents a more formal situation, student behavior tends to be more formal. By comparison, the more casual atmosphere of the apparatus room puts students at ease and minimizes the formality of the student–instructor relationship. This opens up opportunities for the discussion to go more in the direction of the students' interests.

The concept of tailboard chats is not a new one. These discussions have been used for many years and can be an effective method of educating fire fighters. The **tailboard chat** is an informal gathering of fire fighters at the back of an engine where the company talks about various subjects. The tailboard is the equivalent to the water cooler in a business setting. It puts all members of the company at ease and on the same level when you instruct them there. For example, you might use the previous call as an opportunity to reinforce a learning objective. These tailboard chats can happen either back at the station or on the scene after the call is over.

Some instructors use the structure that the company was just at during a call as an example and "simulate" a fire to reinforce learning objectives. The tailboard chat may begin with you saying, "If there were a fire on the third floor of this building, in the B-C corner, where would we place the engine and the truck? What would the first engine company be responsible for doing? What would the first truck company do? What if this fire was at 2:00 AM? At 4:00 PM?" This is tactics and strategy training at its best.

COMPANY-LEVEL INSTRUCTOR TIP

To maximize the learning experience, add realism to a lesson. It helps if the lesson is based on a local area or one that is otherwise known to the students and relevant to their field. This strategy improves both leaning and retention. Real-life examples and experiences are more compelling than far-fetched scenarios.

The Indoor Classroom

Perhaps the most common setting for conducting a class is in a traditional classroom. Thus, when an instructor thinks of a "classroom environment," he or she probably thinks of a classroom in a building. Most often, classes start in an indoor setting and either remain there for the entire class or, once introductory material is covered, move outside to a training ground.

An important consideration in many classrooms today is the addition of new technology that affects the learning process. Most classrooms today have projectors and computers that are used for presenting lesson material. Many agencies have provided wireless internet service to assist students with the learning process or to complete assignments online. Of course, with this technology comes the possibility that the student might be distracted by "surfing" the internet or go to websites that are not class related. Issues related to classroom internet use can be addressed with agency policies or by turning the wireless access on or off as appropriate.

Temperature is very important to the learning process. If a room is too hot or too cold, students will focus more intently on the temperature than on what is being taught. You cannot make every student happy, so you must go with the majority opinion. If possible, lean toward keeping the room cooler versus warmer. In a colder environment, students are less likely to become drowsy. Also, if the temperature is too cool, students can always put on a sweater or light jacket.

You must also provide time for breaks so that students can attend to their personal needs. An old instructor's rule states, "The brain can learn only as long as the bottom will allow it." Some instructors (and students) may consider these breaks to be a waste; nevertheless, they are necessary both for the students and for you. In addition to enhancing students' personal comfort, the informal conversations that take place during a break can actually enhance the learning process.

Classroom Setup

Setting up the classroom is as important to the learning process as copying handouts or creating a slide presentation. Arranging the classroom sets the tone for the learning process. The first question you need to ask is, "Which type of learning do I want to accomplish?" If you plan to lecture to the students, then the room can be set up in rows facing a monitor or dry erase board (**FIGURE 3-8**). **TABLE 3-2** lists various classroom setups, along with their advantages and disadvantages (**FIGURE 3-9**).

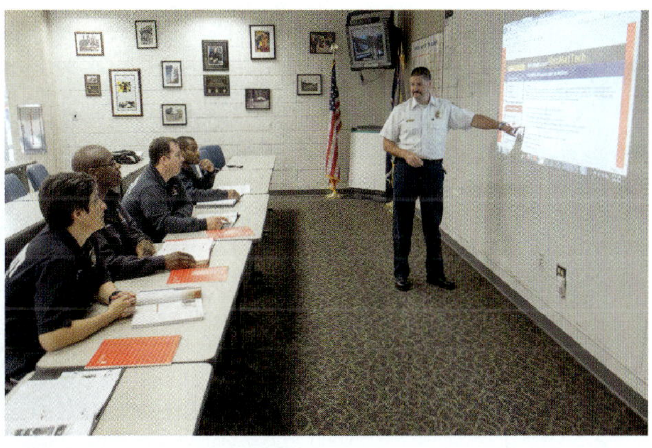

FIGURE 3-8 Your style of presentation will determine the best classroom setup.

TABLE 3-2 Classroom Setups

Method of Instruction	Learning Environment	Advantage	Disadvantage
Lecture	■ Auditorium, traditional, or theater	■ Good choice when students are able to see the front of the room ■ Instructor has more control in this setting ■ Can be effective for demonstrating skills	■ Difficult for students to see one another ■ Depending on how close chairs and tables are, the instructor may be very limited in moving around the classroom ■ Depending on the size of the room, students may have a difficult time hearing the instructor or other students
Discussion	■ Small U-shaped arrangement ■ Hollow square ■ Conference table	■ Students have the opportunity to see one another ■ Good environment for small-group interaction ■ Good environment for instructors to work in smaller groups with students	■ Students can easily be distracted by one another ■ Difficult for all students to see the front of the room ■ Difficult for instructors to control the teaching environment
Demonstration	■ Large U-shaped/ horse-shoe arrangement	■ Allows students to see the demonstration of skills ■ Allows the instructor to move about the room and interact with students	■ Students can easily be distracted by one another ■ Difficult for all students to see the front of the room

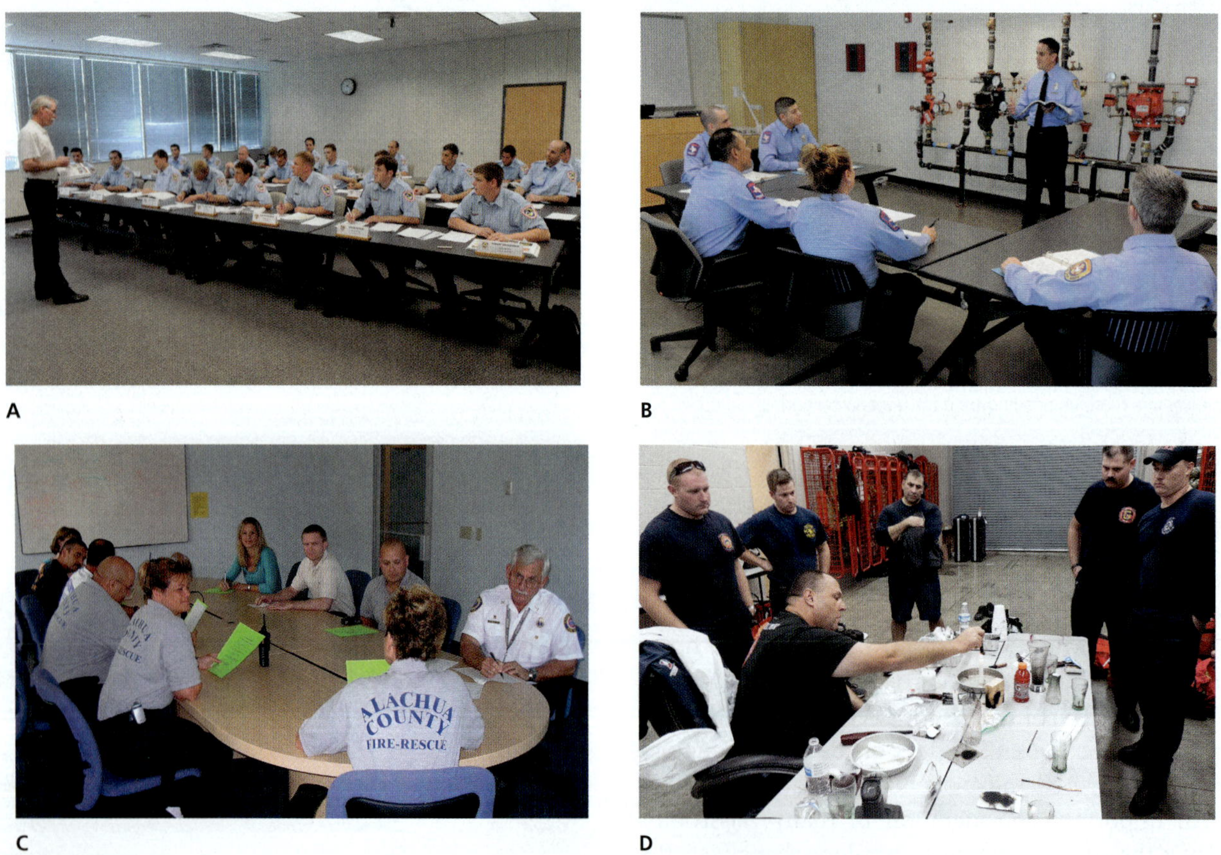

FIGURE 3-9 Sample classroom configurations. **A.** Traditional. **B.** U-shaped (horse shoe). **C.** Conference table. **D.** Tabletop.

A & B: © Jones & Bartlett Learning; C: Courtesy of L. Charles Smeby, Jr./University of Florida; D: © Jones & Bartlett Learning. Photographed by Glen E. Ellman.

Safety

After the basic needs are met, the next-highest-priority needs are those relating to safety. In a classroom environment, the term *safety* is used frequently.

Safety in the classroom is just as important as safety on the fire ground, but the hazards are much different. Ensuring that a classroom is safe involves removing both physical hazards (e.g., the trip hazard of a cord, book-bags around students' feet, wet floors from rain or spilled coffee). Physical hazards need to be controlled to ensure a safe classroom environment.

The second type of safety provided in the learning environment is emotional safety of the students. Students need to have an environment free of judgment or harassment, which will allow them to learn and express their thoughts and opinions. For example, students in a learning environment need to feel that if they make a mistake, there is an opportunity to learn from the mistake. In training, whether in the confines of a classroom or on the expanse of the drill ground, students must feel confident that if they make a mistake, you as the instructor will not belittle or otherwise demean them. Your task is to support students and to help them learn from their mistakes. Football coach Vince Lombardi once said that a person is not measured by how many times he is knocked down, but rather by how many times he gets back up. Your students must believe that you will help them get back up, and this sense of comfort can be provided in the right learning environment.

Lighting

In addition to the arrangement of tables and chairs, having the proper lighting for the room is important. Depending on the type of presentation that you are giving, you may need to adjust the lighting. In some cases, lights may be left on during a PowerPoint presentation or during other projected presentations. In the ideal classroom, the lights will be split, allowing lights in the front of the room to be dimmed while lights in the back of the room remain on to allow students to take notes. Your podium should have a light source so that you can read your notes. If the classroom does not have split lighting or adjustable lighting over the students, then you need to decide which type of lighting is best for your students.

Minimizing Distractions

Proper selection of the learning environment will determine the success or failure of the class in meeting the learning objectives. One challenge that all instructors face is the variety of distractions offered by today's communications technology. Phones, text messaging, pagers, and station alarms—all of these ubiquitous devices can cause students to be distracted from learning. Many of these distractions can be eliminated at the beginning of class by asking students to turn off or silence all electronic devices. If you have on-duty crew members in class, then make arrangements with them to turn down their pagers or radios.

Other distractions, such as people entering and leaving the classroom during a lecture, can be addressed before the class begins by posting a sign on the door stating that class is in session. Request that latecomers wait until a break to enter the classroom. If training is to occur with on-duty crews, consider having one student monitor a portable radio with the volume turned low.

If training is taking place outdoors, then controlling the learning environment is more difficult. Noise and distractions can disrupt the learning environment, so try to conduct your training in an isolated place.

Classroom Arrangement for Testing

The setup of the indoor classroom typically changes when students are required to take a test. Specifically, the classroom should be arranged to provide each student with enough space to put both the testing booklet and the answer key on a writing surface. It should also be designed to minimize the chance of wandering eyes, while simultaneously allowing the instructor to observe all students. Given that most testing is individualized, the classroom should remain quiet. If the testing is group based, you must be able to distinguish between testing noise and distractions from a group. The personal needs of students should be recognized. If a student needs to leave the room to attend to personal needs, the security of the testing process should be maintained. Because testing and evaluating the learning process are important to the fire service, having the right testing environment will ensure that students can focus on the test.

The Outdoor Classroom

Although it might appear that the work conducted in the outdoor classroom is more important than the instruction that occurs in the indoor classroom, both are needed to ensure that students achieve the learning objectives. Your challenge is to match the environment to the learning objectives to make sure that the student is always in the correct environment in which to learn.

Outdoor classrooms differ in more respects than just their location (**FIGURE 3-10**). When moving the learning process to an outdoor venue, the instructor needs to address issues such as weather, training

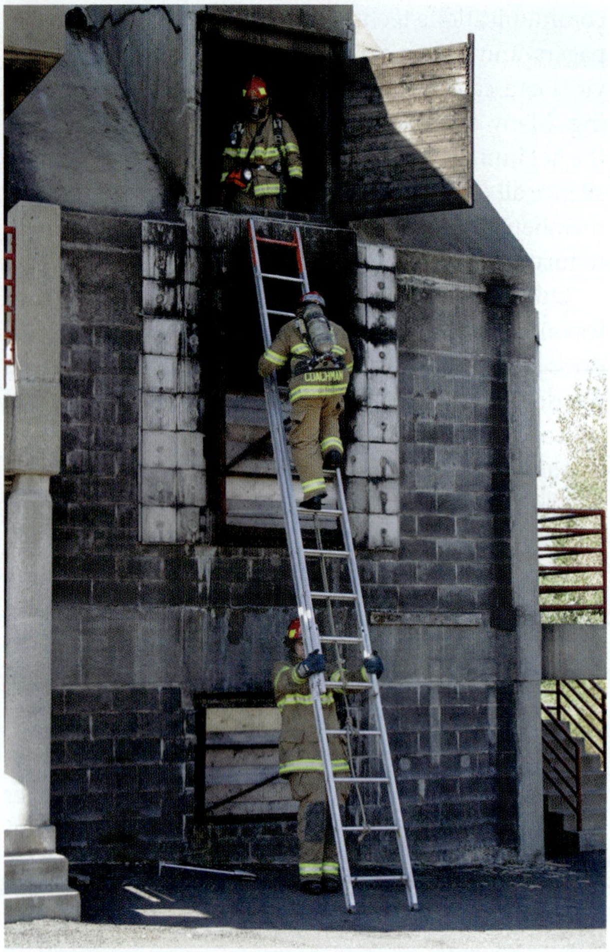

FIGURE 3-10 Outdoor locations can present a set of challenges for the instructor.

and ambient noise, and logistical issues such as equipment needs, parking, or rehabilitation facilities. The key to training outdoors is to plan ahead and to conduct the proper pretraining assessment to ensure a safe and effective learning experience for your students.

When curriculum or training needs require an outdoor training environment, the instructor needs to be prepared to teach in this environment. These outdoor classrooms can be organized on a developed and organized training ground, which could contain a fixed burn building to teach interior fire attack, a mobile prop used to teach fire behavior, or a pond to teach drafting skills. Another type of outdoor classroom could be an off-site location such as a mountain or a slope used to teach high-angle rope rescue skills (**FIGURE 3-11**).

Outdoor locations, whether on a training ground or an off-site location, pose similar challenges and considerations for the instructor to address in order to facilitate the learning process. These challenges include the weather, outside noise, logistics/resources,

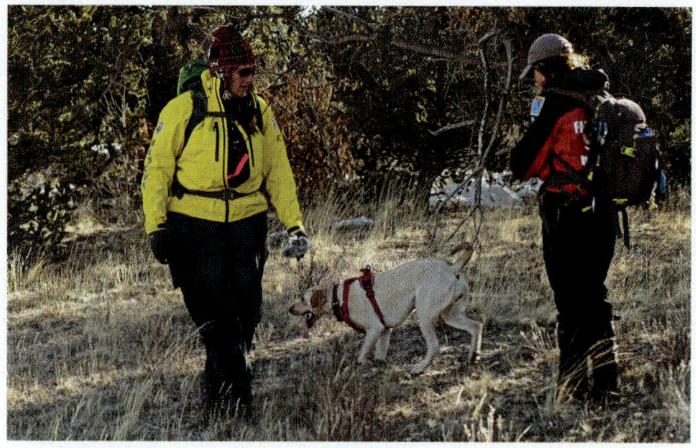

FIGURE 3-11 Technical rescue training environments are often found in the areas where the skills will be used.

and the ability to teach so that students can learn in the outdoor classroom. As mentioned previously, distractions are a common factor in the outdoor setting. To help with this, keep your groups small, so that every student is more closely engaged in the learning process with the oversight of an instructor.

A classic example of an outdoor learning environment that would present several challenges would be training at an acquired structure. These buildings present a great learning opportunity for students, but also create many difficulties for instructors. Following NFPA 1403: *Standard on Live Fire Training Evolutions* will assist the instructor in correctly preparing for such a training event.

Communicating Outdoors

Communicating in the outdoor classroom can be a challenge to any instructor. Learning to establish an environment that will allow you to teach outdoors is just as important as it is when in a traditional classroom.

For example, when teaching in a live fire training scenario, communication can be difficult. In this environment, you first need to be cognizant of your own safety. Taking off your self-contained breathing apparatus (SCBA) mask to communicate in a smoke-filled environment not only puts you at risk but also sends a message to the students that the use of a SCBA mask is not important. Communication in the live fire environment is essential, however, and can be accomplished by first gaining the students' attention and then by using a calm and controlled voice to communicate what you are attempting to teach.

A live fire training scenario is also an environment in which teaching is a constant process. You need to be close enough to the students to observe their behaviors and far enough back to observe the scene and allow the students to perform and learn.

Learning how to communicate in the outdoor classroom is a skill that you will need to develop and always be mindful of when outdoors. Observing your students will be critical to determining whether your voice and the content of your message are reaching everyone. Observing students' body language will be a good indicator of whether your message is getting to everyone.

Safety

One point cannot be emphasized enough: Safety should be your greatest concern in the outdoor classroom. During outdoor training, the stakes become higher and the attention to detail becomes more intense. When performing live fire training, for example, the environment needs to be as safe as possible while allowing learning to take place. You hold students' lives in your hands, and students need reassurance that you take this responsibility seriously. It is important to follow standards such as NFPA 1403, among others. Having the right number of personnel, in the right positions, doing the right things, with an emphasis on safety, makes the learning environment the safest place for fire fighters in which to work and learn.

The purpose of many outdoor training sessions is to teach or evaluate students' psychomotor skills; these skills are the ones that fire fighters use to protect the lives and property of citizens. For that reason, when training and evaluating students, you need to be in the most realistic situation possible while maintaining a safe environment for students. In rope rescue, this concept is called being "redundantly redundant"—that is, there is a safety for everything.

Make sure that students' psychomotor skills are practiced and completed perfectly. A skill is either acceptable or unacceptable—there is no middle ground. If a fire fighter is asked to don a full protective ensemble and forgets to put the hood up, he or she has failed in that skill. Vince Lombardi said, "Practice doesn't make perfect; perfect practice makes perfect." Another relevant saying is, "The more we sweat in training, the less we bleed in battle."

Weather

A major consideration outdoors is the weather. Obviously, outdoor classrooms are subject to the weather conditions. The physical location of your outdoor classroom can determine how you prepare for and handle the class. If you are in the South or Southwest, you may need to deal with high heat levels. If you are in the Northeast or Midwest, you may be more concerned about cold temperatures and snow. No matter where you are, the threat of rain is a consideration when an outdoor classroom will be used for instruction.

The safety of your students should always be your highest concern. Many fire departments use either a temperature/humidity (heat) index or a wind chill index as a guide when determining whether outdoor training is feasible or acceptable within department policy. NFPA 1584: *Standard on the Rehabilitation Process for Members During Emergency Operations and Training Exercises* offers guidelines on temperature and physical exertion levels relating to how much training, PPE, and rehabilitation is required during extreme temperature and weather.

Always have a "plan B" in case inclement weather forces the class to use an alternative location that is unaffected by the weather, such as an apparatus bay floor or a large, unused warehouse. Plans to use these areas should be put into place before the training occurs, rather than decisions being made spontaneously during the training as an emergency measure. Rain is a fact of life. A small amount of rain may not be an issue during outdoor training, but torrential downpours and lightning are definitely reasons to seek an alternative environment. Warming or cooling areas and shelter from wind, rain, or other weather phenomena are necessities for your students' safety.

Noise

Noise in the outdoor environment is also a concern during training. In most cases, you will need to project your voice so that all of the students can hear you without the use of an electronic device such as a microphone. Environmental factors such as wind can be a deterrent in allowing your voice to carry. Other distractions—such as vehicle traffic, ambient noise from the field, or other training activities going on around you—can add to the difficulty of communicating in outdoor environments. During your preplanning of the outdoor classroom, look for locations in which you can present verbal information effectively. Many training grounds have outdoor pavilions that are designed for teaching and for sharing information. Shielding yourself near a fire apparatus can help minimize noise and project your voice. It might not be possible to eliminate all outside noise, so it falls on you as an instructor to use your voice and other teaching skills to help communicate the information and knowledge you are attempting to teach.

Logistics and Resources

When the classroom moves to the outdoors, there are several other issues to address. As part of your classroom setup, ensure that all logistical arrangements have been secured prior to moving outdoors. Reviewing your lesson plan and ensuring that all required equipment and materials are in place before class are steps that are expected of you as the instructor. Knowing the location of restroom facilities and having a rehabilitation area established are just as important as having the right equipment ready for your class. At an established training ground, these resources are usually in place and have been designed into the facility. The real challenge comes when training moves to an off-site location, because you need to convey all of your resources to that site. Making arrangements before class to address the physical needs of your students for restroom facilities and rehabilitation becomes an important challenge when moving to an off-site location. The need to take required and extra equipment with you is also important so downtime is minimized if something breaks or additional equipment is needed.

Contingency Plans

You must have a plan B regardless of the environment. What do you do if the projector fails to work? What do you do if lightning begins to flash in the sky on a live fire training day? What happens if an assistant instructor does not arrive on a practical skill day? All of these contingencies need to be considered and planned for. Many times the solutions are simple—for example, keeping a spare projector bulb or a spare projector, or having a rain date for outdoor training. In any event, you as the instructor need to be able to adjust your training plan so that your training plan can continue. If an evolution or training session cannot continue due to some type of issue, many rescheduling or make-up logistics will be involved in finishing the training. Without question, safety and proper delivery will always take precedence over any of these considerations. A best practice may be to have a set of "ready-to-go" backup drills in the case that training must be stopped. You do not want to lose momentum or the opportunity to train when your department meets only a few times per month.

Another way to look at this situation is much like you would approach an emergency scene. Do you have the resources in place if something should go wrong? For example, suppose you are teaching a psychomotor drill and a trainee gets hurt. Is there an ambulance available? Who is notified? Which forms must be completed? How will the training continue if you are missing one student? On an emergency scene, fire fighters constantly plan for contingencies. Always have a contingency plan. Things can and will go wrong, and having at least considered these issues will allow you to adapt to the changing circumstances quickly.

Teamwork and Self-Actualization

In Maslow's hierarchy of needs, Maslow speaks of the issue of belonging. A main focus of fire training is teamwork, and the learning environment you create must be one that supports and recognizes the crucial nature of teamwork. Many of the best friends you have in the fire service are likely to be people whom you met as you trained to become a fire fighter. During your training, you built a strong sense of camaraderie, which ultimately helped you in completing a very difficult task. An important part of the instruction should be providing time either before, during, or after the formal instruction to allow students to network.

The next level in Maslow's hierarchy of needs is the need for self-esteem or accomplishment in the student. You should create an environment that celebrates students' victories as they are accomplished. Status and recognition can be very powerful motivators in the learning environment. In his book *The One-Minute Manager*, Ken Blanchard talks about catching people doing things right (Blanchard and Johnson, 1982). In a good learning environment, this idea is expanded to not only catching students doing things right but also recognizing and celebrating that accomplishment. People want to be in an environment where they can succeed.

The highest-priority need in Maslow's hierarchy is the need for self-actualization. At this level, the student is able to synthesize material by taking multiple learning situations and putting them together to solve a problem. The need for self-actualization is satisfied in the environment where you perform live fire simulations or even live fire training. Look to challenge your students to take your message and use it to solve a problem.

COMPANY-LEVEL INSTRUCTOR TIP

As an instructor, you should be aware of how demographics affect the classroom. Always exercise caution and common sense in the classroom. Never make a comment that refers to someone's background, such as where they attended school, their marital status, or their ethnicity.

Demographics in the Learning Environment

Demographics include the age, gender, marital status, family size, and educational background of a fire fighter. Demographic considerations extend beyond issues of race and national origin; in the fire service, they require looking in a more holistic manner at everything a fire fighter brings to the department.

Assess a fire fighter's demographics and ask yourself a few questions: Which type of skills does this fire fighter bring? Could these skills be a benefit to the others in the learning environment? Are you dealing with a highly educated individual or a fire fighter who has met only the basic educational requirements? Does the same class include a mix of experienced and inexperienced fire fighters? Determining the answers to these types of questions will help you grasp the basic demographics of your students, shaping your teaching approach.

Another demographic consideration unique to the fire service is the different types of staffing encountered among fire departments. The fire service includes career, volunteer, combination, and paid-on-call fire fighters. The learning objectives for paid-on-call or volunteer fire fighters do not differ, but the presentation to these groups does. Because volunteer and paid-on-call fire fighters generally have full-time jobs, training accommodations must be made to fit their schedules. By gearing instruction toward the demands of the students' schedules, you allow each student to focus fully on the subject at hand and not be distracted. For example, if a class is made up of all career fire fighters, the class may be 6 to 8 weeks long, 8 hours a day. By contrast, if the same class is made up of all volunteers, the class may meet Tuesday and Thursday nights for 3 hours and all day on Saturdays for 6 months. Both classes should cover the same learning objectives to the same levels of proficiency, but the differing demographics of the participants require different schedules.

COMPANY-LEVEL INSTRUCTOR TIP

Today's public safety learning environments are made up of a highly diverse group of students. A major area of focus for the instructor is to identify the characteristics of each learner and build a lesson that will meet the needs of each of these students.

Gender Considerations

Gender is a hot-button issue today. One change that has affected the fire service in the last few years is the abandonment of the term *fireman*. Many qualified women have joined the ranks of this once male-dominated profession, so it is more appropriate to refer to students as *fire fighters*. Firefighting does not, according to the fire, have a gender. Although learning objectives do not change with the gender of the student, you do need to be cognizant of students' gender. If you use the term *guys* to address your students, your students need to understand that "guys" includes both men and women. Remember to be gender neutral when developing learning objectives. The key is to be respectful of all your students at all times.

Offensive Language, Gestures, and Dress

The use of offensive language should be avoided—period. Some people may contend that to make a point, sometimes you must swear or use slang terms; others contend that this is part of the fire service culture. This is not the case. Jokes and language of a sexual or explicit nature are unacceptable in the learning environment. As an instructor, you should have a mastery of the English language. You should be able to make your point without the use of profanity. You will find that students gain a deeper respect for you when you demonstrate eloquence in the classroom.

Do not participate in improper situations. A wise instructor once shared a key piece of wisdom when he said, "If you hear an off-color joke and grin, you're in." If you hear an offensive joke, show that you do not agree with what was said. It is your responsibility to stop any unsafe or inappropriate behavior immediately. It is important to take pride in your department, and one source of that pride involves showing respect to everyone.

Sometimes, regardless of our awareness and best intentions, we inadvertently offend one another. If it happens that you offend a student, apologize to the student in private and then in front of the class. This can go a long way toward making amends.

An equally important step is to establish a policy that covers acceptable behavior and language. Your organization should have a harassment policy that addresses these issues, including remedies for offenses, reporting of incidents, and conduct. The best policy is to understand the audience to whom you are speaking. Ensure that your presentation occurs in a context that is appropriate for your audience. A wise instructor

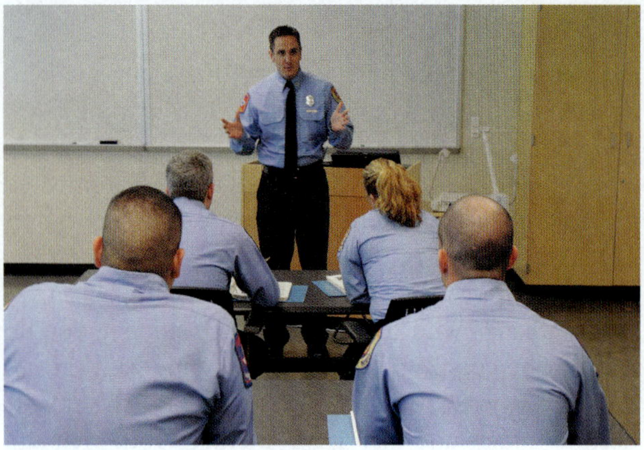

FIGURE 3-12 How you present yourself is a reflection on the fire department.

used to say, "Make sure that your language would be acceptable to your grandmother."

Like words, gestures and dress can sometimes be offensive. How you dress and how you move are representations of your position (**FIGURE 3-12**). Always maintain a neutral position, which allows the student to feel free to express his or her opinion and concerns in a safe environment.

Adapting the Lesson Plan Based on Demographics

The information that you learn as a result of students' verbal introductions may require slight modifications to the lesson plan. Perhaps students will need to spend more time in one area of the class and less time in another. The information gained in this way can also help you decide the depths you need to go to in the various areas of the presentation, perhaps allowing you to lengthen parts of the program and shorten others to meet the needs of the class. For example, if you are presenting a disaster preparedness course in Arizona, you may not need to spend an entire hour on blizzards. Even in a small company training setting, you should be aware of the skill, experience, and ability levels of the members of the class to gain the best results.

If a student requests that you cover a certain topic, you should not rewrite the entire course; however, you should keep the student's request in mind. If time and circumstances permit, you could briefly present the topic and then ask the student, "Did that meet your need?" By doing so, you ensure that students know you are available to instruct them on whatever they need to know to meet the learning objectives of the course. Bear in mind that as an instructor, you must be prepared either to adapt your lesson plan or to tell the student that the topic is outside the scope of the class.

If you indicate that you will cover an area or an objective, you need to ensure that you fully address any concerns or questions about that topic. Meeting this goal requires knowing and understanding your audience. Many fire departments have target hazards or situations that are unique to their locations. For example, many communities in the Northeast include row houses, whereas these structures are rarely found in the Midwest. When asked, "How would you handle this situation?" you should be prepared to render an opinion. By anticipating what the questions will be, you will be prepared to offer an opinion because you have had time to research the question and present an intelligent response. If you do not know the answer, do not—under any circumstance—make up the answer. It is completely acceptable to say, "I do not know, but I will try to find out for you." Fire fighters respect honesty in their instructors.

Training BULLETIN

JONES & BARTLETT FIRE DISTRICT

TRAINING DIVISION

5 Wall Street, Burlington, MA, 01803

Phone 978-443-5000 Fax 978-443-8000

Instant Applications: Methods of Instruction

Drill Assignment

Apply the chapter content to your department's operation, training division, and your personal experiences to complete the following questions and activities.

Objective

Upon completion of the instant applications, fire and emergency services instructor students will exhibit decision making and application of job performance requirements of the instructor using the text, class discussion, and their own personal experiences.

Suggested Drill Applications

1. Identify several NIOSH fire fighter fatality reports that utilized rapid intervention team activations or identified survivors that used skills learned in a fire fighter safety and survival program and discuss them with your shift.
2. Review your department's Rapid Intervention/Safety and Survival SOG and discuss it with your shift, identifying strengths and weaknesses and ways that it can be incorporated into your company-level training.
3. Evaluate the culture of your department's training and identify ways that it can be improved.
4. Discuss the challenges of conducting a fire fighter safety and survival course outdoors and what can be done to make the training more realistic, relevant, and results oriented.

Incident Report: USFA Technical Report, USFA-TR-015/October 1987

Drill Assignment

Review the information in this incident report and prepare a practice presentation for class delivery at the direction of your instructor. Your presentation should include a summary of the incident facts and a review of the NFPA 1403 compliance and noncompliance findings. Use an outline to organize your thoughts. You may be evaluated on your communication skills during your presentation.

Hollandale, Minnesota—1987

Search and rescue drills had been conducted for some time in a small two-bedroom house without problems. Leaves burning in a 35-gallon (132.5-liter) drum were used to create smoke. The drum had a metal cover to reduce the danger of fire spread, and the drum was situated above the floor. Caution was exercised to prevent fire from spreading from the container. Two fire apparatus were on scene with 1400 gallons (5299 liters) of water on one of the fire units and 1000 gallons (3785 liters) in a portable tank. The participants carried a charged 1½" (38.1-mm) hose line.

After the interior search evolutions, the intent was to destroy the house by burning it down. Four crew members wearing full protective clothing, equipped with breathing apparatus, and protected by a charged 1½" (38.1-mm) hose line entered the structure using the east entry that had been used during the drill (**FIGURE 3-A**). They attempted to light a fire in the back bedroom but were unable to get it to ignite, most likely due to the dampness from the water. They moved to the living room and splashed #2 fuel oil on the wall and carpet. Two of the fire fighters moved to the kitchen while another used a propane torch to ignite the fire in the living room. The entire room flashed, and a third fire fighter crawled out, thinking his partner was with him. Three of the fire fighters crawled to the outside. The fourth made it to the kitchen and stopped, where he apparently removed his SCBA mask to call for help and then reentered the fire area and was killed. His Nomex hood, propane torch, and fuel can are later found in the kitchen. The three fire fighters that had exited the house reported the emergency and entry was immediately forced into the front entrance. The fire was quickly extinguished, and the victim was found dead.

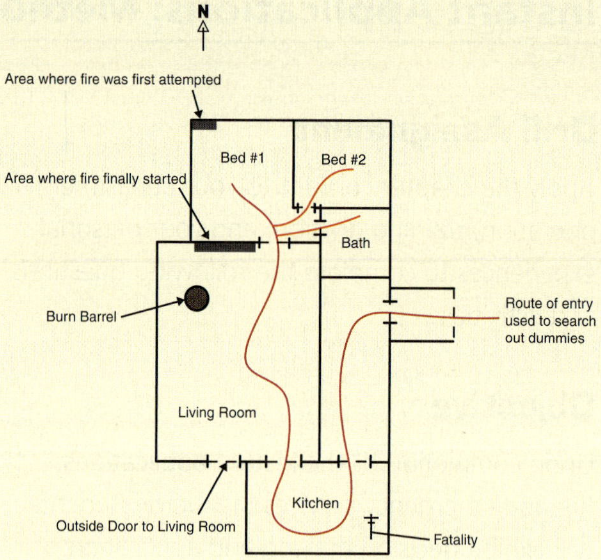

FIGURE 3-A Floor plan of the Hollendale structure.
Reproduced from the Minnesota Department of Labor and Industry, Minnesota OSHA Compliance.

It was uncovered in the investigation that the living room paneling was made of a lightweight combustible material found in mobile homes at the time. The smoke barrel with live fire may have preheated the combustibles in the living room (**FIGURE 3-B**). The report noted that the NFPA 1403 standard should have been followed. Investigators believed that if the deceased had remained in the kitchen, he most likely would have survived.

The fire department was cited by the state OSHA for failure to "examine the building more closely, failure to brief the participants on the building's layout, failure to have a building evacuation plan, and failure to have a qualified instructor on the scene." This was the first fire fighter fatality after the release of NFPA 1403.

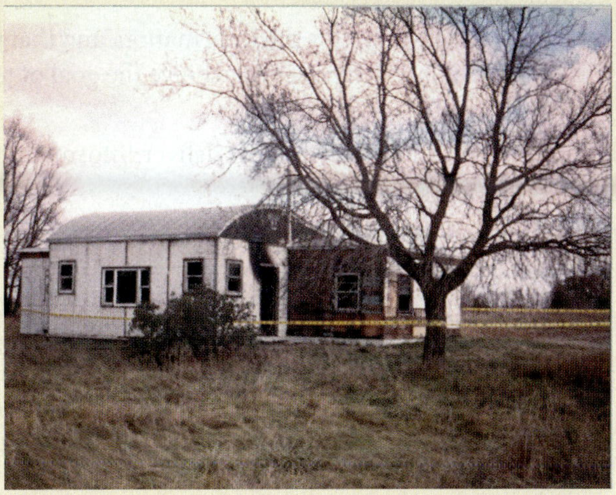

FIGURE 3-B Photo of rear of house in the Hollandale fire. The kitchen is below the area with the flat roof. Note the minor amount of smoke and heat damage above door.
Courtesy of the Minnesota Department of Labor and Industry, Minnesota OSHA Compliance.

Postincident Analysis Hollandale, Minnesota

NFPA 1403 Noncompliant

- Combustible wall paneling and carpeting contributed to rapid fire spread
- Flammable and combustible liquids used
- Flashover and fire spread unexpectedly
- No direct egress from living room
- No formal evacuation plan including evacuation signal
- No incident safety officer
- No interior hose line
- No EMS on scene
- No written emergency plan
- Participants not informed of emergency plans and procedures
- No preburn plan
- No walkthrough performed with students and instructors

After-Action REVIEW

IN SUMMARY

- Adult students need realistic, practical, and knowledgeable lessons that deliver information in a variety of ways to accommodate their differing learning characteristics.
- When you can communicate to students that you know the information, and that you understand their unique needs and motivations, you will find that it is much easier to achieve the goal of teaching the information and having the students learn.
- Determining which method of instruction should be used to deliver information is accomplished using several factors:
  - The experience and educational level of the students
  - The classroom setting or training environment
  - The objectives of the material to be taught
  - The number of students to be taught
- Ask yourself three basic questions when reviewing and planning for the delivery of a lesson plan:
  - What are the goals of the lesson?
  - Who is the intended audience?
  - What are the resources and learning environment characteristics?
- Methods of instruction vary among disciplines, but for the fire service the following are most common and effective in teaching new and in-service personnel:
  - Lecture
  - Demonstration/skill drill
  - Discussion
  - Role play
  - Labs/simulations
  - Case studies
  - Out-of-class assignments
  - Online learning, independent study, and blended learning
- While reviewing and preparing for class with a lesson plan, the four-step method of instruction is the primary process used to relate the material contained in the lesson plan to the students:
  - Preparation
  - Presentation
  - Application
  - Evaluation
- Five effective transition techniques are delineation, words/phrases, pictures, voice, and body language.
- An important part of the learning process is to assess the knowledge gained during class. This is most commonly done by asking the students questions about the material you have presented. Several types of questions may be used:
  - Direct questions
  - Rhetorical questions
  - Open-ended questions
  - Closed-ended questions

- Disruption in the classroom can significantly reduce or limit the amount of learning time for students. It can also lead to unsafe and negative learning that could have serious implications when students apply what they have learned in the field. As the instructor, you are responsible for providing a safe learning environment and proper, safe instruction to all students.
- When you develop your lesson plan, it should be detailed and complete enough to achieve the identified goals and desired outcomes, yet flexible enough that it can be adjusted to meet students' needs on the fly.
- Because learning can take place in many locations—such as a traditional classroom, fire-ground training facilities, or another location such as an acquired structure—you as the instructor need to be keenly aware of your environment.
- When making a presentation or teaching a class, you must be aware of both the audience and their departmental culture.
- Some programs require that students take prerequisite classes before attending certain advanced classes. The fact that students have completed these preliminaries ensures that the students taking your course have a certain base level of training and education.
- Establishing a learning environment is just as important as having a lesson plan. Without the proper environment, the learning process will be limited and can be ineffective.
- Matching the correct classroom arrangement to the needs of the lesson plan will allow students to learn.
- When presenting a lesson in an indoor classroom, consider the classroom environment and setup, safety, lighting, and ways to minimize distractions. Adjustments may need to be made for testing.
- When presenting a lesson in an outdoor classroom, considerations include communication, safety, weather, background noise, logistics, and resources.
- You must have a plan B when using any environment. All potential contingencies need to be considered and planned for.
- Understanding demographics extends beyond issues of race and national origin. In the fire service, taking demographics into account during instruction requires looking in a more holistic manner at everything a fire fighter brings to the department.

KEY TERMS

Access Navigate for flashcards to test your key term knowledge.

Asynchronous learning An online course format in which the instructor provides material, lectures, tests, and assignments that can be accessed at any time. Students are given a time frame during which they need to connect to the course and complete assignments.

Blended learning An instruction method that combines online/independent study with face-to-face meetings with the instructor.

Demographics Characteristics of a given population, possibly including such information as age, race, gender, education, marital status, family structure, and location of agency.

Four-step method of instruction The primary process used to relate the material contained in a lesson plan to the students; the steps are preparation, presentation, application, evaluation.

Independent study A method of distance learning in which students order the course materials, complete them, and then return them to the instructor.

Learning environment A combination of a physical location (classroom or training ground) and the proper emotional elements of both an instructor and a student.

Method of instruction Various ways in which information is delivered to student, both in a classroom and on the training ground. (NFPA 1041)

Synchronous learning An online class format that requires students and instructors to be online at the same time. Lectures, discussions, and presentations occur at a specific hour and students must be online at that time to participate and receive credit for attendance.

Tailboard chat An informal gathering where fire fighters discuss various issues.

REFERENCES

Bear, George G. 1990. "Models and Techniques That Focus on Prevention." In *Best Practices in School Psychology*, edited by Alex Thomas and Jeff Grimes, 652. Silver Spring, MD: National Association of School Psychologists.

Blanchard, Kenneth, and Spencer Johnson. 1982. *The One-Minute Manager*. New York: William Morrow and Company, Inc.

Dale, Edgar. 1969. *Audiovisual Methods in Teaching*. 3rd ed. New York: Dryden Press.

National Fire Protection Association. 2019. *NFPA 1041: Standard for Fire and Emergency Services Instructor Professional Qualifications*. Quincy, MA: National Fire Protection Association.

National Fire Protection Association. 2018. *NFPA 1403: Standard on Live Fire Training Evolutions*. Quincy, MA: National Fire Protection Association.

National Fire Protection Association. 2015. *NFPA 1584: Standard on the Rehabilitation Process for Members During Emergency Operations and Training Exercises*. Quincy, MA: National Fire Protection Association.

Walker, J. E., and Shea, T. M. 1991. *Behavior management: A practical approach for educators*. 5th ed. New York: Macmillan.

CHAPTER PRESENTATION EXERCISE

Instructions: Your course instructor will assign individual or group discussions on the key points and teaching tips of this chapter. You or your group will review the chapter teachings and identify the major learning points from the chapter. You should be able to discuss the points, why they are important, and how/where they apply to your responsibilities at your level of instructor training.

REVIEW QUESTIONS

1. Describe some of the communications techniques that will help you improve the delivery of information to your class.
2. Describe the steps that make up the four-step method of instruction.
3. Describe asynchronous learning.

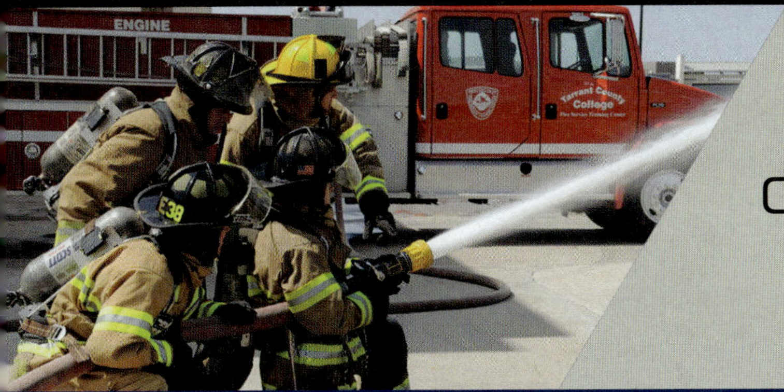

CHAPTER 4

Communication Skills

NFPA 1041 JOB PERFORMANCE REQUIREMENTS

Note: An asterisk denotes that the 1041 standard contains further information in its annex section.

4.4.3 Present and adjust prepared lessons, given a prepared lesson plan that specifies the presentation method(s), so that the method(s) indicated in the plan are used and the stated objectives or learning outcomes are achieved, applicable safety standards and practices are followed, and risks are addressed.

(A)* Requisite Knowledge.

The laws and principles of learning, methods and techniques of instruction, lesson plan components and elements of the communication process, and lesson plan terminology and definitions; learner characteristics; student-centered learning principles; instructional technology tools; the impact of cultural differences on instructional delivery; safety rules, regulations, and practices; identification of training hazards; elements and limitations of distance learning; distance learning delivery methods; and the instructor's role in distance learning.

(B) Requisite Skills.

Oral communication techniques, methods and techniques of instruction, ability to adapt to changing circumstances, and utilization of lesson plans in an instructional setting.

KNOWLEDGE OBJECTIVES

After studying this chapter, participating in a structured learning environment, and completing assigned assessments, you will be able to:

- Identify and describe the elements of the communication process. (**NFPA 1041: 4.4.3**, p 101)
- Compare and describe the different types and styles of communication. (pp 102–105)
- Describe communication techniques that will improve your presentation. (**NFPA 1041: 4.4.3**, pp 102–106)

SKILLS OBJECTIVES

After studying this chapter, participating in a structured learning environment, and completing assigned assessments, you will be able to:

- Demonstrate the ability to use various communication styles in the classroom. (**NFPA 1041: 4.4.3**, pp 102–105)
- Demonstrate effective oral communication techniques. (**NFPA 1041: 4.4.3**, pp 103–105)
- Demonstrate effective written communication techniques. (**NFPA 1041: 4.4.3**, pp 106–110)

You Are the Fire and Emergency Services Instructor

While studying several National Institute for Occupational Safety and Health (NIOSH) fire fighter fatality reports, you notice that a common theme among both the contributing factors and key recommendations is the continued mention of communication issues and recommended training. Communications plays a very important role in most everything we do in the fire service, from training to occupancy inspections to emergency incidents. Understanding this, you have decided to conduct a training session for your department on emergency scene communications.

1. Identify and describe the elements of the communication process.
2. Describe the role of communications in both the learning (training) process and emergency incident response.
3. Compare and describe the different types and styles of communications.
4. Identify barriers to effective communications, both in the classroom and on the emergency incident scene.

Introduction

Communication is the most important element of the learning process. Communication in and of itself is a process that you must master to become an effective fire and emergency services instructor. When you have mastered communication skills, the environment in which you are teaching becomes less of a factor in the learning process. Even if the environment is less than perfect, strong communication skills will enable you to be an effective and dynamic instructor. Your goal is to make sure that your students leave the classroom with a greater knowledge base than they had when they came in.

According to professional educator Leah Davies:

> Being able to communicate is vital to being an effective educator. Communication not only conveys information, but it encourages effort, modifies attitudes, and stimulates thinking. Without it, stereotypes develop, messages become distorted and learning is stifled.

An instructor must be an effective communicator. One of the keys to the learning process is the conveyance of information. When you demonstrate effective communication skills, you can take the learning process to even greater heights by encouraging effort, modifying attitudes, and stimulating thinking.

This chapter addresses both the spoken and written communication processes as well as the environment's effect on communication. Students have different learning styles and use different cues when learning. Knowing how to access these diverse cues and take advantage of them to enhance the learning experience will make you a more effective instructor. See Chapter 2, *The Learning Process*, for more information on different learner characteristics.

The fire service classroom encompasses so much more than four walls, tables and chairs, and a dry erase board. It can also include the back of an engine after the call, a burn building, and even a kitchen table at the station surrounded by members who have just completed an emergency response. No matter what the environment, the end objective is the same: that the student learns and that the student's safety and ability to do his or her job improve. The instructor must have excellent communication skills and must be able to read the students' comprehension of the training through verbal and nonverbal cues. Although the fire service is certainly steeped in tradition, the means of communication used by fire fighters have changed dramatically over the years. The first fire officers used speaking trumpets to communicate to the members of their department at a fire scene. Even with today's many avenues for the rapid transmission of messages, the message itself remains the critical piece of the communication puzzle.

The Basic Communication Process

The basic **communication process** consists of five elements: the sender, the message, the medium, the receiver, and feedback (**FIGURE 4-1**). Surrounding these elements is the environment. The five elements of the communication process act like the links of a chain. For the chain to function properly, all the links must be attached to one another. If any one of the links breaks, then the chain falls apart.

The Sender

In the communications chain of the fire service classroom, the **sender** is you, the instructor. As the sender, you must know which style of communication to use. The choice of the style of communication is based on many factors, including your comfort level. If you are more comfortable using oral (verbal) communication, then you are likely to use that style most often. Many other methods of instruction that center on the sender and how he or she delivers training material are discussed in Chapter 3, *Methods of Instruction*.

The Message

The next link in the communication chain is the **message**. What are you trying to communicate to your students? You must encode the point of the lesson and then transmit it. This may sound simple, but it is actually the most complex part of the communication process. For students to understand your message, they must hear it, decode it or put it into their own terms, and then ensure that their terms match your terms. Consider the command, "Put out that fire now." A student might hear this message as "Get a hose and spray some water right now," when the message really was "Get a fire extinguisher and suppress those sparks."

The Medium

How the message is transmitted is as important as the message itself. The means of conveying a message constitutes the **medium**. For example, your tone of voice, volume, speed of voice, and other qualities all convey information. If you give a lecture about a new piece of personal protective equipment (PPE) while sitting behind a desk, fiddling with a paper clip, and speaking in a very relaxed manner, you will convey to the students the message, "This new piece of PPE really isn't that important," even though the message you are stating verbally might be "This piece of equipment will save your life."

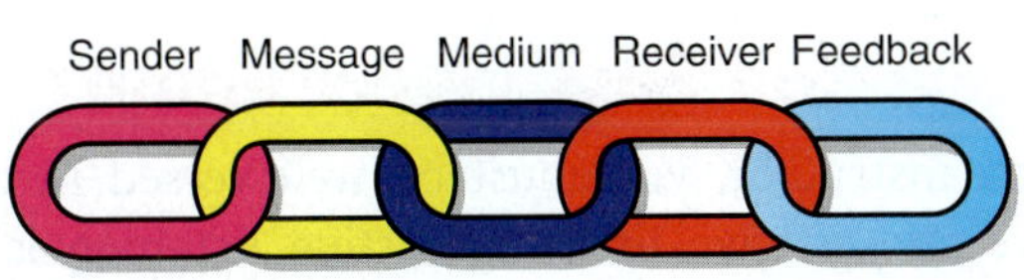

FIGURE 4-1 The five elements of the communication process act like the links of a chain.

The Receiver

The next link in the communications chain is the **receiver**. In the learning environment, this link is the student. The receiver plays an important, active role in the communication chain; that is, the student needs to listen actively and maintain focus to decode your message. At the start of each training session, remind students of their role in the communications chain and continue to keep them engaged throughout the learning process. Fulfilling this role means leaving all distractions at the door and focusing solely on the information you present. Ensure that all students understand their active role in the communications process.

A student's previous experience and knowledge base play a major role in determining whether the student is able to receive your message. Adapt your style and presentation for your students. If you "talk down" to students or if the presentation goes over their heads, the message is not in a form that they can receive.

Feedback

Feedback is the link that completes the communication process. It is often considered the most important step in the communication process because it allows the sender to determine whether the receiver understood the message. Feedback can take the form of either verbal or nonverbal response. An example of the verbal feedback process is when orders are given over the radio. Consider this example:

> **Incident Commander:** Engine 2, stretch a line to Division C and provide exposure protection.
> **Engine 2:** Engine 2 copies—we are stretching a line to Division C for exposures.

An example of nonverbal feedback would be blank stares from students, indicating that they do not understand the message. Collectively asking a classroom of students if they understand is not the best method of determining whether the message was properly received. The natural response is "yes," because no student wants to admit that he or she does not understand. Asking a student to describe your message in his or her own words may be an effective way to make sure that the student understands your message. However, this can depend significantly on the dynamics of the class. If the student's description is incorrect, gently explain that it's not quite right and ask for other students to offer the information.

Face-to-face conversation is the most effective means of conveying many types of information. With this approach, the sender and the receiver can engage in a two-way exchange of information that incorporates body language, facial expressions, tone of voice, and inflection. In contrast, when verbal communication must be conducted over radio or telephone, supplementary expressions are sacrificed. When discussing communication in the fire service, particularly within the incident command system, face-to-face communication is considered the preferred method. Usually, a face-to-face exchange is required if there is a transfer of command so that the sender and the receiver can pick up on any nonverbal indicators of confusion.

Another type of feedback may be apparent when you are giving feedback on a research paper. Writing notes in the margins of the paper allows the student to review and process your comments carefully, as opposed to just saying, "Nice job," and handing the student the paper.

The Environment

Surrounding all of the links of the communication chain is the environment. The environment—which includes physical, social, and environmental factors—can dramatically affect the communication process.

The physical environment is the room or area in which communication is taking place. It could be a classroom, the training ground, or even cyberspace. The physical environment can either inhibit or enhance the learning process. Teaching in a classroom with radios blaring and phones ringing directly outside, for example, will inhibit the communication process. When students cannot hear or see you, your message has a limited chance of being understood. Whether you are working in a classroom or on a busy training ground, make sure that all your students can see and hear you.

The social environment is the context in which the communication takes place. If the class is not enthusiastic about the message, the message will have a limited chance of being received. Mandatory training usually has this effect. You must make sure that your students want or need to receive your message—this is the art of motivation. Show your students why they need your message. Instructors must also expect the students to ask why and must not react by getting defensive. This challenges the instructor to find additional methods of explaining the material. Although students may ask why for different reasons, keep in mind that they have been engaged in what you were saying and participating in the preparation step of the learning process.

The final component is the environmental factor. The receiver must first feel that his or her needs are being met. An environment that is physically difficult for its inhabitants to tolerate is distracting for students. For example, if the room is too cold or too hot, then your message will not be received properly. Select an appropriate location for instruction. Having an impromptu lesson in a truck bay with heaters running may distract students and cause them to lose interest in your message quickly. Lessons that continue too long may also cause discomfort for students and negatively impact the learning process.

Nonverbal Communication

According to Charles R. Swindoll (2003), an American writer and clergyman, "Life is 10 percent what happens to you and 90 percent how you react to it." The same can be said about nonverbal communication: Communication is 10 percent what you say and 90 percent how you say it.

Nonverbal communication is a difficult communication skill to control because you generally do not watch yourself in the mirror all day. This type of communication includes the tone of your voice, your eye movement, your posture, your hand gestures, and your facial expressions. For example, eye contact can show sincerity. If you can look a student in the eye, you are demonstrating trustworthiness and caring. If you cannot maintain eye contact, you lessen the feeling of trust. You can also use your eyes to elicit a reaction: If you continue to look at a student, then that student is compelled to focus on you.

Standing straight and tall is a sign of confidence. You should work on your posture for this reason alone (**FIGURE 4-2**). In addition to showing confidence, such a stance helps maintain your back in good health during long days of instruction.

Hand gestures can express either aggression or enthusiasm. Rapid hand movements or repeated movements of the hands to the face can be signs of deception or uncertainty.

Active and Passive Listening

As an instructor, you must be well versed in both active and passive listening. **Active listening** is the process of hearing and understanding the communication sent and demonstrating that you are listening and have understood the message. It requires you to

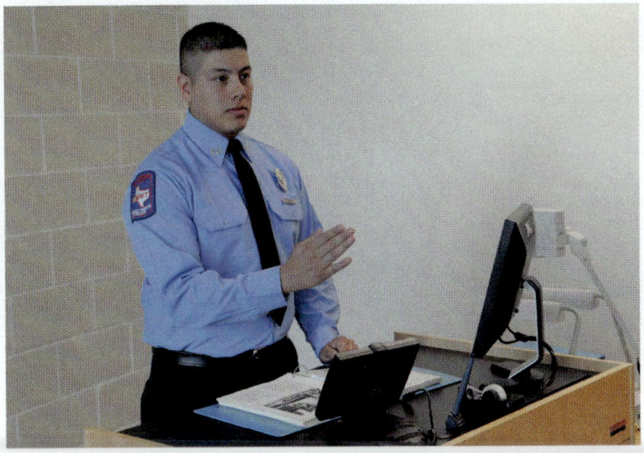

A

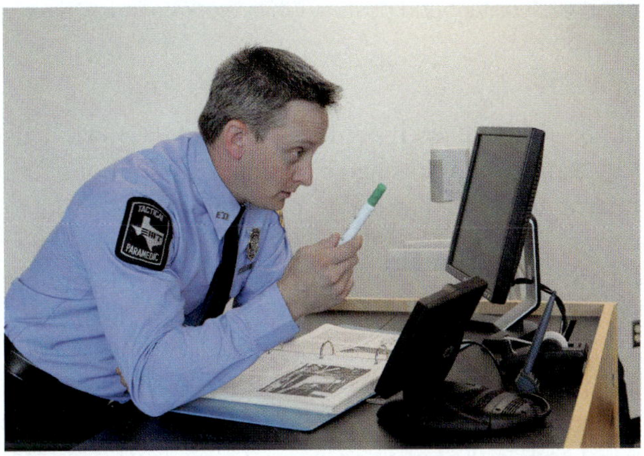

B

FIGURE 4-2 **A.** Good posture is critical for good communication. **B.** Poor posture is unprofessional.

keep your mouth closed and your ears wide open. As part of active listening, it is also very important that you hear the entire message. All too often, instructors formulate an answer before the student finishes asking the question. If you find yourself jumping in with an answer, try restating the student's question before answering. "Why do we use foam on a chemical fire? We use foam on a chemical fire because . . ."

Passive listening is listening with your eyes and your senses without reacting to the message. Observe the student's body language and facial expressions **FIGURE 4-3**. Nervous movements can be indicative of misunderstanding or confusion, whereas a relaxed brow and alert eyes can indicate comprehension and interest.

Carefully monitor what you are communicating nonverbally. Unknowingly, you may communicate through your body language or your attire that students should take unnecessary risks on the training ground. One of the best ways to develop your communication skills is straightforward: Practice them. One method is to have another instructor sit through

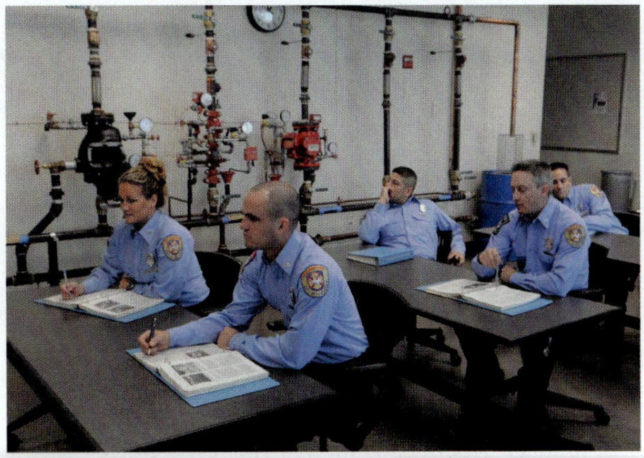

FIGURE 4-3 Pay attention to what your students are telling you with their body language.

your presentation and evaluate you. This evaluation should include how you communicated your message, which nonverbal cues you gave, and how your tone of voice affected the delivery of your message. Through such a peer evaluation, you can see the student's perspective of you.

Another technique is to make a video of your presentation. Watch the recording and look for any nonverbal cues that do not match your message. Many of the nonverbal cues you project become more obvious when you play the recording back at a faster-than-normal speed. Finally, close your eyes and listen to your voice at normal speed. Is your voice really sending your intended message?

COMPANY-LEVEL INSTRUCTOR TIP

Always strive to improve your presence in the learning environment by avoiding habitual and annoying distractions such as the use of repetitive words or physical gestures like playing with keys in your pocket.

Verbal Communication

Verbal, or oral, communication is more than just talking. Many people talk, yet never actually communicate. Great communicators, by contrast, use many tools to convey their message. Watch and listen to the speeches of John F. Kennedy and Martin Luther King, Jr.—both were highly effective communicators, inspiring their followers to take action. At his inauguration in 1961, Kennedy said, "And so, my fellow Americans, ask not what your country can do for you; ask what you can do for your country" (Kennedy, 1961). The inflection in his voice added emphasis to his words and reinforced his message. In his "I Have a Dream" speech at the Lincoln Memorial in 1963, King used personalization so that the entire audience would put themselves in his shoes for a moment (King, 1963).

Many factors, including language and tone, affect verbal communication. The volume of your speech is important. By lowering or raising your voice, you can emphasize a point. You can also use volume to gain the attention of your students. A loud, forceful tone will let the class know that you are very serious. Thus, when a student faces imminent danger, your voice must be loud and forceful.

Likewise, the importance of speaking softly cannot be overstated. When speaking to a student privately, maintain both a level of decorum and a softer tone to your voice. In addition, a softer voice is less threatening and does not put the student on the defensive. If the student is defensive, he or she is less likely to receive your message.

Bringing your voice to a loud crescendo and then making it softer can serve to emphasize your message. This technique is especially effective when you are using compare-and-contrast strategies. For example, during a discussion of tone of voice with fire officers, you might want to compare a dominant tone versus a supportive tone. You would speak loud and forcibly to show dominance, and then speak calmly and softly to show support. The same technique can also be used when describing an escalating event. For example, when describing a flashover, you would speak at normal volume to describe the fire building. As the fire builds, your volume would increase until the flashover occurs, with your voice booming.

COMPANY-LEVEL INSTRUCTOR TIP

When posing questions, an effective practice is to call on a student for the answer before asking the question. This allows the student the opportunity to focus on the question and formulate a response. In most instances, early engagement in the active listening process produces effective results.

The learning environment is also a factor when it comes to voice volume. If you are instructing outside or in a noisy environment, the volume of your voice may have to increase to project it over any **ambient noise**. Of course, sometimes ambient noise is chattering students. In those cases, you should use volume to gain your students' attention and silence.

Projecting your voice is important. If you are stationary or do not have the ability to walk around, be aware of the need to make your voice carry to the back of the room to each student (**FIGURE 4-4**). This feat can be accomplished by using a microphone. If a microphone is not available, use your voice as a tool to convey your message. If you are more mobile, you may be behind or among the students, so be sure to project your voice so that everyone in the class can hear you.

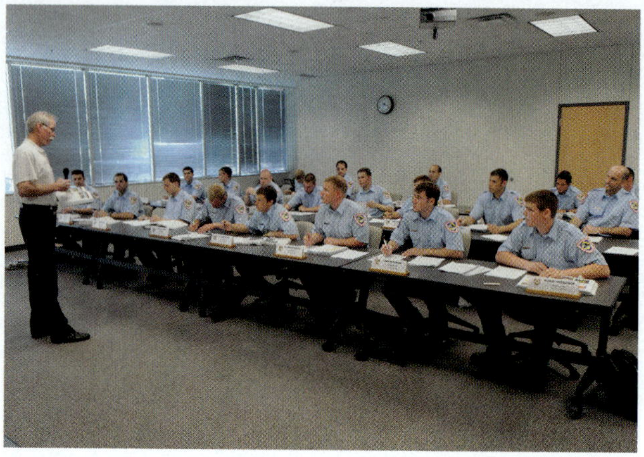

FIGURE 4-4 Project your voice and maintain good eye contact and posture while working in large classrooms.

The difference between instructors can sometimes be as simple as the level of enthusiasm projected through the voice. Enthusiasm breeds enthusiasm. It creates interest both in the topic and in you. Focus on teaching the courses that fascinate you—this will add passion to your presentation. For those topics that may not be as exciting, research why the topic is important. Understanding the underlying value of the topic will help you make it more interesting for the students. The dynamic use of voice is one of the most effective methods of holding students' attention. Knowing when and how to change your voice is a skill learned through practice. Practice making a conscious effort to really use your voice to convey your message until it becomes automatic.

It is important to be aware of any students who have any level of hearing impairment. For a student with hearing difficulty, you may need to consider your body positioning so that the student is able to see your face while you are speaking, or use an auxiliary device to assist the student in hearing the lesson.

Language

The fire service has its own unique language. We use terms that mean something completely different to the general public. For example, when we say "company," we mean a group of personnel assigned to perform a task; by contrast, the general public defines *company* as a business. Within the fire service, terminology can change from department to department and from region to region. A rescue in one department is called an ambulance in another. It is imperative that you use the terminology of your own department when discussing equipment, apparatus, or procedures. Use words that are familiar to your audience and explain new terms thoroughly. Mentioning the problems of fighting a fire in a "group home," for instance, may not be effective if the students do not understand what a group home is.

The use of appropriate language is critical. Avoid language that does not put you or your department in the best light. Ask yourself if you would use the same language around the family dinner table. Once spoken, words cannot be taken back. Exercise restraint and caution when speaking. Always be on guard with your speech: As an instructor, you are held to a higher standard. Many students have expectations of what an instructor should say and do, so never let your guard down.

The tone of your voice can express more than your words. The purpose of tone is to express emotion. Your tone should always be positive, while expressing the passion of conviction. If your words say that you believe in something but your tone expresses apathy, the students will hear apathy, no matter what your words say. To see how this effect works, watch an actor on stage. He may be having a bad day, but when he steps on stage, he portrays good humor and joy. As the instructor, you must put your personal feelings aside and use your tone of voice to express the message properly. Ethically speaking, fire fighters routinely use language that they would never use in front of their grandmothers. Is it ethical to use that same language when instructing? While your first instinct may be to communicate directly in the students' everyday language, it is inappropriate to do so in the classroom. You are judged by your actions. Always take the high road.

The fire service classroom can be as simple as a room with chairs, tables, and any number of audiovisual devices to enhance the learning experience, or it can be as complex as a state-of-the-art "techno-heaven" with multimedia consoles that respond to your requests with only a touch of a button. Sometimes the classroom may be a bunkroom that serves as a multipurpose room with an overhead projector and slide projector, but it can also be the back of a fire engine or the base of the training tower. Many facilities have "dirty" classrooms—that is, designated areas allowing fire fighters in full turnout gear to discuss the training session before or after it occurs.

The purpose of the classroom is to facilitate the learning process. Consequently, the physical location is less important than the communication process. The back of an engine can be a great learning environment if the proper communication skills are used. Many company officers take time after a call to discuss how the call went. This mini-critique can be of great value to the company, even without the traditional classroom or the audiovisual devices; only good communication is necessary for this kind of education.

Audience Analysis

As a good instructor, you need to determine how your message needs to be communicated before deciding on the appropriate format for your presentation. You also need to evaluate your audience to determine how they will best receive your message.

At the most basic level of firefighting, the lecture is usually the most appropriate presentation method. Because students at the entry level have very little experience to draw upon, it is best to use an informative lecture to communicate concepts and objectives. You need to pass the information to the student in a very direct manner. It will be repetitive in nature—some would say almost rote memorization.

In speaking to more experienced fire fighters, the lecture is more persuasive in nature. With these students, you may be taking a skill learned in basic training and discussing it in finer detail at a higher level. This type of class requires students to be convinced about the importance of the message; otherwise, they might tune out the lecture because they mistakenly believe that they already know everything possible about the skill.

Another type of audience encountered by fire instructors is made up of experienced fire fighters and fire officers. These students tend to require discussions rather than informative lectures. Discussions engage these experienced students and encourage them to incorporate their knowledge and experiences into the learning process. This concept, which is sometimes referred to as a "tailboard chat," is used with more experienced fire fighters because it takes their existing knowledge and experience and melds it to a new concept (**FIGURE 4-5**). By examining and reexamining the way we do things, and by discussing experiences and options, new ideas and new ways of doing things are developed. This sort of exchange can be very exciting and rewarding because you can witness an idea developing in front of you. In fact, many of the tools used in the fire service today evolved out of discussions that arose when fire fighters saw a problem or a situation that needed to be improved and made adaptations to rectify the need. This style of instruction is sometimes referred to as facilitation.

Alternative communication methods should also be considered. For example, role playing can often reinforce learning objectives. In role playing, you can

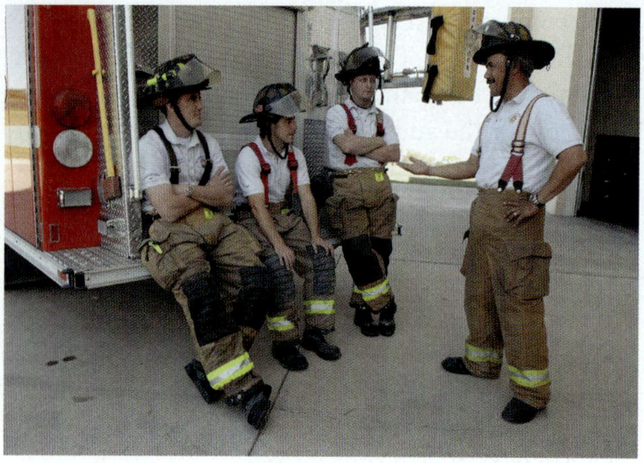

FIGURE 4-5 The tailboard chat can provide an opportunity for a quick training exercise or to analyze the recent response.

take the position of someone with whom the student interacts. This method requires you to have an idea of how a student will respond in this situation and to be prepared for that response. You should be prepared for several potential responses from the student and be able to lead the student toward the learning objective. At the end of the role playing, you should explain the learning objective of the exercise.

Another possible communication method consists of group exercises. With this method, you use the collaborative efforts of the group to benefit all members of the group. Such a technique exploits the natural tendency of fire fighters to work in groups. With group work, you can evaluate whether students can work collaboratively to solve a problem. In most cases, this is the way a fire company solves problems in the field. It is imperative that you listen to the conversations in the groups. Walk around to each group and stand near or actually sit down with the group and listen. You can see if the group is moving in the right direction or needs to be redirected. If necessary, help the group along by saying, "Have you considered . . ." Steering the discussion is not equivalent to giving students the answer, but rather assists them in remaining focused on the message. Be sure to solicit outcomes from each group involved in the exercise; adult learners will want to have their work discussed and will not appreciate "busy work" during a class.

Your communication style will be situational, such that you may have to use several different styles during the same presentation. When teaching a class on fire extinguishers, for example, you might begin with a lecture style and then move into a psychomotor session. When giving the lecture, you are simply presenting facts: There is no pressure and no sense of danger. When you move into the psychomotor session, however, it may be necessary to speak authoritatively to ensure that the students understand the issues of safety.

Issues of safety will inevitably affect your communication style. When you explain to new recruits that they must stay down in a fire situation, they generally nod their heads as you explain the science of thermal layering. When you get on the fire ground, be more forceful in your tone and action to keep your students focused on safety.

When an important objective needs to be reinforced, you can highlight it by changing your communication style. For example, by adding a group exercise in the middle of a lecture, you highlight the learning objective.

Time is another factor when considering communication styles. If students spend 2 hours straight sitting and listening to a lecture, retention of the material can diminish. Nothing is worse for a student than to have a monotone instructor lulling him or her to sleep with an endless lecture. Retention of material is increased by adding activities. Engaging the student in the learning will pay big dividends. For example, if a student has to speak and do something, the information will be retained longer and more completely. This consideration is especially important after a meal. The more activities you can provide to students after a lunch break, the more likely they are to retain the information. The cone of learning illustrates the importance of communication skills and how students are able to remember information (**FIGURE 4-6**). The more active the student is in the learning, the more effective and real the learning is to them. Lesson plans are discussed in Chapter 5, *Using Lesson Plans*; activities or chances for student practice or participation are incorporated in the application step of a lesson plan.

Written Communications

Written communication is needed to document both routine and extraordinary fire department activities. It establishes institutional history and is the foundation of any activity that the fire department wishes to accomplish. As a senior chief explained, "If it is not written down, it did not happen." The instructor is responsible for many types of written communications, including narratives, which are included in training records, and more comprehensive training reports, such as annual reports of training activities. Although e-mail has replaced many formal written letters and other communications, a written communication

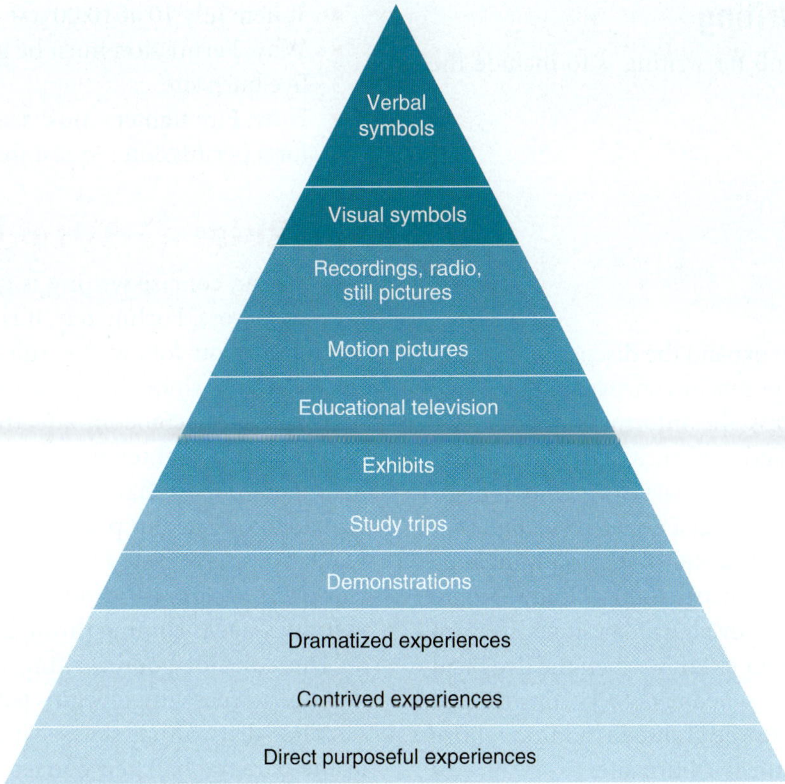

FIGURE 4-6 Cone of learning.

Modified from: Dale, Edgar. *Audio-Visual Methods in Teaching*, 1E. © 1969 Wadsworth, a part of Cengage Learning, Inc.

serves as a permanent record of an event or happening. Each agency should specify guidelines that outline which types of written documentation are necessary for specific occurrences, such as reports of injuries and documentation of training issues.

Reading Level

Most newspapers in the United States are written at approximately a sixth-grade reading level to allow for understanding by the general public. The newspaper does not intend to talk down to its readers who have a higher level of education; instead, it is simply ensuring that the majority of readers can easily understand the information presented.

Do you know the reading levels of each of your students? Most fire fighters are required to have a high school education or a GED, so the expectation is that all students can read and write at the high school level. Most educational textbooks are written at a reading level that the majority of fire fighters should understand. Technical editors and select fire service personnel review textbooks to establish their readability before they are printed and bound.

Most word processing programs can perform an evaluation of the document's reading level based on the Flesch–Kincaid readability index. With this index, a higher number indicates that the document is easier to read. Therefore, the higher the Flesch–Kincaid number, the lower the reading level. The index is based on the average number of words per sentence and the number of syllables per 100 words. Be aware of the length of your sentences and the complexity of the words you use. Always keep your students' reading levels in mind when writing.

Writing Format

It is also important to know which format you should use when writing. In general, when writing to individuals within your organization, you can use a memo (short for *memorandum*). Such a document is designed for in-house communications only. For example, a memo from the chief of your training division to all instructors might inform them of an upcoming training drill. Written communications intended for readers outside the organization should appear in letter format, using departmental letterhead, and should be signed by the sender. A letter would be the appropriate form of communication to Mr. Jones confirming a preincident planning appointment at his coffee shop, for example.

The Five Ws of Writing

The basic rule of thumb for writing is to include the "five Ws":

1. Who
2. What
3. Where
4. When
5. Why

Add an "H"—How—to expand the discussion further.

By including these points in your writing, you will ensure that you address the information necessary for readers to understand your message properly. For example, suppose you need to write a memo about a live burn that will take place at a donated structure on the outskirts of town (**FIGURE 4-7**). You want your students and additional instructors to know where and when to meet on the live burn day. You also want the entire fire department to know when the live burn is taking place, who is scheduled to be onsite, and whether permission must be granted if additional fire fighters want to be on the live burn site.

The memo in Figure 4-7 contains all five Ws (plus H) of writing:

- Who: Lavalle Fire Department
- What: Live burn training exercise
- Where: 1015 Willow Way
- When: July 10 at 10:00 AM
- Why: Permission must be granted to be on the live burn site
- How: Fire fighters must see Officer Archie Reed for a permission request form

> To: Lavalle Fire Department
> Cc: Chief Michael Deforge
> From: Officer Archie Reed
> Date: May 23
> Subject: Live Burn on July 10
>
> On July 10, the Lavalle Fire Department will conduct a live burn at 1015 Willow Way. Fourteen students from the Fire Suppression Course will be present. Students will participate in supervised training using medium-diameter hose lines during defensive operations.
>
> Students and Fire Service Instructors Thomas, Kelly, Hinkler, and Andrews will assemble at the South Street Fire Station at 10:00 a.m. to be transported to the live burn structure. Safety procedures will be reviewed at the site prior to the live burn. In addition to the students and the fire service instructors, Engine Company 3 will be on site.
>
> If you are not a student in the Fire Suppression Course, an assigned fire service instructor, or a member of Engine Company 3, you may not be on the live burn site without written permission. Please see Officer Archie Reed for a permission request form.

FIGURE 4-7 A sample memo using the five Ws of writing.

The Rules of Writing

Good, clear, concise writing is critical to getting your message across. Fortunately, it is easy to improve your writing: If you follow the rules of good writing in step-by-step fashion and practice for 15 minutes each day, you can become an effective written communicator. As a fire fighter, you train on a regular basis to maintain your firefighting skills. Similarly, as an instructor, you need to practice your writing skills on a regular basis. This step involves writing and allowing fellow instructors to read your writing to ensure that your message is coming through loud and clear.

The rules of good writing begin with the paragraph. Each paragraph begins with an introduction—a sentence or two that states what you plan to discuss in the paragraph. Then comes the main body of the paragraph—the frame. Like the frame of a structure, the frame of the paragraph is the support that holds everything together. The conclusion reviews what was discussed in the paragraph and reinforces the frame, as explained here:

> The fire officer must first consider the intended audience for the report before writing. For example, a fire officer may be assigned to prepare a study that proposes closing three companies and using quints that can respond as either engine or ladder companies. If the report is intended for internal use, the technical information would use normal fire department terminology. Conversely, if the report is intended for the fire chief to deliver to the city council, with copies going to the news media, many of the terms and concepts would need to be explained in simple terms for the general public. Always consider who your audience is before writing a report.

To practice constructing a solid paragraph, consider writing a two- to three-paragraph summary after every class. What was your message for the class? Did your students receive it?

Once you have mastered the building of a paragraph, you are on your way to constructing a complete written structure—anything from a two-paragraph memo, to a full-page letter, to a 10-page report for the city council. The paragraph is your basic building block of writing. All good writing has an introduction, a frame, and a conclusion. In an eight-paragraph report that is intended for the city council and explains why the fire department's training budget should be increased by 10 percent, for example, the report would be broken down in the following way:

- Paragraphs 1 and 2: Introduction. These paragraphs give an overview of why the fire department needs to increase the training budget.
- Paragraphs 3 through 7: Frame. These paragraphs discuss in depth the specific reasons why the training budget should be increased. For example, the city might have grown by 20 percent in 3 years and needs more fire fighters to provide good service.
- Paragraph 8: Conclusion. This paragraph summarizes the arguments for increasing the fire department's training budget.

Style

Most of the writing you do as a fire fighter and as an instructor will be technical in nature. In such a case, your sole objective is to convey information—not to express emotion or to inspire passionate feelings. Writing in the fire service should not be boring or uninspiring, but it should remain true to the premise that you write to impart facts.

Once words are printed, they are difficult to retract. Read an editorial column in a newspaper to see how writing can affect people's thoughts and emotions. Words can be construed in different ways by different people, so it is extremely important to choose your words carefully. The meaning of words can change based on geographical location. A person's individual experiences also can change the meaning of a word. Know your audience before you begin to write. Your goal is to make certain that your message is clearly and properly conveyed to every reader. Choose your words carefully when writing. Make every effort to ensure that alternative interpretations cannot occur. Failure to do so can mislead students and ultimately lead to undesired performances.

Informal Communications

Informal communications include internal memos, e-mails, instant messages, and messages transmitted via mobile data terminals. Informal reports have a short life and are not archived as permanent records. Instead, they are used primarily to record or transmit information that will not be needed for reference in the future. Be aware that some agencies, as public agencies, are required to keep archived records of even informal records, and such communications may be subject to freedom of information requests.

Some informal reports are retained for a period of time and may become a part of a formal report or investigation. For example, a written memo could document an informal conversation between a fire instructor and a fire fighter regarding a training drill attendance issue. The memo might note that the student or crew member was warned that corrective action is required by a particular date. If the issue is corrected, the warning memo is discarded after 12 months. If the fire fighter continues to demonstrate poor attendance, the memo becomes part of the formal documentation of progressive discipline.

In recent years, the storage and recall of e-mails has been a topic of much discussion. Policies will vary from agency to agency, so know your department's policy about e-mails, instant messages, and related informal communication. Ignorance will not usually work as a defense in a court of law, so know your agency's policy regarding the use of this type of informal communication.

Formal Communications

A **formal communication** is an official fire department document printed on business stationery with the fire department letterhead. If it is a letter or report intended for someone outside the fire department, the document is usually signed by the fire chief or a designated staff officer to establish that it is an official communication. Subordinates often prepare these documents and submit them for an administrative review to check the grammar and clarity. A fire chief or the staff officer who is designated to sign the document performs a final review before it is transmitted.

The fire department maintains a permanent copy of all formal reports and official correspondence from the fire chief and senior staff officers. Formal reports are usually archived.

Standard Operating Procedures

Standard operating procedures (SOPs) are written organizational directives that establish or prescribe specific operational or administrative methods to be followed routinely for the performance of designated operations or actions. SOPs are intended to provide a standard and consistent response to emergency incidents as well as personnel supervisory actions and administrative tasks. They serve as a prime reference source for promotional exams and departmental training.

SOPs are formal, permanent documents that are published in a standard format, signed by the fire chief, and widely distributed. They remain in effect permanently or until they are rescinded or amended. Many fire departments conduct a periodic review of all SOPs so they can revise, update, or eliminate any that are outdated or are no longer applicable. Any changes in the SOPs must also be approved by the fire chief. SOPs should always be referenced as part of a training session, especially when demonstrating skills and ability.

General Orders

General orders are formal documents that address a specific subject, policy, condition, or situation. They are usually signed by the fire chief and can be in effect for various periods, from a few days to permanently. Many departments use general orders to announce promotions and personnel transfers. Copies of the general orders should be made available for reference at all fire stations.

Announcements or Communications

The formal organization may use announcements, information bulletins, newsletters, websites, or other methods to share additional information with fire department members. These methods are generally used to distribute short-term and nonessential information that is of interest.

Legal Correspondence

Fire departments are often asked to produce copies of documents or reports for legal purposes. Instructors must always remember that training records are also legal documents and, as such, are available for scrutiny through the legal system. Sometimes the fire department is directly involved in the legal action, whereas in other cases the action involves other parties but relates to a situation in which the fire department responded or had some involvement. It is not unusual for a fire department to receive a subpoena—a legal order demanding all of the documentation that is on file pertaining to a particular incident or person. Gathering such documents is a task that can require extensive time and effort. In any situation for which there is a request for reports or documentation, consult with legal counsel.

The fire fighter or officer who prepared a report may be called on, sometimes years later, to sign an affidavit or appear in court to testify that the information provided in the report is complete and accurate. He or she might also have to respond to an **interrogatory**, which is a series of written questions asked by someone from an opposing party. The fire department must provide written answers to the interrogatories, under oath, and produce any associated documentation. If the initial incident report or other documents provide an accurate, factual, objective, complete, and clear presentation of the facts, the response to the interrogatory is often a simple affirmation of the written records. The task of dealing with the interrogatory can become much more complex and embarrassing if the original documents are vague, incomplete, false, or missing.

Reports

Reports should be accurate and present the necessary information in an understandable format. All reports should be proofread before being submitted. The purpose of the report might be to brief the reader, or it might provide a systematic analysis of an issue. If the fire chief wants only to be briefed on a new piece of equipment and the fire officer delivers a fully researched presentation, both parties would be frustrated.

Some reports are prepared on a regular schedule, such as daily, weekly, monthly, or yearly. Other types of reports are prepared only in response to specific occurrences or when requested. To create a useful report, you must understand the specific information that is needed and provide it in a manner that is easily interpreted.

Some reports are presented orally; others are prepared electronically and entered into computer systems. Some reports are formal, whereas others are informal. The most common form of reporting is verbal communication from one individual to another, either face-to-face or via a telephone or radio. To be effective, the transfer of information must be clear and concise, using terminology that is appropriate for the receiver.

Monthly Activity and Training Report

The monthly activity and training report documents the company's activity during the preceding month. These reports typically include the number of emergency responses, training activities, inspections, public education events, and station visits that were conducted during the previous month. Some monthly reports include details such as a list of the number of feet of hose used and the number of ladders deployed during the month. The number of training hours completed, members who receive certifications or attend classes, and any number of training-related projects or meetings should be documented in a regular format to highlight the role and importance that training plays in an organization.

In many cases, the officer delegates the preparation of routine reports that do not involve personnel actions or supervisory responsibilities to subordinates. In such a case, the officer is still responsible for checking and signing the report before it is submitted.

Some fire companies or municipal agencies post a version of their monthly reports on their public website. These reports often include digital pictures of the incidents and the people involved.

Special events or unusual situations that occurred during the month might also be included in the report. For example, the monthly report might note that the company provided standby coverage for a presidential visit or participated in a local parade.

COMPANY-LEVEL INSTRUCTOR TIP

Both instructors and administrative staff share the responsibilities for completing written documentation. Instructors should be aware of any written documentation that is required for their program and the timeline in which these forms need to be submitted.

Infrequent and Special Reports

Infrequent reports usually require a fire instructor's personal attention to ensure that the report's information is complete and concise. Such reports include the following types of documents:

- Fire fighter injury report
- Student complaints
- Property damage or liability-event report
- Vehicle accident or equipment damage report
- New equipment or procedure evaluation
- Suggestions to improve fire department operation
- Response to a grievance or complaint
- Fire fighter work improvement plans
- Research report or recommendation

A chronological statement of events is a detailed account of activities, such as a narrative report of the actions taken at an incident or accident. A **recommendation report** is a document that suggests a particular action or decision.

Some reports incorporate both a chronological section and a recommendation section. For example, the fire fighter line-of-duty death investigations produced by NIOSH include a chronological report of the event, followed by a series of recommendations that could prevent the occurrence of a similar situation.

Writing a Decision Document

The goal of a decision document is to provide enough information and persuasion, so the intended individual or body accepts your recommendation. This type of report includes recommendations for employee recognition or formal discipline, for a new or improved procedure, or for adoption of a new device. A decision document usually includes the following elements:

- **Statement of problem or issue:** One or two sentences.
- **Background:** Brief description of how this became a problem or an issue.
- **Restrictions:** Outline of the restrictions affecting the decision. Factors such as federal laws, state regulations, local ordinances, budget or staff restrictions, and union contracts are all restrictions that could affect a decision.
- **Options:** Where appropriate, provide more than one option and the rationale behind each option. In most cases, one option is to do nothing.
- **Recommendation:** Explain why the recommended option is the best decision. The recommendation should be based on considerations that would make sense to the decision maker. If the recommendation is going to a political body and involves a budget decision, it should be expressed in terms of lower cost, higher level of service, or reduced liability. The impact of the decision should be quantified as accurately as possible, with an explanation of how much money it will save, which new levels of service will be provided, or how much the liability will be reduced.
- **Next action:** The report should clearly state the action that should be taken to implement the recommendation. Some recommendations may require changes in departmental policy or budget. Others could involve an application for grant funds or a request for a change in state or federal legislation.

Training BULLETIN

JONES & BARTLETT FIRE DISTRICT

TRAINING DIVISION

5 Wall Street, Burlington, MA, 01803

Phone 978-443-5000 Fax 978-443-8000

Instant Applications: Communication Skills

Drill Assignment

Apply the chapter content to your department's operation, training division, and your personal experiences to complete the following questions and activities.

Objective

Upon completion of the instant applications, fire and emergency services instructor students will exhibit decision making and application of job performance requirements of the instructor using the text, class discussion, and their own personal experiences.

Suggested Drill Applications

1. Review a recent NIOSH fire fighter fatality report that involves communications in either the Contributing Factors or Key Recommendations areas and identify what your department could do to address the issue.
2. Evaluate a recent training session you conducted or participated in during which you experienced communication difficulties. Identify solutions for avoiding the communications pitfalls in future sessions.
3. Identify the different means of written communications employed by your organization and discuss ways to improve the communications process.
4. After conducting a training session with your shift, discuss your own personal communications traits and ask for feedback on how you can improve your delivery during training.

Incident Report: NIOSH Report: F2003-28

Drill Assignment

Review the information in this incident report and prepare a practice presentation for class delivery at the direction of your instructor. Your presentation should include a summary of the incident facts and a review of the NFPA 1403 compliance and noncompliance findings. Use an outline to organize your thoughts. You may be evaluated on your communication skills during your presentation.

Poinciana, Florida—2002

Just 10 months after the incident in Lairdsville, and less than 3 weeks after the sentencing of the Lairdsville chief officer, a live fire training session trapped two fire fighters in Poinciana, Florida, near Kissimmee.

The 1600-ft^2 (148.6-m^2) cement block house had three bedrooms, one of which was converted from a one-car garage with the large door removed, the wall blocked up, and a window installed (**FIGURE 4-A**).

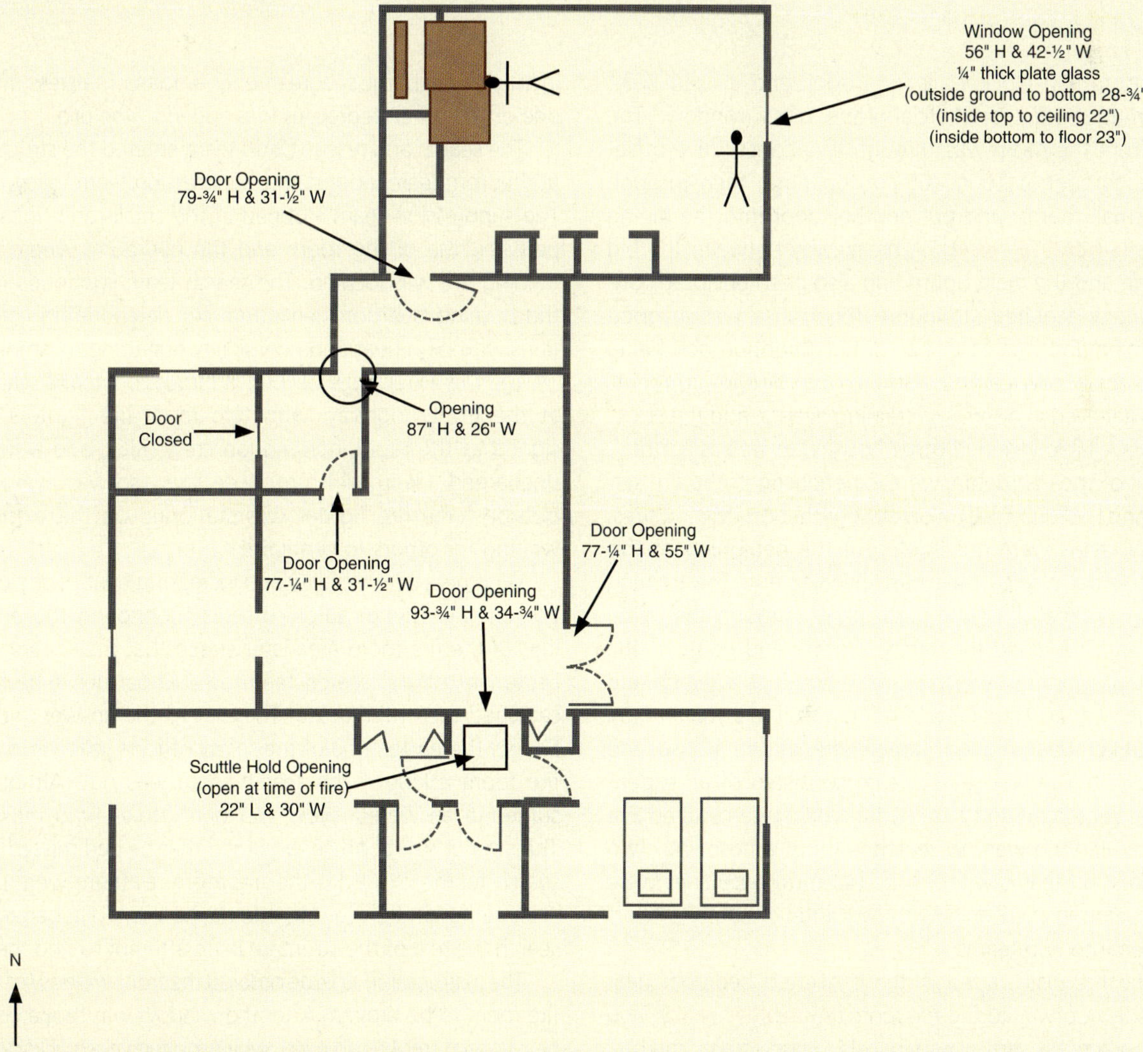

FIGURE 4-A Poinciana floor plan.
Courtesy of the Florida State Fire Marshal.

Incident Report continued

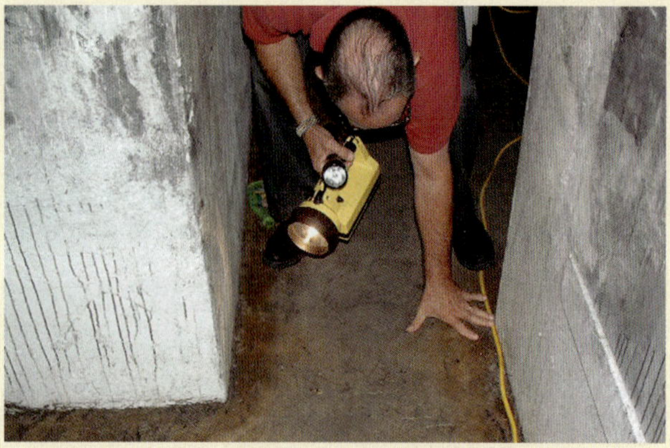

FIGURE 4-B Two consecutive offset turns and this narrow hallway made it difficult for fire fighters to maneuver.
Courtesy of the Florida State Fire Marshal

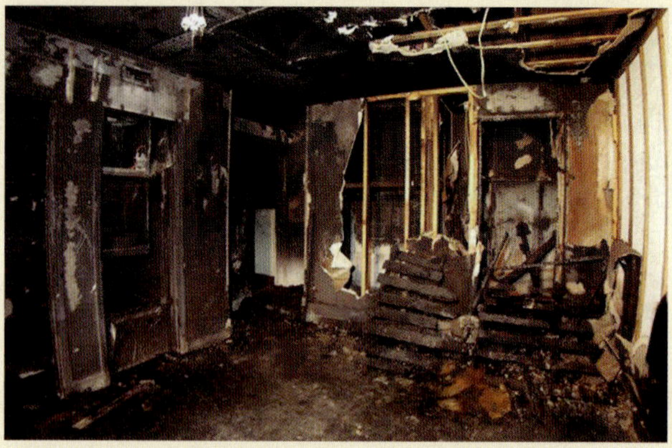

FIGURE 4-C Interior of fire room in Poinciana.
From the NIOSH Fire Fighter Fatality Investigation and Prevention Program, Investigation Report F2002-34.

The room had block walls, one door, and a fixed ¼-in. (6.4-mm) thick, commercial-grade glass window. The exit from the room was through two consecutive offset turns, through a 26-in. (65-cm) opening, then through two small rooms, and out another door into the dining room (**FIGURE 4-B**). A breezeway between the old garage and the main house had also been enclosed. Unlike many acquired structures, this house was in good condition and was part of an entire neighborhood being razed for a new campus. Several area fire departments were involved in a series of training events, and the structures available included other houses, as well as a motel.

All of the instructors were experienced in the fire service and had previously worked together on training fires. Safety crews were not briefed at the beginning of this exercise because of their past involvement. The training officer walked all of the participants through the structure and explained the safety aspects and goals of the training evolution, which were to conduct a search and rescue with an actual fire burning and find a mannequin in bunker gear hidden somewhere in the house and remove it. The first search team consisted of an experienced lieutenant and a trained recruit (state-certified Fire Fighter II), who were to search without a hose line. Two suppression teams with 1¾-in. (44-mm) hose lines were in position in the house with four interior safety officers broken into two teams.

The fire was started in the converted bedroom near the only doorway to the fire room (**FIGURE 4-C**). Two piles, practically vertical with pallets, wood scraps, and hay, were almost adjacent to each other, one inside and one outside the open closet. After the fire started, and with the instructor-in-charge's agreement, a foam mattress from one of the other bedrooms was added to the pile.

The search and rescue (SAR) team entered the structure at the front (east) door with a suppression team following. The suppression team stopped in the small room located between the dining room and the bedroom, where the training fire was located. The search team continued into the burning bedroom, encountering deteriorating conditions with high heat and no visibility due to heavy smoke.

On the exterior, a second suppression team waited at the front doorway, with two more fire fighters assigned as the rapid intervention crew (RIC), and a third, uncharged 1¾-in. (44-mm) hose line also was available outside. One fire fighter was stationed on the exterior waiting for orders to ventilate.

With near zero visibility and increasing heat conditions, two of the interior safety officers monitoring the activities of the fire room area later stated that they heard the lieutenant of the search team ask his partner if he had searched the entire room. They heard the answer "yes." Shortly thereafter, one of the safety officers yelled into the fire room asking if the search team was out. Although someone answered "yes," no one knows who replied. The interior safety officer assumed that he had missed the search team's exit from the fire room, as there were several fire fighters present by the dining room. He began to search the rest of the structure in an attempt to find them.

The instructor-in-charge ordered the front window of the fire room to be broken. After the window was broken out, heavy black smoke followed, which ignited very quickly with flames forcibly venting from the window. The suppression crew closest to the fire room applied water in short bursts, but increasing heat and steam forced the safety officers and the suppression crew to back out. Both safety officers were forced to exit the structure, after receiving burn injuries.

The second suppression team was ordered to replace the first team and engage the fire. The second team and an interior safety officer entered the fire room and extinguished the fire.

During this time the instructor-in-charge called the missing fire fighters several times and received no answer.

While the second suppression team was overhauling the fire area, they found a body in fire fighter bunker gear facedown on the floor. Both of the suppression team fire fighters initially thought it was the rescue mannequin, not realizing it was the lieutenant of the SAR team.

After no radio response from the SAR team, the instructor-in-charge ordered a personnel accountability report (PAR) and ordered the RIC to enter the structure and find the SAR team.

The suppression team that found the lieutenant dragged him to the front window of the fire room and removed him to the outside. The missing fire fighter was also found inside that window, and he too was removed to the outside. The entire event, from the time the SAR crew entered to when the first of the two fire fighters was located, was under 14 minutes. The two fire fighters died despite working in teams with experienced instructors, two interior staffed hose lines, two interior safety teams, an RIC with its own hose line, a participant walk-though, and other safeguards in place.

NIOSH investigated the fire. Two separate investigations were conducted by the state fire marshal: one for criminal violations, and an administrative investigation of state training codes. No criminal charges were filed; however, the findings included the following:

- "All of the participants stated . . . they did not have any concerns regarding the conditions of the fire inside the structure and it appeared to them as normal fire behavior."
- Although NFPA 1403 was already required in state code, it was under the environmental laws and so the law enforcement department of the state fire marshal's office did not have the authority to enforce it.
- The fire was started in a room with too much fuel for the size of the room, including a foam mattress that was added after ignition. Flashover was precipitated by too high a fuel load and inadequate ventilation.
- National Institute of Standards and Technology (NIST) determined that the mattress was contributory to considerable smoke production; however, in testing, the room flashed over in roughly the same time without the mattress present.

Postincident Analysis Poinciana, Florida

NFPA 1403 Noncompliant

- No written preburn plan prepared
- Accountability was not maintained at the point of entry to the fire room
- Safety crews did not have specific assignments or emergency procedures
- Fire started near the only doorway in and out of the fire room
- Excessive fuel loading
- No communications plan in place

NFPA 1403 Compliant

- Experienced instructors had worked together on training fires before
- Primary and secondary suppression crews inside with hose lines
- A walk-through of the structure was conducted
- Crews were alerted of the possibility of a victim
- Structure in good condition

Other Issues

- Radio communications less than optimal
- Egress limited by offset turns, a 26" (66-cm) opening, and multiple rooms and turns

After-Action REVIEW

IN SUMMARY

- Communication is the most important element of the learning process.
- The basic communication process consists of five elements: the sender, the message, the medium, the receiver, and feedback.
- Be aware of the message that you are sending to students nonverbally through your body language.
- Your communication style must be adapted to match the situation. You may have to use several different styles during a presentation.
- As an instructor, you must be well versed in both active and passive listening.
- Many factors, including language and tone, affect verbal communication.
- Written communication is needed to document both routine and extraordinary fire department activities. It establishes institutional history and serves as the foundation of any activity that the fire department wishes to accomplish.
- The most common form of reporting is verbal communication from one individual to another, either face-to-face or via a telephone or radio. To be effective, the transfer of information must be clear and concise, using terminology that is appropriate for the receiver.
- Reports should be accurate and present the necessary information in an understandable format. The purpose of the report might be to brief the reader, or it might provide a systematic analysis of an issue.
- Most presentations for an instructor involve informative speeches, or lectures. As a good instructor, you must determine how your message needs to be communicated before selecting the appropriate format for your presentation.

KEY TERMS

Access Navigate for flashcards to test your key term knowledge.

Active listening The process of hearing and understanding the communication sent; demonstrating that you are listening and have understood the message.

Ambient noise The general level of background sound.

Communication process The process of conveying an intended message from the sender to the receiver and getting feedback to ensure accuracy.

Feedback The fifth and final link of the communication chain. It allows the sender (the instructor) to determine whether the receiver (the student) understood the message.

Formal communication An official fire department communication. The letter or report is presented on stationery with the fire department letterhead and generally is signed by a chief officer or headquarters staff member.

General orders Short-term documents signed by the fire chief that remain in force for a period of days to 1 year or more.

Informal communications Internal memos, e-mails, instant messages, and computer-aided dispatch/mobile data terminal messages. Informal reports have a short life and are not archived as permanent records.

Interrogatory A series of formal written questions sent to the opposing side of a legal argument. The opposition must provide written answers under oath.

Medium The third link of the communication chain, which describes how you convey the message.

Message The second and most complex link of the communication chain; it describes what you are trying to convey to your students.

Passive listening Listening with your eyes and other senses without reacting to the message verbally.

Receiver The fourth link of the communication chain. In the fire service classroom, the receiver is the student.

Recommendation report A decision document prepared by a fire officer for the senior staff. The goal is support for a decision or an action.

Sender The first link of the communication chain. In the fire service classroom, the sender is the instructor.

REFERENCES

Davies, Leah. "Effective Communication." Kelly Bear. http://www.kellybear.com/TeacherArticles/TeacherTip15.html. Accessed August 17, 2018.

Kennedy, John F. 1961. "Inaugural Address." John F. Kennedy Presidential Library and Museum. http://www.jfklibrary.org/Asset-Viewer/BqXIEM9F4024ntFl7SVAjA.aspx

King, Martin Luther Jr. 1963. Martin Luther King's speech: "I have a dream"—the full text. http://abcnews.go.com/Politics/ martin-luther-kings-speech-dream-full-text/story?id= 14358231&page=2

National Fire Protection Association. 2019. *NFPA 1041: Standard for Fire and Emergency Services Instructor Professional Qualifications*. Quincy, MA: National Fire Protection Association.

National Fire Protection Association. 2018. *NFPA 1403: Standard on Live Fire Training Evolutions*. Quincy, MA: National Fire Protection Association.

Swindoll, Charles R. 2003. *Strengthening Your Grip*. Cengage.

CHAPTER PRESENTATION EXERCISE

Instructions: Your course instructor will assign individual or group discussions on the key points and teaching tips of this chapter. You or your group will review the chapter teachings and identify the major learning points from the chapter. You should be able to discuss the points, why they are important, and how/where they apply to your responsibilities at your level of instructor training.

REVIEW QUESTIONS

1. The communication process consists of five elements. Explain what each of these is.
2. Explain passive and active listening.
3. Describe some of the elements that are in a report or decision document.

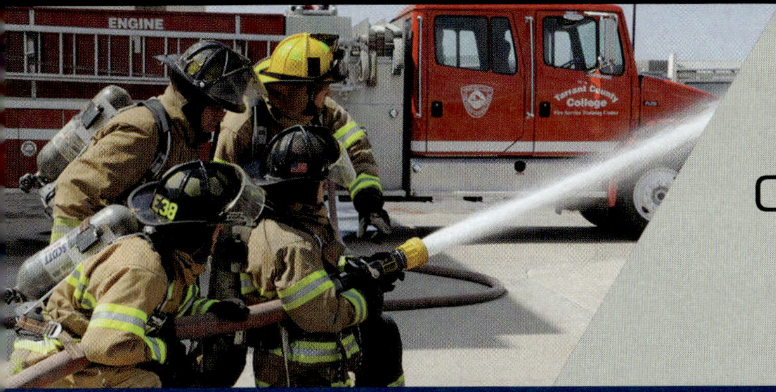

CHAPTER 5

Using Lesson Plans

NFPA 1041 JOB PERFORMANCE REQUIREMENTS

Note: An asterisk denotes that the 1041 standard contains further information in its annex section.

4.2.2 Assemble course materials, given a specific topic, so that the lesson plan and all materials, resources, and equipment needed to deliver the lesson are obtained.

(A) Requisite Knowledge.

Components of a lesson plan, policies and procedures for the procurement of materials and equipment, and resource availability.

(B) Requisite Skills.

None required.

4.2.3 Prepare requests for resources, given training goals and current resources, so that the resources required to meet training goals are identified and documented.

(A) Requisite Knowledge.

Resource management, sources of instructional resources and equipment.

(B) Requisite Skills.

Oral and written communication, forms completion.

4.2.4* Schedule single instructional sessions, given a training assignment, AHJ scheduling procedures, instructional resources, facilities and timeline for delivery, so that the specified sessions are delivered according to AHJ procedure.

(A) Requisite Knowledge.

AHJ scheduling procedures and resource management.

(B) Requisite Skills.

Training schedule completion.

4.3.2* Review instructional materials, given the materials for a specific topic, target audience, learner characteristics, and learning environment, so that elements of the lesson plan, learning environment, and resources that need adaptation are identified.

(A) Requisite Knowledge.

Recognition of student learner characteristics and diversity, methods of instruction, types of resource materials, organization of the learning environment, and policies and procedures.

(B) Requisite Skills.

Analysis of resources, facilities, and materials.

4.3.3* Adapt a prepared lesson plan, given course materials and an assignment, so that the needs of the student and the objectives of the lesson plan are achieved.

(A)* Requisite Knowledge.

Elements of a lesson plan, selection of instructional aids and methods, and organization of the learning environment.

(B) Requisite Skills.

Instructor preparation and organization techniques.

4.4.3 Present and adjust prepared lessons, given a prepared lesson plan that specifies the presentation method(s), so that the method(s) indicated in the plan are used and the stated objectives or learning outcomes are achieved, applicable safety standards and practices are followed, and risks are addressed.

(A)* Requisite Knowledge.

The laws and principles of learning, methods and techniques of instruction, lesson plan components and elements of the communication process, and lesson plan terminology and definitions; learner characteristics; student-centered learning principles; instructional technology tools; the impact of cultural differences on instructional delivery; safety rules, regulations, and practices; identification of training hazards; elements and limitations of distance learning; distance learning delivery methods; and the instructor's role in distance learning.

(B) Requisite Skills.

Oral communication techniques, methods and techniques of instruction, ability to adapt to changing circumstances, and utilization of lesson plans in an instructional setting.

KNOWLEDGE OBJECTIVES

After studying this chapter, participating in a structured learning environment, and completing assigned assessments, you will be able to:

- Identify and describe the components of learning objectives. (**NFPA 1041: 4.3.3**, p 122)
- Describe the parts of a lesson plan. (**NFPA 1041: 4.3.2, 4.4.3**, pp 124–126)
- Describe the instructional preparation process. (**NFPA 1041: 4.2.2, 4.2.3, 4.3.2, 4.3.3**, pp 128–129)
- Describe the lesson plan adaptation process and limits for the Fire and Emergency Services Instructor I. (**NFPA 1041: 4.3.1, 4.3.3**, pp 129–132)
- Identify the factors to consider when scheduling a training session. (**NFPA 1041: 4.2.4**, pp 128–129)

SKILLS OBJECTIVES

After studying this chapter, participating in a structured learning environment, and completing assigned assessments, you will be able to:

- Prepare to teach a lesson. (**NFPA 1041: 4.2.2, 4.2.3, 4.3.2**, pp 127–128)
- Review a lesson plan and identify the adaptations needed. (**NFPA 1041: 4.3.3**, pp 129–132)
- Adapt a lesson plan so that it meets the needs of the students and ensures that learning objectives are met. (**NFPA 1041: 4.3.3**, pp 129–132)

You Are the Fire and Emergency Services Instructor

Recently, your community has annexed a neighboring area of the county that is more rural in nature than your primary response area. As a result, your shift captain has asked for you to deliver a training session to your shift on water shuttle operations, a subject you haven't trained on before primarily because your jurisdiction is fully covered with a municipal water distribution system. While researching the internet for training materials, you have encountered a lesson plan published by an established training academy in another state that appears to suit your needs.

1. Identify and describe the parts of a lesson plan.
2. Describe the lesson plan adaptation process for the Instructor I.
3. Identify the learning objectives necessary for the training session that you found.
4. Describe how you, as an Instructor 1, can adapt the lesson plan you found to better suit the needs of your department and ensure that learning objectives are met.

Introduction

When most people think about the job of a fire and emergency services instructor, they picture the actual delivery of a presentation in front of the classroom. Although lectures are an important aspect of instruction, they are not the only part of the job. Most instructors spend many hours planning and preparing for a class before students ever arrive in the classroom. There are several details to address when planning a class:

- What are the expected outcomes (objectives) of the training session?
- How much time will the class take?
- How many students will attend the class?
- Are there student prerequisites required to understand the objectives?
- Which training aids and equipment will be needed?
- In what order will the instructional material be presented?
- Will the delivery schedule be affected by availability of specific resources?

All of these questions and more are answered during the planning and preparation for the class. This information is compiled into a document called a **lesson plan**. A lesson plan is a detailed guide used by the instructor for preparing and delivering instruction to students. An instructor who uses a well-prepared and thorough lesson plan to organize and prepare for class greatly increases the odds of ensuring quality student learning. An Instructor I uses a lesson plan that is already developed, usually by an instructor who is certified as an Instructor II or higher. The Instructor II has received training in how to develop his or her own lesson plan and may be responsible for developing all parts of the lesson plan, including objectives, lesson outline, suggested student activities, methods of evaluation, and many other components of a properly crafted class session.

As an Instructor I, you are responsible for delivering training from a prepared lesson plan. An Instructor I is able to **adapt** a lesson plan to meet specific student-centered needs but will not modify the *content* of the lesson plan—that remains the responsibility of an Instructor II or above. Instructing from a prepared lesson plan is the core outcome of your instructor training. You already understand the learning process, various methods of instruction, and communication skills. That knowledge will allow you to use the lesson plan as a tool to influence a change in behavior. This chapter sets the stage for you to be successful in delivering effective training by using a standard form and content layout to ensure you meet the lesson goals.

Why Use a Lesson Plan?

Many fire fighters who are assigned to instruct a class have a lot of emergency scene experience and may have even participated in group discussions on department operations, personnel evaluations, or the budget process. However, working from prepared lesson plan materials is a process with which many fire fighters have no experience, as they may have participated as students and not in delivering information *to* students.

Many people without experience in the field of education may not understand the importance of a lesson plan. Attempting to deliver instruction without a lesson plan is like driving in a foreign country without a map (**FIGURE 5-1**). The goal in both situations is to reach your intended destination. In a lesson plan, the learning objectives are the intended destination. Without a map (the lesson plan), you most likely will not reach the destination. If you attempt to shoot from the hip without a prepared lesson plan that details the expected outcomes, content may be skipped, safety points may be omitted, and inconsistency between deliveries will occur. Also, without a lesson plan that contains learning objectives, you may not even know what the destination for the class is. In other words, if you do not have clearly written learning objectives for your class and a plan for how to achieve them, there is a high probability that you will not be successful.

Occasionally, an instructor may use a lesson plan from an established or ongoing training program. Such lesson plans may have been adapted for previous deliveries based on a specific audience and factors related to that class. If an instructor becomes complacent and fails to check the existing lesson plans fully against his or her own class requirements, the result may be an inferior lesson delivery for the students.

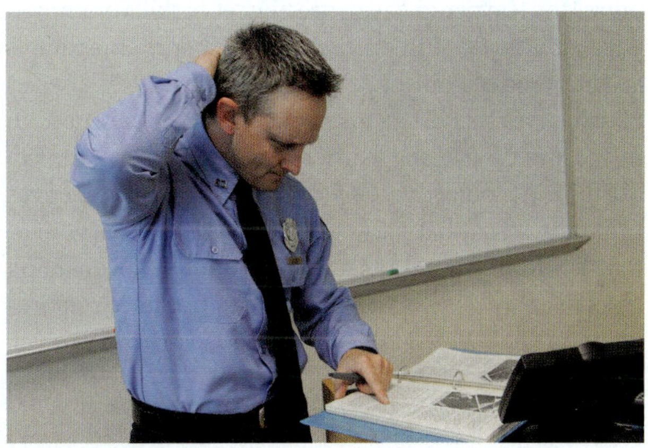

FIGURE 5-1 Using a lesson plan keeps the instructor organized and provides a clear direction for the class.

Written lesson plans also ensure consistency of training throughout the various companies of a large fire department, or when a class is taught multiple times, especially by different instructors. In such cases, a common lesson plan ensures that all students receive the same information. Lesson plans are also used to document what was taught in a class. When the class needs to be taught again in the future, the new instructor will be able to refer to the existing lesson plans and achieve the same learning objectives.

COMPANY-LEVEL TRAINING TIP

In the case of legal action against the instructor or educational institution, the lesson plan may become a critical piece of documentation. When writing a lesson plan, you must ensure the information is technically correct, not just for educational purposes, but potentially for legal reasons.

Understanding Learning Objectives

All instructional planning begins by identifying the desired outcomes. What do you want the students to know or be able to do by the end of class? These desired outcomes are called objectives. A **learning objective** is defined as a goal that is achieved through the attainment of a skill, knowledge, or both, and that can be observed or measured. Sometimes these learning objectives are referred to as performance outcomes or behavioral outcomes, for a simple reason: If students are able to achieve the learning objectives of a lesson, they will achieve the desired outcome of the class. Effective instructors always start their presentations by discussing and reviewing the objectives of the presentation with the students.

A **terminal objective** is a broader outcome that requires the learner to have a specific set of skills or knowledge after a learning process. An **enabling objective** is an intermediate objective and is usually part of a series of objectives that direct instructors on what they need to instruct and what the learners will learn to accomplish the terminal objective. Consider the enabling objectives to be the steps that allow you to reach the top floor—that is, the terminal objective. Terminal and enabling objectives are developed from job performance requirements (JPRs), which is covered at the Instructor II level.

The Components of Learning Objectives

Many different methods may be used for writing learning objectives. One method commonly employed in the fire service is the **ABCD method**, where the acronym stands for **A**udience (Who?), **B**ehavior (What?), **C**ondition (How or using what?), and **D**egree (How well?). (Learning objectives do not always need to be written in that order, however.) The ABCD method was introduced in the book *Instructional Media and the New Technologies of Education* written by Robert Heinich, Michael Molenda, and James D. Russell (1998).

Audience

The **audience** of the learning objective describes who the students are. Are your students experienced fire fighters or new recruits? Fire service learning objectives often use terms such as *fire fighter trainees*, *cadets*, *fire officers*, or *students* to describe the audience. In the case of this class, you will see objectives with an audience of *fire and emergency services instructor.* Some lesson plans will contain multiple objectives to meet the course goal. In this case, it is acceptable to reference the audience once at the beginning of the objective listing, as long as all of the objectives relate to the same audience members. If the objective is written correctly, the audience demographics will be evident in the structure of the objective.

Behavior

Once the students have been identified, typically the **behavior** is listed next. The behavior must be an observable and measurable action. A common error in writing learning objectives is using words such as *know* or *understand* for the behavior. Is there really a method for determining whether someone understands something? It is preferable to use words such as *state*, *describe*, or *identify* as part of learning objectives—these are actions that you can see and measure. It is much easier to evaluate the ability of a student to identify the parts of a portable fire extinguisher than to evaluate how well the student understands the parts of a portable fire extinguisher. The importance of the behavior portion of the objective will be discussed later in the chapter.

The behavior may identify the type of presentation or class that will be conducted. Words such as *describe* or *state* in the objective imply that the student will know something, whereas words such as *demonstrate* or *perform* indicate that the student will be able to do something. This is where the terms **cognitive objective** or **psychomotor objective** are applied in a properly formatted objective (**TABLE 5-1**). Instructors should blend presentation styles to enhance the learning environment whenever possible. Appealing to multiple senses and allowing for many application opportunities enhances learning.

TABLE 5-1 Examples of Learning Objectives and Their Parts

	Complete Objective	Parts
Cognitive Objectives	The fire fighter will identify hose loads used by the department from photos of finished hose beds with 100 percent accuracy.	▪ Audience • Fire fighter ▪ Behavior • Identify hose loads ▪ Condition • Examples of finished hose beds ▪ Degree • 100 percent accuracy
Psychomotor Objectives	The fire fighter will rebed a flatbed using a minimum of 300 ft (91 m) of 3-in. (76-mm) supply hose according to department hose manual without errors.	▪ Audience • Fire fighter ▪ Behavior • Rebed flat load ▪ Condition • 300 ft (91 m) of 3-in. (76-mm) supply hose ▪ Degree • 100 percent accuracy

Condition

The **condition** describes the situation in which the student will perform the behavior. Items that are often listed as conditions include specific equipment or resources given to the student, personal protective clothing or safety items that must be used when performing the behavior, and the physical location or circumstances for performing the behavior. For example, the following phrases in an objective specify the condition:

> ". . . in full protective equipment, including self-contained breathing apparatus (SCBA)."
> ". . . using the water from a static source, such as a pond or pool."

Degree

The **degree** is the last part of the learning objective; it indicates how well the student is expected to perform the behavior in the listed conditions. With what percentage of completion is the student expected to perform the behavior? Total mastery of a skill would require 100 percent completion—this means perfection, following every step on the skill sheet. For example, a student performing a ladder raise needs to complete all of the steps on the skill checklist to raise the ladder safely. Skipping any step (failing the skill) may result in a serious injury, damage to the ladder, or death. In contrast, many times knowledge-based learning objectives are expected to be learned to the degree stated in the passing rate for written exams, such as 70 percent or 80 percent. Another degree that is frequently used is a time limit, which can be included in learning objectives dealing with both knowledge and skills.

Using the ABCD Method

Strictly speaking, well-written learning objectives should contain all four elements of the ABCD method. Nevertheless, learning objectives are often shortened because one or more of the elements are assumed to be known. If a lesson plan is identified as being used for teaching potential fire and emergency services instructors, for example, every single objective may not need to start with "the fire and emergency services instructor trainee." The audience component of the ABCD method may be listed once, at the top of all the objectives, or not listed at all.

The same principle applies to the condition component. If it is understood that a class requires all skills to be performed in full personal protective gear, it may not be necessary to list this condition in each individual learning objective. It is also common to omit the degree component, as many learning objectives are written with the understanding that the degree will be determined by the testing method. If the required passing grade for class written exams is 80 percent, it is assumed that knowledge learning objectives will be performed to that degree. Similarly, if the skill learning objectives for a class are required to be performed perfectly, a 100 percent degree for those learning objectives can be assumed.

Learning objectives should be shortened in this way only when the assumptions for the missing components are clearly stated elsewhere in the lesson plan. Of course, a learning objective is unlikely to omit the behavior component because it is the backbone of the learning objective. Some curricula do require the ABCD to be stated each time, in sequence, and in complete form. For enabling objectives, a shortened form may sometimes be permitted; otherwise, many of the components in the series of objectives would simply be restated over and over again, which may confuse or frustrate a learner trying to identify course expectations.

ABCD learning objectives do not need to contain all of the parts in the ABCD order. Consider the following example:

> In full protective equipment including SCBA, two fire fighter trainees will carry a 24-foot (7-m) extension ladder 100 feet (30 m) and then perform a flat raise to a second-floor window in less than 1 minute and 30 seconds.

Here the audience is "the fire fighter trainees." The behaviors are "carry a 24-foot (7-m) extension ladder" and "perform a flat raise." Both carrying and raising are observable and measurable actions. The conditions are "full protective equipment including SCBA," "100 feet (30 m)," and "to a second-floor window"; they describe the circumstances for carrying and raising the ladder. The degree is "less than 1 minute and 30 seconds." The fire fighter trainees must demonstrate the ability to perform these behaviors to the proper degree to meet this learning objective successfully.

The ABCD method is a clear and appropriate way to address objectives. Inclusion of all four of its elements is essential in the construction of the terminal objective, which is the main idea for the lesson. This objective should contain all the components to inform the students what will be taught, the method of evaluation, and the resources consulted for the information presented. Subsequent (enabling) objectives may assume certain points previously stated in the main objective, such as audience, degree, and references, as long as these points are clarified in the main objective. Each enabling objective allows the student to meet the intent or goal of the terminal objective.

Parts of a Lesson Plan

Many different styles and formats for lesson plans exist. No matter which lesson plan format is used, however, certain components should always be included. Each of these components is necessary for you to understand and follow a lesson plan (**FIGURE 5-2**).

Lesson Title

The **lesson title** or lesson topic describes what the lesson plan is about. For example, a lesson title may be "Portable Fire Extinguishers" or "Fire Personnel Management." Just by the lesson title, you should be able to determine whether a particular lesson plan contains information about the topic you are planning to teach. A title page may be used to highlight or preview the content of the lesson plan package (**FIGURE 5-3**). It may serve as a summary of all of the contents and help prepare you for the class.

Level of Instruction

It is important for a lesson plan to identify the **level of instruction**, because your students must be able to understand the instructional material. Just as an elementary school teacher would not use a lesson plan developed for high school students, so you as an instructor must ensure that the lesson plan is written at an appropriate level for your students. Often the level of instruction in the fire service corresponds with National Fire Protection Association (NFPA) standards for professional qualifications. If you are teaching new recruits or cadets, you would use lesson plans that are designated as having a Fire Fighter I or II level of instruction. If you are teaching fire service professional development classes, you may use lesson plans that are specified as having a Fire Officer I or II level of instruction. Another method of indicating the level of instruction is by labeling the lesson plan with terms such as *beginner*, *intermediate*, or *advanced*. No matter which method is used to indicate the level of instruction, you should ensure that the material contained in a lesson plan is at the appropriate level for your students.

Another component of the level of instruction is the identification of any prerequisites. A **prerequisite** is a condition that must be met before the student is permitted to receive further instruction. Often, a prerequisite is another class. Ensure that the proper prerequisites are met by each of your students. Failure to do so may mean that a student performs tasks that he or she is not qualified or prepared to perform.

For example, a Fire Service Administration class would be a prerequisite for taking an Advanced Fire Service Administration class. A certification or rank may also be a prerequisite. Before being allowed to receive training on driving an aerial apparatus, for example, the department may require a student to hold the rank of a Driver and possess Driver/Operator—Pumper certification.

Instructor Guide

Lesson Plan

Lesson Title: Use of Fire Extinguishers
Level of Instruction: Fire Fighter I

Method of Instruction: Demonstration

Learning Objective: The student shall demonstrate the ability to extinguish a Class A fire with a stored-pressure water-type fire extinguisher. (NFPA 1001, 4.3.16)

References: Fundamentals of Fire Fighter Skills, 4th Edition, Chapter 7

Time: 50 Minutes

Materials Needed: Portable water extinguishers, Class A combustible burn materials, skills checklist, suitable area for hands-on demonstration, assigned PPE for skill

Step #1 Lesson Preparation:
- Fire extinguishers are first line of defense on incipient fires
- Civilians use for containment until FD arrives
- Must match extinguisher class with fire class
- FD personnel can use in certain situations, may limit water damage
- Review of fire behavior and fuel classifications
- Discuss types of extinguishers on apparatus
- Demonstrate methods for operation

Step #2 Presentation

A. Fire extinguishers should be simple to operate.
   1. An individual with only basic training should be able to use most fire extinguishers safely and effectively.
   2. Every portable extinguisher should be labeled with printed operating instructions.
   3. There are six basic steps in extinguishing a fire with a portable fire extinguisher. They are:
      a. Locate the fire extinguisher.
      b. Select the proper classification of extinguisher.
      c. Transport the extinguisher to the location of the fire.
      d. Activate the extinguisher to release the extinguishing agent.
      e. Apply the extinguishing agent to the fire for maximum effect.
      f. Ensure your personal safety by having an exit route.
   4. Although these steps are not complicated, practice and training are essential for effective fire suppression.
   5. Tests have shown that the effective use of Class B portable fire extinguishers depends heavily on user training and expertise.
      a. A trained expert can extinguish a fire up to twice as large as a non-expert can, using the same extinguisher.
   6. As a fire fighter, you should be able to operate any fire extinguisher that you might be required to use, whether it is carried on your fire apparatus, hanging on the wall of your firehouse, or placed in some other location.

B. Knowing the exact locations of extinguishers can save valuable time in an emergency.
   1. Fire fighters should know what types of fire extinguishers are carried on department apparatus and where each type of extinguisher is located.
   2. You should also know where fire extinguishers are located in and around the fire station and other work places.
   3. You should have at least one fire extinguisher in your home and another in your personal vehicle, and you should know exactly where they are located.

C. It is important to be able to select the proper extinguisher.
   1. This requires an understanding of the classification and rating system for fire extinguishers.
   2. Knowing the different types of agents, how they work, the ratings of the fire extinguishers carried on your fire apparatus, and which extinguisher is appropriate for a particular fire situation is also important.
   3. Fire fighters should be able to assess a fire quickly, determine if the fire can be controlled by an extinguisher, and identify the appropriate extinguisher.
      a. Using an extinguisher with an insufficient rating may not completely extinguish the fire, which can place the operator in danger of being burned or otherwise injured.
      b. If the fire is too large for the extinguisher, you will have to consider other options such as obtaining additional extinguishers or making sure that a charged hose line is ready to provide back-up.
   4. Fire fighters should also be able to determine the most appropriate type of fire extinguisher to place in a given area, based on the types of fires that could occur and the hazards that are present.
      a. In some cases, one type of extinguisher might be preferred over another.

Step # 3 Application

Slides 7–10

Ask students to locate closest extinguisher to training area

Review rating systems handout—Have students complete work book activity page #389

What happens if wrong type or size extinguisher is used?

FIGURE 5-2 The components of a lesson plan (indicated in bold print).

D. The best method of transporting a hand-held portable fire extinguisher depends on the size, weight, and design of the extinguisher.	
1. Hand-held portable fire extinguishers can weigh as little as 1 lb to as much as 50 lb.	
2. Extinguishers with a fixed nozzle should be carried in the favored or stronger hand. a. This enables the operator to depress the trigger and direct the discharge easily.	*Display available types of extinguishers*
3. Extinguishers that have a hose between the trigger and the nozzle should be carried in the weaker or less-favored hand so that the favored hand can grip and aim the nozzle.	
4. Heavier extinguishers may have to be carried as close as possible to the fire and placed upright on the ground. a. The operator can depress the trigger with one hand, while holding the nozzle and directing the stream with the other hand.	
5. Transporting a fire extinguisher will be practiced in Skill Drill 8-1.	
E. Activating a fire extinguisher to apply the extinguishing agent is a single operation in four steps.	
1. The P-A-S-S acronym is a helpful way to remember these steps: a. Pull the safety pin. b. Aim the nozzle at the base of the flames. c. Squeeze the trigger to discharge the agent. d. Sweep the nozzle across the base of the flames.	*Have students demonstrate steps using empty extinguisher*
2. Most fire extinguishers have very simple operation systems.	
3. Practice discharging different types of extinguishers in training situations to build confidence in your ability to use them properly and effectively.	
4. When using a fire extinguisher, always approach the fire with an exit behind you. a. If the fire suddenly expands or the extinguisher fails to control it, you must have a planned escape route. b. Never let the fire get between you and a safe exit. After suppressing a fire, do not turn your back on it.	*Complete skills sheet #7–9 for each student*
5. Always watch and be prepared for a rekindle until the fire has been fully overhauled.	
6. As a fire fighter, you should wear your personal protective clothing and use appropriate personal protective equipment (PPE).	
7. If you must enter an enclosed area where an extinguisher has been discharged, wear full PPE and use SCBA. a. The atmosphere within the enclosed area will probably contain a mixture of combustion products and extinguishing agents.	*Review PPE required for extinguisher use*
F. The oxygen content within the space may be dangerously depleted.	*Discuss hazards of extinguishing agents*
Step #4 Evaluation: 1. Each student will properly extinguish a Class A combustible fire using a stored-pressure type water extinguisher. (Skill Sheet x-1) 2. Each student will return extinguisher to service. (Skill Sheet x-2) **Lesson Summary:** • Classifications of fire extinguishers • Ratings of fire extinguishers • Types of extinguishers and agents • Operation of each type of fire extinguishers • Demonstration of Class A fire extinguishment using a stored pressure water extinguisher **Assignments:** 1. Read Chapter 7 prior to next class. 2. Complete "You are the Firefighter" activity for Chapter 7 and be prepared to discuss your answers.	

FIGURE 5-2 *Continued*

Method of Delivery

As addressed in Chapter 3, *Methods of Instruction*, the method in which the lesson plan is intended to be delivered is an important element in the lesson plan. At a quick glance, you can see whether the lesson plan will be a classroom lecture or a hands-on training class. Some agencies who review training delivery will actually measure the number of hands-on sessions (psychomotor, manipulative) compared to classroom (cognitive, knowledge) to ensure that there is balance in the types of training delivered by the department. Some examples of methods of instruction include lecture, demonstration, and small group discussion.

Learning Objectives

As mentioned earlier in this chapter, learning objectives are essential to the lesson plan. These may also be called behavioral objectives, performance objectives, or learning outcomes. All lesson plans must have learning objectives. Many methods for determining and listing learning objectives are available. The specific method used to write the learning objectives is not as important as ensuring that you understand the learning objectives for the lesson plan that you must present to your students. The Instructor II will use JPRs to develop the learning objectives in the ABCD format, and the Instructor III will write course objectives.

JBL Fire Department
Division of Training

Lesson Title

Training Date: | **Location of Training:**

Firehouse Code: | **Safety Plan Required? Y ☐ N ☐**

Topic:	**Instructor(s):**
Teaching method(s):	**Time allotted:**
Handouts:	
AV needs:	**Teaching resources:**
Level of instruction:	**Evaluation method:**
NFPA JPR's:	**Equipment needed:**
LEARNING OBJECTIVES: *Upon completion of the class and study questions, each participant will independently do the following with a degree of accuracy that meets or exceeds the standards established for their scope of practice:*	
General class activities for student application	
Safety Briefing 1.	**SAFETY RED FLAGS** **ALL STOPS:**

FIGURE 5-3 A sample cover sheet for a lesson plan. This gives the user an "at-a-glance" view of the presentation they will deliver.

References

Lesson plans often contain an outline of the information that must be understood to deliver the learning objectives. Instructors who are not experts in a subject may need to refer to additional references or resources to obtain further information on these topics. The references/resources section may contain names of books, websites, or even names of experts who may be contacted for further information. By citing references in the lesson plan, the validity of the lesson plan can be verified.

Materials Needed

Most lesson plans require some type of instructional materials to be used in the delivery of the lesson plan. Instructional materials are tools designed to help you present the lesson plan to your students. For instance, audiovisual aids are the type of instructional material most frequently listed in a lesson plan—that is, a lesson plan may require the use of a computer. Other commonly listed instructional materials include handouts, pictures, diagrams, and models. Also, instructional materials may be used to indicate whether additional supplies are necessary to deliver the lesson plan. For example, a preincident planning lesson plan may list paper, pencils, and rulers as the instructional materials needed. The actual equipment students will be using or operating could be shown and passed around during the classroom portion of the lesson (e.g., nozzles, hand tools, personal protective equipment [PPE]).

Some lesson plans will indicate the approximate time it will take to deliver the lesson. This is a subjective estimate in most cases as there are many factors that influence delivery time, including the amount of questions or discussions that take place during the training. Additionally, knowing the number of slides used in a cognitive lesson may be helpful to the instructor.

COMPANY-LEVEL TRAINING TIP

Instructors are the "building contractors" for their courses. The construction materials or tools are the items the instructor needs to compile to make a presentation effective. As the instructor, you must design and make lesson plans work for you.

Lesson Outline

The **lesson outline** is the main body of the lesson plan. This element is discussed in detail later in this chapter. The lesson outline comprises four main elements: *preparation*, *presentation*, *application*, and *evaluation*, which are the components of the four-step method of instruction. Each area fulfills a specific purpose in the delivery of instruction. Instructors who engage their students effectively use each part to ensure that the objectives of the lesson plan are properly met to the level intended. See Chapter 3, *Methods of Instruction*, for more information on the four-step method of instruction.

Lesson Summary

The **lesson summary** simply summarizes the lesson plan. It reviews and reinforces the main points of the lesson plan. The lesson summary plays an important role in the overall lesson, allowing you to enhance the application step by asking summary questions on key objective and lesson points. You may view this as the instructor asking the student, "What did I just teach you or show you?"

Assignment

Lesson plans often contain an **assignment**, such as a homework-type exercise that will allow the student to further explore or apply the material presented in the lesson plan. Be prepared to explain the assignment, its due date, the method for submitting the assignment, and the grading criteria to be used.

Instructional Preparation

Once you have a lesson plan, the instructional preparation begins. Which materials are needed for the class? Which instructional technology tools will be used? Where will the class be conducted? How much time will be needed? These and many other questions must be answered during instructional preparation. The information contained in the lesson plan should be used as a guide for instructional preparation.

Student Preparation

Students should prepare for instruction by coming to a class prepared and ready to learn. Certain classroom or drill-ground rules may exist that prohibit bringing cell phones, newspapers, or other reading materials into the learning environment. The instructor should monitor the preparedness of the students as they come to the classroom or drill ground, and may enhance their readiness to learn by providing class information and objectives ahead of time. The expectations and outcomes may be better if the students take the time to prepare before the class. Bringing textbooks, notebooks, and writing supplies is another important part of the student's preparation.

Organizational Techniques

Identify the time available for you to plan and prepare for the class. The time available for preparation is usually the amount of time from the point when the lesson plan is identified until the day when the class is scheduled to be taught. Identify the milestones that must be accomplished as part of this timeline. Depending on the lesson plan, milestones may include obtaining audiovisual equipment, purchasing materials, reserving a classroom, or previewing audiovisual aids.

Procuring Instructional Materials and Equipment

Most classes take advantage of instructional materials or equipment. The method of obtaining these instructional materials and equipment differs from fire department to fire department. A common method of procuring materials is for the instructor to contact the person in the fire department who is responsible for purchasing training materials, such as a training officer or someone assigned to the training division. You may be required to provide a list of needed materials to the training officer. Often, this list of materials must be submitted well in advance of when the class is scheduled to begin, due to the purchasing requirements of your agency. The key is to know your agency's time frame and to work within it to allow you to follow policy. The training officer, in turn, compiles the materials either by purchasing new materials or by securing materials already available at the training division. The training officer contacts the instructor when all class-related materials are available.

Another common method for procuring class equipment is the equipment checkout process, which is typically managed by the fire department's training division. For example, if you need a multimedia projector for a class, you would submit a request for the projector in which you indicate the date and time when it is needed. The training division would then reserve the projector for you. Depending on the organizational procedures, you might be required to pick up the projector and set it up, or the training division might set up the projector at the class location for you. Regardless of how you obtain your projector, you should make sure you understand how to use it and how to troubleshoot any problems before class begins.

Preparing to Instruct

The most important part of the instruction's preparation is preparing for actual delivery of the lesson plan in the classroom or on the drill ground. If you obtain the necessary materials, equipment, apparatus, drill tower, or classroom, but you do not prepare to deliver the lesson plan, the class will not be successful. You should be thoroughly familiar with the information contained in the lesson plan, which may require you to consult the references listed in the lesson plan and research the topic further.

No matter which method of instructional delivery is used, you should always rehearse your presentation before delivering it to a training session full of students. A class is destined for failure if you are seeing the presentation material for the first time in front of the class. Successful instructors have a sound understanding of the information that they are delivering and can adapt to the particular needs of their class because they always know what is coming next.

Scheduling

An Instructor I may be called upon to schedule a single instructional session. This type of instruction may focus on a subject that is covered only one time based on a needs assessment, or it may be part of an overall training program. Address the following factors when scheduling a single instructional session:

- Define and understand the goal of the session.
- Determine the time necessary to deliver the session and the department scheduling process.
- Identify and locate all training materials for the session, including lesson plans, skill sheets, and equipment needed to meet the objectives. Prepare requests for resources through the proper channels and ensure that expendable materials are replaced and accounted for in the agency.
- Gain approval from supervisors as necessary for members to attend the session. Make sure that members can attend. Determine response procedures with supervisors and officers.
- Schedule and deliver sessions according to the authority having jurisdiction. Make sure notice is given to any instructors who will assist.
- Complete training record reports as required by department policy. Create a through training record report, with all required data, objectives, and narratives of the session. Once complete, forward all reports through the proper channels for recordkeeping purposes.

Adapting Versus Creating a Lesson Plan

One of the most important distinctions between an Instructor I and an Instructor II is the Instructor II's ability to create and modify a lesson plan. A lesson plan is a guide or a roadmap for delivering instruction, but rarely is it implemented exactly as written. To understand what can and cannot be changed by each level of instructor, let us review what the JPRs for NFPA 1041: *Standard for Fire and Emergency Services Instructor Professional Qualifications*, say about creating and adapting a lesson plan:

> **Fire and Emergency Services Instructor I**
>
> **4.3.2** Review instructional materials, given the materials for a specific topic, target audience, learner characteristics, and learning

environment, so that elements of the lesson plan, learning environment, and resources that need adaptation are identified.

4.3.3 Adapt a prepared lesson plan, given course materials and an assignment, so that the needs of the student and the objectives of the lesson plan are achieved.

The Instructor I should not alter the *content* or the lesson objectives. Prior to the beginning of the class, the instructor should be able to evaluate local conditions, assess facilities for appropriateness, meet local standard operating procedures (SOPs), and recognize students' limitations. As the Instructor I, you should be able to change the *method of instruction* and the *course materials* to meet the needs of the students and accommodate their individual learner characteristics, including making adaptations as necessary due to the learning environment, audience, capability of facilities, and types of equipment available. NFPA 1041 charges the Instructor II with creating a lesson plan, which includes making modifications to the plan as needed.

Fire and Emergency Services Instructor II

5.3.2 Create a lesson plan, given a topic, learner characteristics, and a lesson plan format, so that learning objectives, a lesson outline, course materials, instructional technology tools, an evaluation plan, and learning objectives for the topic are addressed.

Put simply, an Instructor II can create and make basic or fundamental changes to the lesson plan, whereas an Instructor I can adapt only to local conditions without altering objectives. Fundamental changes include changing the performance outcomes, rewriting the learning objectives, modifying the content of the lesson, and so on.

As the Instructor I, you can make the lesson plan fit the situation and conditions. These conditions include the facility, the local SOPs, the environment, limitations of the students, and other local factors.

NFPA 1041 specifically states that an Instructor I may adapt the method of instruction and course materials to meet the needs of the students and accommodate the individual instructor's style. Here are a few real-life examples:

- An Instructor I *may change a lesson plan's method of instruction* from lecture to discussion if he or she determines that the latter method would be a better presentation format because of the students' level of knowledge.
- An Instructor I *may adapt the classroom setting* if the facility cannot meet the seating arrangement listed in the lesson plan.
- An Instructor I *may adapt the number of fire fighters* performing an evolution in a lesson plan from three to four to meet local staffing SOP requirements.
- An Instructor I *cannot* modify a lesson plan learning objective that states a fire fighter must raise a 24-ft (7.3-m) extension ladder because he or she feels the task is too difficult for one fire fighter.
- An Instructor I *cannot* change the JPR of developing a budget in a Fire Officer lesson plan because he or she does not feel comfortable teaching that subject.

As with all other positions within the fire service, it is important that instructors perform only those actions within their level of training. As an Instructor I, you must recognize what you can and cannot do. Acting outside your scope of training may lead to legal liability. If you are ever unsure whether you have sufficient knowledge or skills to teach a topic, discuss this issue with your superior.

Lesson plans must remain dynamic in both the short term and the long term. In the short term, you should understand when it is appropriate to adjust a lesson plan during its delivery based on students' learning styles, changing conditions, timing considerations, and students' progress. In the long term, you should provide input to your supervisor regarding the success of the delivery. If problems occurred or improvements are needed, report this feedback as well.

One critical component of lesson plan adaptability is the break times. Break times are built into course schedules and may need to be adjusted to reflect the training environment or to accommodate other classes being conducted at the same time.

If you make adjustments to the delivery of a lesson plan, it is critical that you ensure that all learning objectives are still covered. For example, many times activities must be scheduled around the activities of other courses. Scheduling use of resources in the field with other instructors can help reduce conflicts. The program coordinator should be advised if an instructor intends to move portions of the program around so that the coordinator can ensure the change does not affect other programs and shared resources.

Reviewing Instructional Materials for Adaptation

There are many ways for an Instructor I to obtain a lesson plan: fire service websites, commercially published curriculum packages, the National Fire Academy, the instructor's fire department's training library, or other fire departments. No matter which method is used, the lesson plan must be reviewed, and any areas that need adaptation must be identified. This is true even for lesson plans that were originally developed within your own fire department. Over time, standards and procedures change; a lesson plan that was completely correct for your department when it was created may be out-of-date in just a few months.

After obtaining a lesson plan, you must review the entire lesson plan and determine whether adaptations are needed to make it usable for your class. As part of the class planning and preparation process, lesson plan adaptations must be scheduled and completed before you deliver the presentation to the class. A lesson plan might need adaptations for many reasons, such as differences related to the learning environment, the audience, the capability of facilities, and the types of equipment available. Always be prepared to adapt the lesson plan to accommodate last-minute classroom or equipment changes. While these occurrences should be rare, they do happen.

Instructors may find they need to adapt a lesson plan in situations where all members of the audience do not come from one department, as in a regional or academy delivery. If you are teaching from a prepared lesson plan within your department only, the audience factors, prerequisite knowledge, and abilities are likely already known, so you may have to adapt the lesson plan only if it is from an outside source or to tailor it to the available delivery time.

Evaluating Local Conditions

The main focus when adapting a lesson plan is to make minor adjustments so it fits your local conditions and your students' needs. To accomplish this, you must first be familiar with your audience. The Instructor I should contemplate the following questions when reviewing a lesson plan for any adaptations needed to accommodate the intended audience:

- Which organizational policies and procedures apply to the lesson plan?
- What is the current level of knowledge and ability of your students?
- Which types of tools and equipment will your students use in performing the skills within the lesson plan?

The second area pertaining to the local conditions that must be considered is you, the Instructor I:

- What is your experience level and ability? Can you identify resources and materials to improve your knowledge and background? If not, be prepared to ask for assistance from another instructor.
- How familiar are you with the topic that will be taught? Teaching material you are not familiar with can pose severe safety and credibility hazards. If you are not familiar with the topic, do not attempt to fake it, as wrong or incomplete information could be dangerous.
- What is your teaching style?

The answers to these types of questions will allow you to adapt the lesson plan so that you deliver the lesson in the most effective way given your own abilities.

Evaluating Facilities for Appropriateness

You should also review and adapt the lesson plan based on the facilities that will be used when delivering the class. Several factors—for example, the equipment available, student seating, classroom size, lighting, and environmental noise—must be considered as part of this evaluation. For example, a lesson plan may call for students to sit at tables that have been moved into a U-shaped arrangement. However, if the local classroom has desks that are fixed to the floor, you will not be able to arrange the seating as indicated in the lesson plan. The lesson plan would then need to be adapted to meet the conditions of the facility and the seating arrangement changed accordingly. You should make this adaptation, keeping in mind the reason for the indicated seating arrangement.

Meeting Local SOPs

A lesson plan must be reviewed to ensure that it meets and follows local SOPs. This is one of the most important considerations when adapting a lesson plan. You should never teach information that contradicts a SOP. Not only would this lesson be confusing for the students, but it would also create a liability for you. If a student were to be injured or killed while performing a skill in violation of a SOP, you would be held responsible. At a minimum, you would be disciplined within the organization—but it is also possible that you might be held legally responsible in either criminal or civil court.

When reviewing a lesson plan, make note of the SOPs that may cover the topics in the lesson plan. After completely reviewing the lesson plan, research the SOPs and ensure that no conflicts exist. If your research turns up conflicting information, you should adapt the lesson plan to meet the local SOPs as long as it does not change the lesson objectives. If you are not familiar with your local SOPs, contact someone within the department who can assist you with ensuring that the lesson plan is consistent with local SOPs.

Evaluating Limitations of Students

The lesson plan should also be reviewed in light of student limitations and adapted to accommodate those limitations if possible. The lesson plan should be at the appropriate educational level for the students, and the prerequisite knowledge and skills should be verified. For example, if you were reviewing a lesson plan to teach an advanced hazardous materials monitoring class, students should have already undergone basic hazardous materials training. If you were training new fire fighters and reviewing this lesson plan, you may not be able to adapt it. Instead, you would most likely have to require students to undergo additional training before the lesson plan would be appropriate to present to them.

Adapting the Method of Instruction

The method of instruction is the one area that an Instructor I may readily modify. Such a modification may be needed to allow you to deliver the lesson plan effectively, but it should not change the learning objectives. For example, you may not be comfortable using the discussion method to deliver a class on fire service sexual harassment as indicated by the lesson plan. Instead, you might adapt the lesson plan and change the method of instruction to lecture. This would allow the same information to be taught, just in a different format, and the same learning objectives would still be achieved.

Instructors regularly adapt material to meet their departmental needs and to improve the curriculum. Is it ethical to alter material to reflect your personal opinions when those opinions run counter to the traditional way of thinking? The solution to this dilemma is not as simple as it may seem. Imagine where the fire service would be today if only a few years ago bold instructors did not step up to the plate and refuse to present material that was not based on safe practices. "Doing the right thing" is what ethical decisions are all about—but there is a fuzzy line between "the right thing" and "my way is the only right way."

For example, changing a course by eliminating the use of fog nozzles because you believe that these nozzles lead to hand burns is as dangerous as another instructor eliminating the use of smooth-bore nozzles from a lesson plan. The reality is that students must understand the appropriate use, benefits, and dangers of each type of nozzle. What might seem like a simple adaptation could have serious consequences for a student who is not trained thoroughly and properly to department standards.

Accommodating Instructor Style

In addition to ensuring that the method of instruction best suits your abilities, lesson plans may be adapted to accommodate your personal style. A lesson plan often reflects the style of the instructor who wrote it. When reviewing and adapting a lesson plan, consider whether the lesson plan—and especially the presentation section—fits your own style. For example, a lesson plan may call for a humorous activity designed to establish a relationship between the instructor and the students. If you are teaching a military-style academy class, this may not be the best style, so you may need to adapt the presentation accordingly.

Meeting the Needs of the Students

All adaptations should be done with one purpose in mind—namely, meeting the needs of the students. As with all lesson plans, the main goal is to provide instruction that allows students to obtain knowledge or skills. This goal should be verified after you review and adapt a lesson plan.

Training BULLETIN

JONES & BARTLETT FIRE DISTRICT
TRAINING DIVISION
5 Wall Street, Burlington, MA, 01803
Phone 978-443-5000 Fax 978-443-8000

Instant Applications: Lesson Plans

Drill Assignment

Apply the chapter content to your department's operation, its training division, and your personal experiences to complete the following questions and activities.

Objective

Upon completion of the instant applications, fire and emergency services instructor students will exhibit decision making and application of job performance requirements of the instructor using the text, class discussion, and their own personal experiences.

Suggested Drill Applications

1. Using a sample lesson plan included in supplemental course material, identify the components of the lesson plan.
2. Using the same sample lesson plan, adjust the lesson plan based on the needs of different audiences.
3. Analyze an existing lesson plan from your department. Are the components complete and accurate?
4. Review the Incident Report in this chapter and be prepared to discuss your analysis of the incident from a training perspective and as an instructor who wishes to use the report as a training tool.

Incident Report: USFA-TR-015/October 1987

Drill Assignment

Review the information in this incident report and prepare a practice presentation for class delivery at the direction of your instructor. Your presentation should include a summary of the incident facts and a review of the NFPA 1403 compliance and noncompliance findings. Use an outline to organize your thoughts. You may be evaluated on your communication skills during your presentation.

Milford, Michigan—1987

Four days after the fatal training fire in Hollandale, Minnesota, a training session that was supposed to teach fire fighters to recognize physical evidence of arson fires trapped six fire fighters on the second floor of a 120-year-old house (**FIGURE 5-A**). The wood-framed house had low-density ceiling tiles with lightweight wood

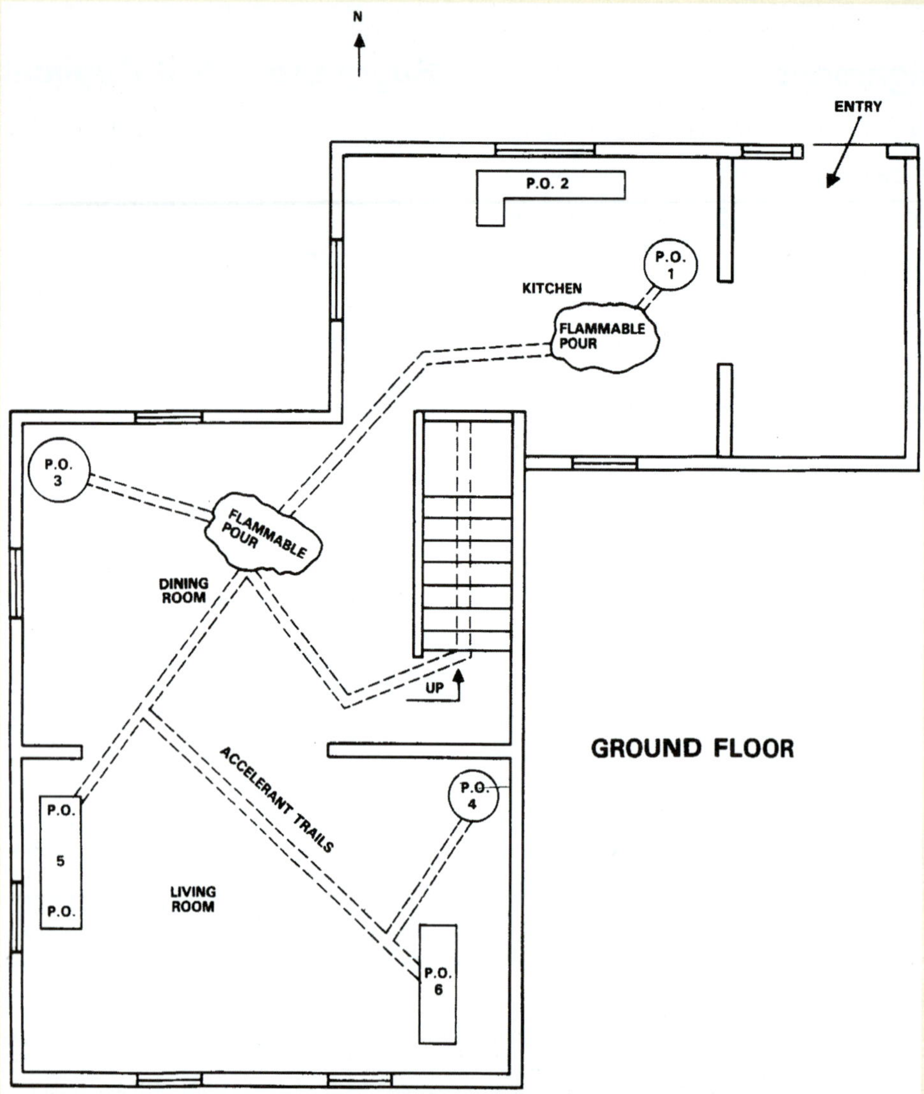

FIGURE 5-A Floor plan of the involved Milford structure.
Courtesy of the U.S. Fire Administration.

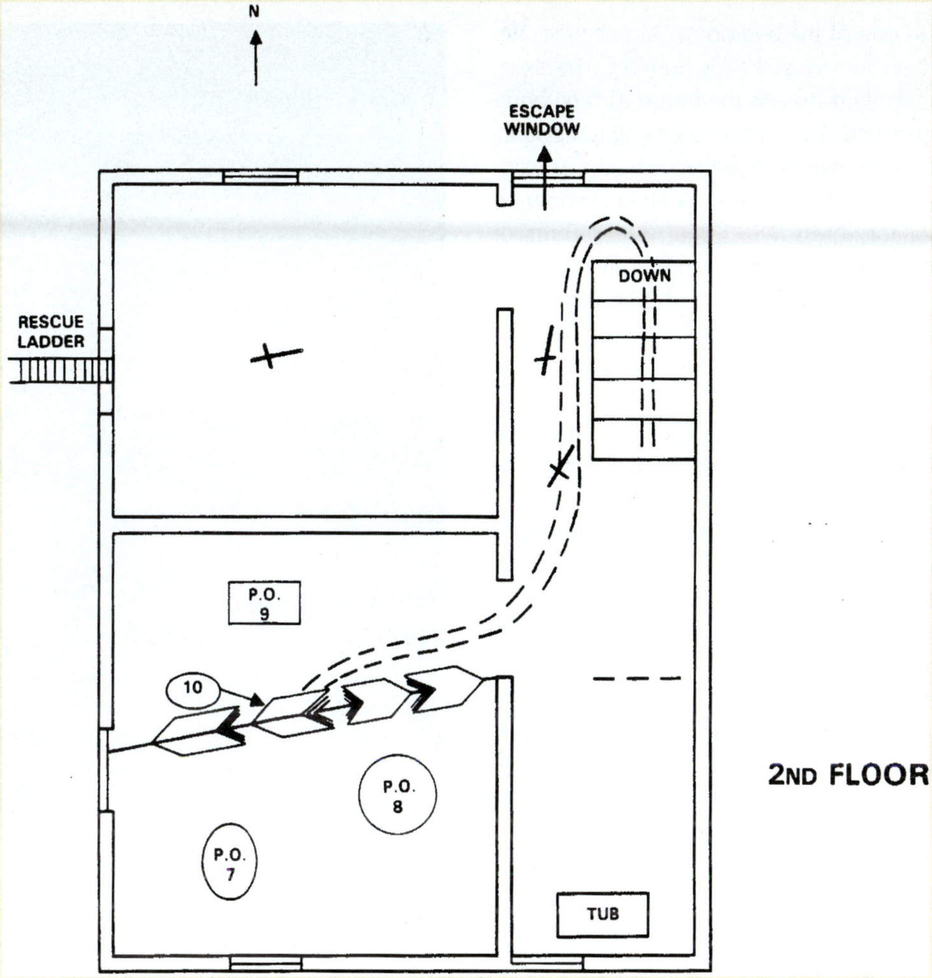

FIGURE 5-A *Continued*

paneling on the first floor. There were numerous holes in the walls and ceilings.

Various arson scenarios were set up in each of the rooms on both floors using furniture, clothing, and other items. Both flammable and combustible fluids were used. Multiple hose lines were charged and ready on the outside of the structure. Portable water tanks were set up and filled with tenders, prepared for a water shuttle operation.

Fire fighters toured the building to see the scenarios before ignition. Initial ignition efforts failed, and several windows on the second floor were broken to improve ventilation. A fire set on a couch in the southwest corner of the living room using flammable or combustible liquids was openly burning and had breached the exterior wall and entered the attic space.

One fire fighter was already inside trying to ignite the fires on the second floor. Four fire fighters were directed to enter the house, along with the assistant chief. Without a hose line, these fire fighters passed multiple burning fire sets that were producing little heat or smoke. Most likely, they did not see the fire in the living room or realize it had spread to the attic. They met with the assistant chief and another fire fighter on the second floor

Incident Report continued

to ignite a fire in one of the bedrooms. At this time, the other upstairs bedroom was already burning. The assistant chief directed them to exit the house as fire conditions rapidly intensified. The escape route down the stairs to the first floor was cut off and, under very adverse conditions, the fire fighters were able to locate a window on the second floor for egress (**FIGURE 5-B**). Three of them were able to exit through the window and onto the first-floor roof below. Reportedly, the SCBA face piece was melting off the last fire fighter able to exit.

Outside, fire fighters observed the change in conditions and the rescue of the assistant chief and the two other fire fighters. They initiated suppression and rescue operations. Ladders were raised to the second-floor windows in the now almost fully involved house.

The first trapped fire fighter was located and removed in approximately 10 minutes. The others were all located on the second floor shortly thereafter. Per the NFPA report, "One of the fire fighters who was able to escape did not know that he would be part of an interior training until he was instructed to 'suit up,' and even then he was unsure of his specific assignment." Three fire fighters died in the fire, which was the first multiple-death training incident in the United States since the release of *NFPA 1403: Standard on Live Fire Training Evolutions* in 1986.

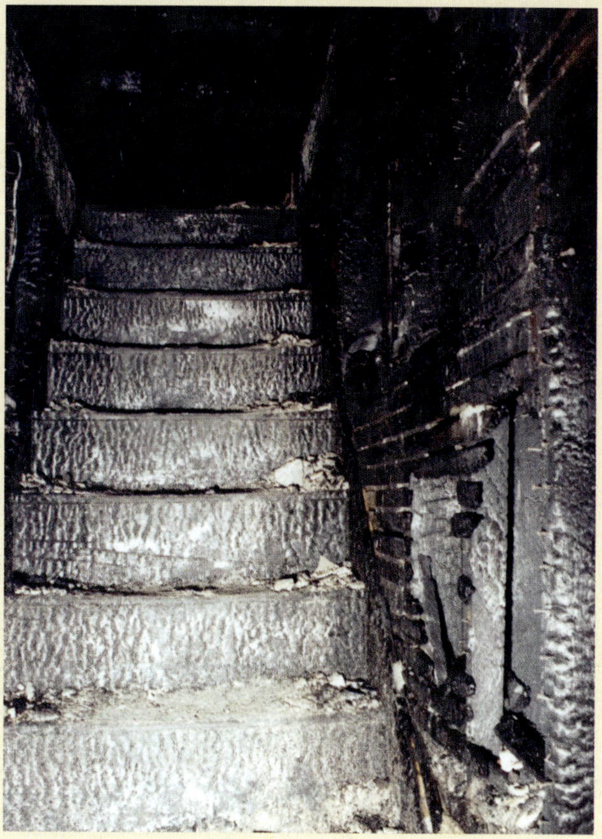

FIGURE 5-B Stairs to the second floor of the Milford house show significant fire involvement that blocked escape from second floor.

Postincident Analysis Milford, Michigan

NFPA 1403 Noncompliant

- Combustible wall paneling and ceiling tiles contributed to rapid fire spread
- Flammable and combustible liquids used
- Multiple simultaneous fires on two floors
- No interior hose line
- Numerous holes in walls and ceilings allowed fire spread
- Interior stairs only exit other than windows (Note: a violation due to the limited normal means of egress, which may have precluded the use of the upper floor without additional provisions put in place)
- Flashover and fire spread unexpected
- Fire chief claimed no knowledge of NFPA 1403

After-Action REVIEW

IN SUMMARY

- An instructor who uses a well-prepared and thorough lesson plan to organize and prepare for class greatly increases the odds of ensuring quality student learning.
- All instructional planning begins by identifying the desired outcomes, called objectives.
- In the ABCD method of writing learning objectives, ABCD stands for **A**udience (Who?), **B**ehavior (What?), **C**ondition (How or using what?), and **D**egree (How well?).
- A lesson plan includes the following parts:
  - Lesson title, or lesson topic
  - Level of instruction
  - Behavioral objectives, performance objectives, and learning outcomes
  - Instructional materials needed
  - Lesson outline
  - References/resources
  - Lesson summary
  - Assignment
- While reviewing and preparing for class with a lesson plan, the four-step method of instruction is the primary process used to relate the material contained in the lesson plan to the students:
  - Preparation
  - Presentation
  - Application
  - Evaluation
- Preparing for instruction is very important. You may need to spend several hours preparing to teach a class, including reviewing the lesson plan, reserving classrooms and instructional aids, and purchasing materials.
- An Instructor I can use a lesson plan to teach a class and may adapt the lesson plan to the local needs of the class.
- The method of instruction is the one area that an Instructor I may readily alter.
- The main focus when adapting a lesson plan is to make minor adjustments so it fits your local conditions and your students' needs. To accomplish this goal, you must be familiar with your audience.
- You should review and adapt the lesson plan based on the facilities that will be used when delivering the class.
- A lesson plan must be reviewed to ensure that it meets and follows local SOPs. After completely reviewing the lesson plan, research the SOPs and ensure that no conflicts exist.
- The lesson plan should be reviewed based on student limitations and adapted to accommodate those limitations if possible.
- Reviewing and adapting a lesson plan should be a formal process. You should document in writing which adaptations have been made.
- All adaptations should be done with one purpose in mind—namely, meeting the needs of the students.

KEY TERMS

Access Navigate for flashcards to test your key term knowledge.

ABCD method A process for writing lesson plan objectives; it includes four components: audience, behavior, condition, and degree.

Adapt To make fit (as for a specific use or situation).

Assignment The part of the lesson plan that provides the student with opportunities for additional application or exploration of the lesson topic, often in the form of homework that is completed outside of the classroom.

Audience Who the students are.

Behavior An observable and measurable action for the student to complete.

Cognitive objective A statement that defines a learning outcome that is based on knowledge and understanding.

Condition The situation in which the student will perform the behavior.

Degree The last part of a learning objective, which indicates how well the student is expected to perform the behavior in the listed conditions.

Enabling objective An intermediate learning objective, usually part of a series that directs the instructor on what he or she needs to instruct and what the learner will learn to accomplish the terminal objective.

Learning objective A goal that is achieved through the attainment of a skill, knowledge, or both, and that can be measured or observed.

Lesson outline The main body of the lesson plan; a chronological listing of the information presented in the lesson plan.

Lesson plan A detailed guide used by an instructor for preparing and delivering instruction.

Lesson summary The part of the lesson plan that briefly reviews the information from the presentation and application sections.

Lesson title The part of the lesson plan that indicates the name or main subject of the lesson plan. Also called the lesson topic.

Level of instruction The part of the lesson plan that indicates the difficulty or appropriateness of the lesson for students.

Prerequisite A condition that must be met before a student is allowed to receive the instruction contained within a lesson plan—often a certification, rank, or attendance of another class.

Psychomotor objective A statement that defines a learning outcome that is based on increasing the learner's ability to perform a specified motor skill.

Terminal objective A broader outcome that requires the learner to have a specific set of skills or knowledge after a learning process.

REFERENCES

Heinich, Robert, Michael Molenda, and James D. Russell. 1998. *Instructional Media and the New Technologies of Education*. 6th ed. Upper Saddle River, NJ: Prentice Hall College Division.

National Fire Protection Association. 2018. *NFPA 1403: Standard on Live Fire Training Evolutions*. Quincy, MA: National Fire Protection Association.

National Fire Protection Association. 2019. *NFPA 1041: Standard for Fire and Emergency Services Instructor Professional Qualifications*. Quincy, MA: National Fire Protection Association.

CHAPTER PRESENTATION EXERCISE

Instructions: Your course instructor will assign individual or group discussions on the key points and teaching tips of this chapter. You or your group will review the chapter teachings and identify the major learning points from the chapter. You should be able to discuss the points, why they are important, and how and where they apply to your responsibilities at your level of instructor training.

REVIEW QUESTIONS

1. Effective instructors always start their presentations by discussing and reviewing what with their students?

2. Explain the components of the ABCD method of a learning objective.

3. Describe the main goal of a lesson plan.

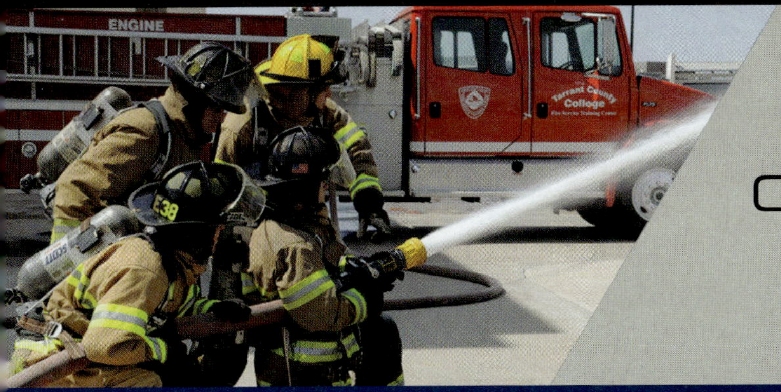

CHAPTER 6

Technology in Training

NFPA 1041 JOB PERFORMANCE REQUIREMENTS

Note: An asterisk denotes that the 1041 standard contains further information in its annex section.

4.3.3* Adapt a prepared lesson plan, given course materials and an assignment, so that the needs of the student and the objectives of the lesson plan are achieved.

(A)* Requisite Knowledge.

Elements of a lesson plan, selection of instructional aids and methods, and organization of the learning environment.

(B) Requisite Skills.

Instructor preparation and organization techniques.

4.4.2 Organize the learning environment, given a facility and an assignment, so that lighting, distractions, climate control or weather, noise control, seating, audiovisual equipment, teaching aids, and safety are addressed.

(A) Requisite Knowledge.

Learning environment management and safety, advantages and limitations of audiovisual equipment and teaching aids, classroom arrangement, and methods and techniques of instruction.

(B) Requisite Skills.

Use of instructional media and teaching aids.

4.4.5 Operate instructional technology tools and demonstration devices, given a learning environment and equipment, so that the equipment functions, the intended objectives are presented, and transitions between media and other parts of the presentation are accomplished.

(A) Requisite Knowledge.

Instructional technology tools, demonstration devices, and selection criteria.

(B) Requisite Skills.

Use of instructional technology tools, demonstration devices, transition techniques, cleaning, and field level maintenance.

KNOWLEDGE OBJECTIVES

After studying this chapter, participating in a structured learning environment, and completing assigned assessments, you will be able to:

- Describe the types of multimedia tools available for the fire and emergency services instructor. (**NFPA 1041: 4.3.3, 4.4.2**, pp 143–148)
- Describe the advantages and limitations of audiovisual equipment and other teaching aids. (**NFPA 1041: 4.4.2**, pp 140–149)
- Describe how to use multimedia tools. (**NFPA 1041: 4.4.5**, pp 143–149)
- Describe when to use multimedia tools in a presentation. (**NFPA 1041: 4.4.2**, pp 143–149)
- Describe how to maintain instructional technology tools. (**NFPA 1041: 4.4.5**, p 149)

SKILLS OBJECTIVES

After studying this chapter, participating in a structured learning environment, and completing assigned assessments, you will be able to:

- Demonstrate how to use multimedia tools during a classroom presentation. (**NFPA 1041: 4.4.5**, pp 143–149)
- Demonstrate how to maintain instructional technology tools. (**NFPA 1041: 4.4.5**, p 149)

You Are the Fire and Emergency Services Instructor

You are a relatively new instructor but have already learned that the methods of instruction used can influence students' retention of material and participation in class. In reviewing the training calendar for the next training period, you notice a variety of instructional opportunities in which you can participate. One class will include primarily young fire fighters who are in the early stages of the fire academy; another class will consist of a mix of new and experienced members. Your experience with technology-based instruction is sound, and you contemplate the methods that might be used to deliver these classes. You can foresee the use of blended learning where the students complete some of the coursework online and other parts in traditional environments.

1. Which type of technology-based instruction is the younger generation of fire fighters accustomed to in their education so far?
2. To which traditional methods of instruction have the experienced members become accustomed?
3. How does a blended learning approach maximize your ability to share information with your students? What are the downfalls of this approach?

Introduction

The use of training aids has been part of the training process, regardless of the discipline, since the beginning of humankind. Ancient warriors learned how to fight with practice swords and shields before they used real ones; commanders would draw scenarios in the sand while trainees would gather around to observe. Table-top simulators were used to run mock battles while commanders looked on and learned what was to happen before ever stepping foot on the battlefield. All of these activities are forms of training aids to assist the instructor in training and the students in learning.

The training aids we use in the fire service have evolved from basic chalkboards and erasers to a presentation platform such as the most commonly used ones like PowerPoint (PPT), Prezi, Apple Keynote, and computer simulations run in a classroom or over the internet. You would be hard pressed to participate in a lecture today without some type of presentation management or presentation delivery system.

Although training aids are fundamental in assisting the instructor in the learning process, they are merely "aids" to help the instructor impart the knowledge the fire fighter needs to know and understand. As an instructor, it is your responsibility to learn how and when to use these tools during your presentations and, when necessary, to be able to troubleshoot or repair them in the field. The key is to remember that these tools are there to "assist" you during your presentation—but ultimately, you are the instructor, and the students learn from you.

Technology-Based Instruction

One of the most dynamic and fast-changing concepts in education and training is **technology-based instruction (TBI)**. TBI may also be called other names, such as *e-instruction*, *internet-based instruction*, or *distance learning*. In general, TBI is defined as presenting training and education using the internet or a cloud-based file management system from a student would download files for their coursework. As is true for traditional methods of instruction, there are both advantages and disadvantages to TBI. TBI tends to be a student-centered instructional method because in most cases students can control the pace, the rate of delivery, and even the time at which they view lessons and information. This flexibility is highly desirable to many busy adults, fire fighters and emergency medical services (EMS) providers included. Learning should be student-centered, and when TBI is used, each student can adapt the material being presented to their individual style. Research also supports the student-centered nature of TBI as being more effective, in that students can repeat lesson areas they are struggling with, while instructors enjoy the ability to monitor each student's participation and progress more closely.

Consider a traditional slide presentation given by even the most dynamic instructor. Some students may disengage from the learning process, while other, more engaged and participatory students carry the load in answering questions and giving examples. Unless the instructor carefully engages and involves everyone, some students could sit through an entire presentation and receive a passing grade simply by attending the session, without truly participating in it. Consider this example: The instructor displays a slide of a house fire. The instructor asks for a student to perform a size-up and initial radio report. In a class of 25 students in a typical classroom-based delivery, chances are that only a few students will be able to participate in answering the question. Using TBI, the instructor can set up a system that shows the same slide, but then requires all students to perform the size-up and initial radio report in a narrative example. The TBI method will certainly involve all students, whereas the more traditional approach may not.

Distance Learning

Distance learning simply consists of instruction "a distance away." A student who may be located at home or in a remote classroom receives instruction and assignments from a training center or college/university. Distance learning can even take place without an instructor being present. Distance learning programs can be as simple as a package of printed materials sent through the mail, or as complex as Flash animation presented during a video conference. Today, the majority of distance learning is accomplished through a combination of reading assignments, online activities and assessments, video conferencing, video presentation, testing with proctors, and written assignments. Student evaluations are processed through an instructor.

Computer-Based Training and Learning Management Systems

Computer-based training (CBT) software provides a virtual course environment with tools for course preparation, delivery, and management. With this software, you have the tools to prepare course materials and efficiently manage day-to-day teaching tasks. Many CBT programs offer features that allow you to facilitate collaborative learning, personalize content based on students' unique needs, and positively affect learning outcomes. CBT is not limited to students in colleges and universities; it has also changed the way in which private industry and public safety agencies train their staff members.

CBT can be a powerful way of teaching. It can inform, illustrate, test, and demonstrate complex concepts simply. For example, students can view Flash animations with a voiceover that explains how a fire pump works internally. They can also click on parts of the fire pump image to see labels or learn more details. If real-world experience is desired, some systems have built-in simulators to enable students to experiment with key concepts while using different parameters. This allows students to benefit from real-world learning while ensuring that they can make mistakes without endangering personnel or equipment.

E-learning (short for "electronic learning") is a form of computer-based training—one that has enjoyed increased popularity and prevalence in recent years. Web-based learning management systems are at the heart of the e-learning experience. The following terms will help you understand the systems that support CBT:

Learning management system (LMS) A learning management system is a web-based software application that allows online courseware and content to be delivered to learners, that also includes classroom administration tools such as activity tracking, grades, communications, and calendars. An LMS is sometimes also referred to as a virtual learning environment (VLE) or learning course management system (LCMS).

Synchronous learning Synchronous learning happens when learners are all engaged in or receiving educational content simultaneously. An example might be a live webcast, webinar, or online chat session.

Asynchronous learning Asynchronous learning simply means that all learners are not consuming content at the same time. In a traditional face-to-face classroom, all learners would hear a lecture simultaneously. In an asynchronous learning environment, however, the same learners might consume educational content at different times, usually at their own pace, provided they adhere to established submission deadlines set by the instructor.

Hybrid learning Sometimes referred to as "blended" or "distributed" learning, hybrid learning occurs when some content is available for completion online and some learning requires face-to-face instruction or demonstration.

Courseware Courseware is any educational content that is delivered via a computer.

Flipped classroom An instructional approach that reverses or "flips" the standard learning environment by delivering online content for self-study and reserving the physical classroom for mentored practice that traditionally would have been assigned as homework. The in-person practice sessions allow for more direct application of class content by the student with instructor involvement versus a traditional homework assignment the student would do alone.

Virtual classroom A virtual classroom is a digital environment where content can be posted and shared, and where instructors can create quizzes and assignments to be completed and tracked online via an internet-connected computer.

Webinar An online meeting, the word *webinar* is the portmanteau of "web" (denoting the online component) and "seminar." These meetings occur in real time and usually allow for participants to share their desktop screens, web browsers, and documents as the meeting is occurring.

Social learning Social learning is an informal method of learning using technologies that enable collaborative content creation. Examples include blogs, social media (e.g., Twitter, Facebook), collaborative discussions, and wikis.

Instructor-led training (ILT) In the world of e-learning, ILT usually refers to a scenario in which a human instructor facilitates both the in-person sections and the online component of the course. Instructors usually set deadlines for submission, create quizzes and assignments, and track student progress.

Self-directed study Prepackaged learning modules can be designed to allow learners to engage in self-directed study—to stop and start as they desire, progress to completion of the module, and submit a final score to determine whether they passed or failed the module, all without an instructor's involvement. An example would be the online Incident Command System (ICS) courses freely available from the Federal Emergency Management Agency's (FEMA's) Emergency Management Institute.

The popularity of e-learning has exploded in the past few years. In fact, many colleges and universities have doubled or tripled their courses offered via the web. All degree levels can now be completed over the internet, from Associate to Doctoral, in many fire and emergency service disciplines. Recognizing this fact, many students now expect courses to be offered in this manner. Colleges, universities, fire departments, and other training organizations are all considering how best to integrate e-learning into the instructional experience.

Of course, no technology can ever replace the wisdom and experience of a seasoned fire and emergency services instructor. E-learning is not a threat to instructors, but rather a tool that can be used to address challenges posed by live training. For example, in the future, virtual reality simulators could be used instead of live burns in the early stages of training. The skill will eventually need to be performed to be truly learned, but work with simulators can increase students' comfort level with the scenarios before encountering them with all dangers present.

An LMS is a web-based software application that acts as both a digital content warehouse and a classroom management tool. Learning objects (content) reside within the LMS and are accessible to any member of a course who has internet access. LMS platforms allow instructors to upload (and thereby save and store) documents into their online classroom and then link those resources in a meaningful way for learners to consume. In this regard, the LMS acts like a repository for your content.

Uploading documents to a website, however, hardly provides the entire solution with regard to managing an online classroom. Just as you would do in a traditional classroom, as the instructor, you need to track *how well* your e-learning students are performing, *what* they are consuming, and *whether* relevant objectives have been met. That is where the classroom management piece of an LMS comes into play. **FIGURE 6-1** shows possible course management tools.

Although an LMS can be used to facilitate fully online learning, in the context of fire service instruction it is critical that students demonstrate comprehension of topics as well as a capability to perform critical tasks. Given this requirement, the hybrid learning approach is preferable.

When you consider the difficulties facing today's instructor—shrinking budgets, departments located at a geographical distance from the nearest training facility, increased hours and curriculum requirements, and the composition of the fire service (70 percent volunteer, meaning they have other primary responsibilities)—a compelling argument for the inclusion of technology begins to emerge.

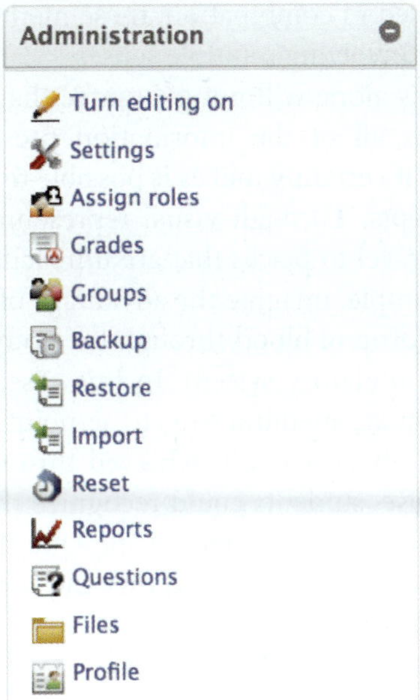

FIGURE 6-1 Course management tools.

An LMS is *not* a replacement for the human instructor, hands-on evolutions, or face-to-face interactions. In the world of public safety education, the LMS should be seen as an extension of the instructor—a tool to augment what you are already doing in the classroom, which is why the concept of hybrid learning is both viable and appealing. It represents an alternative to totally internet/computer-based training. It takes the best parts of the learning environment and partners them with computer-based elements so that the student has greater flexibility in completing assignments. Texts, assignments, and exercises can be completed online, and discussion and hands-on learning can be completed in the classroom. This creative alternative is useful in attempting to meet the needs of both the student and the fire service instructor. It can be difficult for any fire fighter—not just volunteers—to be in a classroom at the same time, 5 days per week.

Multimedia Applications in Instruction

A key element in most presentations is the use of a multimedia tool in some form, ranging from handouts to slide presentations. Using multimedia tools enhances the learning process for students and can make your job easier (**FIGURE 6-2**). At the same time, multimedia tools can be a distraction if they are poorly developed or used improperly. Knowing how to use multimedia tools effectively is just as important as knowing the lesson plan. When preparing to give a presentation, part of your efforts should focus on reviewing the instructional technology tools of the lesson plan.

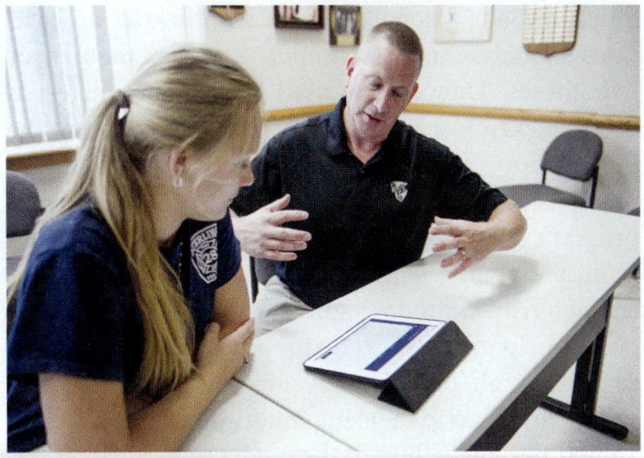

FIGURE 6-2 When used appropriately, multimedia tools enhance the learning process.

Understanding Multimedia Tools

Multimedia tools and applications come in a variety of types and are intended for a variety of uses. There are PowerPoint and Keynote software programs; videos; CBT programs; internet-based training; distance learning; National Fire Academy training programs; tablet computers; digital audio players; and smart phones. It might seem that it would be impossible to choose from such an abundance of multimedia tools, but each fills a specific niche based on the type of learning that is to take place.

Learn how to use multimedia tools before you apply them in the learning environment. It may take a fair amount of preparation to master the tools you choose to make your presentation. Sometimes use is as simple as pressing the "play" button; at other times it is as complicated as learning a whole new "language" or software program or transitioning among various types of media. As an instructor, it is up to you to learn how to use these tools correctly and incorporate them smoothly into your presentation skills.

COMPANY-LEVEL INSTRUCTOR TIP

Don't fall into the trap of blaming a poor presentation on your inability to use the equipment, and don't depend on multimedia tools to instruct for you. Practice with these tools to make them an effective medium that enhances your existing instructional skills.

When to Use Multimedia Presentations

Multimedia presentations enhance student learning by allowing students to see, hear, and (in some cases) touch the educational content. Multimedia applications should be used to simplify complex theories or hypotheses. They can be used to reinforce materials through exercises, pictures, or words that relate to the information you are presenting. They can summarize previously integrated material for use in the current program so that you do not waste a lot of time covering prerequisites. In combination with the learner characteristics of today's students, multimedia presentations help maintain students' interest.

Despite all of these advantages, there are occasional drawbacks to using multimedia in training. Sometimes, the failure of the media to perform as designed can put the user at a loss. As an instructor, you must be versatile enough to be able to overcome these glitches and not let failure impede what you are trying to present. If a technology failure does happen, then you must have a plan B.

One issue facing instructors is determining what type of multimedia to use and when it is appropriate to use. Multimedia resources are not *always* needed. The delivery format must be appropriate for the audience and appropriate to the nature of the content being presented.

The learning environment has long been known as a place where networking and information combine to create the learning experience. This milieu allows the students to learn from one another as well as from the instructor and the materials presented. At its best, this environment tends to encourage students to learn for themselves. Think of the saying, "You can lead a horse to water, but you cannot make it drink." The same is true for students: You can present all the material in the world, but if students do not want to learn, they won't. Multimedia tools try to break down the resistance to learning by engaging the student.

Multimedia should be used whenever its application makes it easier for students to grasp the material. It does not matter if the application means bringing the emergency incident into the classroom, demonstrating a nonthreatening environment, exemplifying safety concerns, or using simulation or distance education. The only reason to use multimedia tools is to help students learn.

Selecting the right media application is critical. When used as an instructional aid, the right tool allows you to clarify the information you present to students. Essentially, the various multimedia features organize the way in which students receive the material. Diagrams, flowcharts, and graphics impart information that can be retained by students who are visual learners. The lecture or audio cues assist auditory learners. Used in combination, these methods engage students by involving multiple senses.

Emphasis alone will not guarantee that every student retains all of the information presented in a course, but it certainly makes it possible to clarify difficult concepts. Through visual representations, students can travel to places that are unreachable in real life. For example, imagine the advantage of being able to follow a drop of blood through the body to understand the circulatory system. In this case, words are not an adequate medium to get the point across, yet the desired effect is easily achieved through simulation. Likewise, students could recognize the different ways that heat is transferred by allowing them to feel the heat from a light bulb to clarify the concept of radiant heat transfer.

Multimedia Presentations: Best Practices

During the course of your career, you will find that the use of multimedia tools can greatly enhance your ability to convey your message. But use of technology can also come with some drawbacks. To minimize the potential pitfalls, consider these issues when using multimedia tools:

- Do not read from the slides. All instructors make this mistake at one time or another. Most slides are outlines of the lesson plan and serve to emphasize critical points. The only time it is acceptable to read from the slide is if you are reading a quote, legal definition, standard operating procedure, or legal statement.
- Select the appropriate level of lighting for the type of multimedia equipment you are using. If you want students to take notes during the presentation, the room must be dark enough to see the slides, yet light enough to write.
- There is an art to transitioning from the lecture to the multimedia technology—and practice makes perfect.
- When lecturing with slides being projected behind you, do not stand in front of the projection screen. It is difficult for students to see what you are talking about if you are in the way.
- Always have your multimedia equipment set up before class and the media queued. Video or audio recordings should be ready to go at the touch of a button.
- If an internet connection is required, test it for access, and confirm that it can adequately handle the media in your presentation.

- Always have a backup plan. What if you have problems with the computer or projector? Always have a plan B.

Technology and Software

Presentation Programs

Presentation programs include a variety of software programs developed by software vendors. Products such as PowerPoint, Keynote, Prezi, SlideDog, and Google Slides are software programs that are used in creating portable presentations for business, education, and government. Each presentation program has its own unique features and benefits that you can use to enhance your instruction. Some are easier to use than others; some allow for greater flexibility. For the purposes of this chapter, we refer to presentation programs with the acronym PPT, reflecting the fact that, at this time, most fire departments use the PowerPoint program (**FIGURE 6-3**). If you use another software program, the basic style rules are still relevant.

The ability to embed video and audio clips into your presentation is one advantage of using PPT, and it adds a new layer of sophistication and professionalism to your presentation. A disadvantage is the potential for over-reliance on technology as part of your instruction. If your computer doesn't work or problems crop up between the computer and projector, then you cannot use the presentation. If your instruction relies solely on your slides and the technology fails, then you may have to reschedule your presentation if you do not have backup technology available.

Another disadvantage associated with these kinds of presentations is the overload factor. Some slide presentation creators tend to include too much information, too many sounds, and too many visual effects on their slides. Keep your presentation simple and concise for greatest effect.

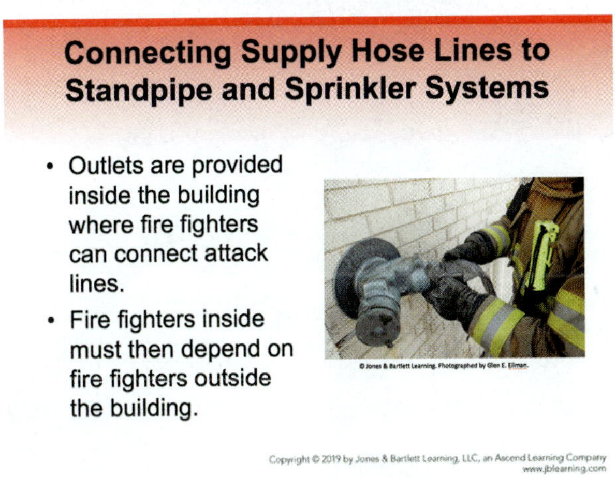

FIGURE 6-3 A sample PowerPoint slide.
© Jones & Bartlett Learning.

Suggestions for Uses of Slides

If you plan to use slides to illustrate or otherwise support a lecture, remember that lecture notes displayed on your slides play a different role in the lecture than handwritten lecture notes that only you can see. Don't try to make them play the same role, or you may find students reading your slides instead of listening to you.

You can use slides in the lecture to list the major points of your presentation. Several major points might stay on the screen as you develop each of them in turn, providing a way for students to place each point within the larger context. Again, one slide with several terms may remain on the screen for some time, allowing you to refer to each term as you introduce it.

In addition, slides can be used to create prompts for group work, being projected for all groups to see as the students do their work. This approach helps students move from one stage to the next when you manually change the slide or through the use of a timer built into the slide presentation. Slides can also contain breakouts that indicate how each group will handle different aspects of a scenario.

Always give credit where credit is due. If materials came from a journal or other publication, remember to credit the authors. Regardless of how you found the material, how long ago the information was developed, and whether you had to obtain permission, give credit to its author. This will assist you in presenting credible and defendable information.

Presentation-Ready Programs

Prepackaged software programs are a valuable resource when you are planning your instruction. Educational publishers provide instructors with presentation-ready programs for use on computers at the local level. This material includes slide presentations, testbanks, handouts, and other course-specific material that will assist the instructor. Thanks to these programs, you do not need to spend valuable preparation time developing your own presentation; instead, you can simply use the professionally developed materials. Of course, you must still familiarize yourself with the presentation before class, rather than seeing it for the first time in front of the class. Professionally developed presentations are intended to be dynamic instructional tools, used to enhance students' learning experience, but will never replace the experienced instructor. No presentation-ready programs should truly be considered ready-to-use. Instead, instructors must review materials ahead of time and adapt them to the students who will use them. Some of the most detailed presentations will customize stock backgrounds with department logos and department scenes to make the material more relevant to the students.

Data Projectors

Liquid crystal display (LCD) projectors and digital light processor (DLP) projectors (also known more simply as data projectors) are used with video players, computers, and visual projectors to project documents, images, and motion pictures so that a group of students can easily view the material simultaneously. Data projectors can present material on screens ranging in size from 2 ft (0.6 m) wide to 30 ft (9.1 m) wide (**FIGURE 6-4**). Important features to consider when selecting a data projector are the ability to show videos directly, audio capabilities, screen resolution, and the brightness of light emitted by the projector (measured in lumens). You should also consider the price of the equipment and the price and lifespan of the bulb.

The size of a data projector is compact, so unless mounted to a wall, it can be moved from among facilities with little effort. The various pros and cons should be examined before purchasing a data projector. As with an overhead projector, having an extra bulb available is a good idea.

You should also consider the issues that can arise in the classroom when you use a data projector. First, make sure that the cables match the output of the computer and the input of the projector, such as VGA, HDMI, or DVI. Also, make sure that the cables are long enough, because short cables will hinder your setup and use of the projector. It is still common to find projectors whose inputs do not work with more current technology, so make sure you have an adapter that works with your equipment.

You must learn the proper start-up procedures for your data projector. Generally, the data projector must be connected to the computer before the computer is turned on. Learn how to get the computer to send its output to the data projector. Some computers will automatically recognize the data projector device, but often you must press a control-function key to activate the connection. Given these caveats, always test your presentation before class.

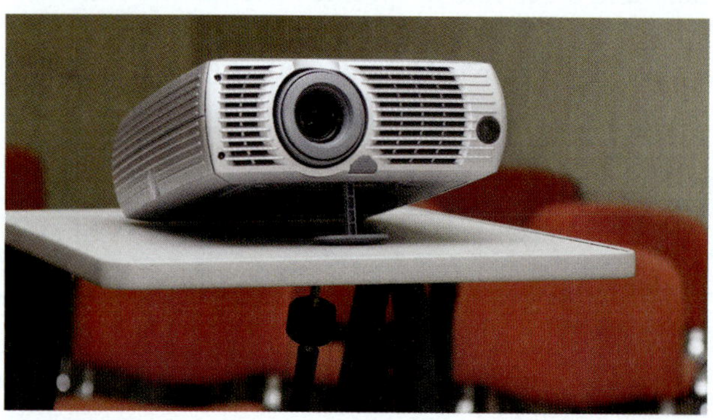

FIGURE 6-4 A data projector can enhance your presentation.

Digital Audio Players and Portable Media Devices

Digital audio players, such as the iPod, are creating a new horizon for digital recording. In the past, the digital audio player was used to download music and music videos. Through the creative work of many instructors, digital audio players are becoming a mainstream technology for students at most universities. These devices are so compact that students can carry them easily and download lectures or pictures that can be reviewed while outside of class (**FIGURE 6-5**).

Some digital audio players allow students to use an audio record feature. Several media outlets are actively engaged in offering downloads, or podcasts, to these

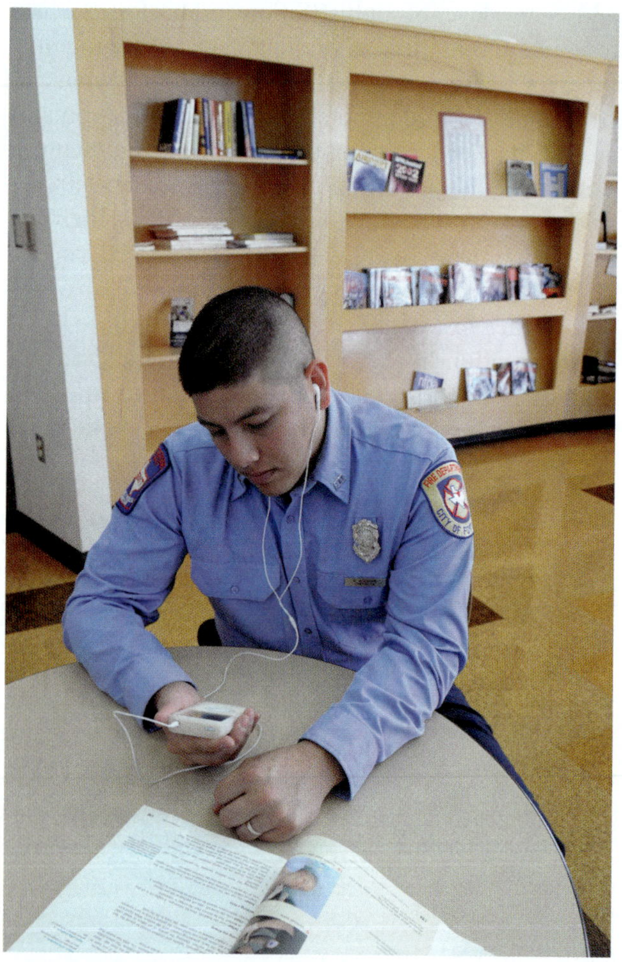

FIGURE 6-5 Digital audio players allow students to listen to lectures and view images outside the classroom.

devices featuring such notable fire service figures as Chief Billy Goldfeder.

Students may also find that digital audio players allow them to complete class assignments. In some courses, students may be able to use desktop video editing software to create and edit projects for course assignments. The results can be uploaded to the training center's computer system for presentation, or content playback can occur immediately via classroom instructional technology equipment. Digital audio player devices can store not only images and audio, but also entire presentations created in PowerPoint, word processing documents, or files created with other software.

As an instructor, you can benefit greatly from these devices. The possibilities for their use are endless: classroom performance and practice, group discussions, field interviews, interviews with content experts, classroom lectures, and discussions or presentations. The possibility of a podcast replacing a webcast allows you to make the materials for a class more widely available, too.

As with other technologies, we must wait to see which benefits this technology will ultimately yield. As more digital systems become available and their costs are driven lower by greater demand, fire service instruction may be transformed from a system of learning confined to a specific locale to one where information can be obtained "on the fly." As technology adapts, improves, and advances, new opportunities will be found to augment educational media.

Tablet Computers

A tablet is a wireless portable computer with a touch screen that generally is smaller than a notebook computer but larger than a smart phone (**FIGURE 6-6**).

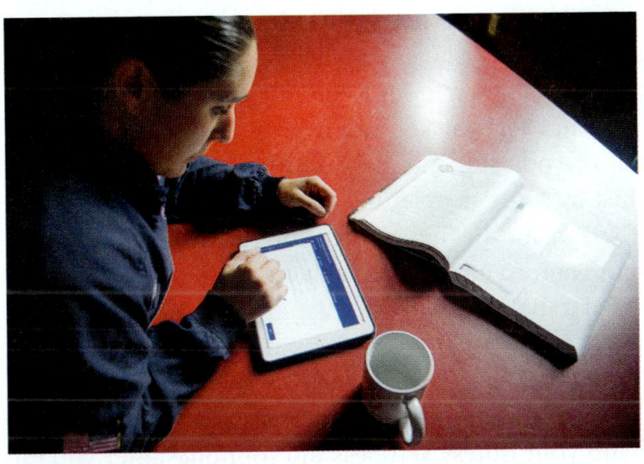

FIGURE 6-6 Students can use tablet devices to take notes, complete assignments and e-mail them to the instructor, view course material, and conduct research during class.

These devices either include the keyboard on the screen or allow an external keyboard to be attached to the device. Such computers offer a wide range of capabilities and features such as cameras, phones, e-books, videoconferencing, and GPS satellite navigation. Many fire and EMS agencies have adopted these devices for fire inspections, preplanning activities, and gathering information during a medical emergency. Students can use these devices to take notes, complete assignments and e-mail them to the instructor, view course material, and conduct research during class. In some instances, instructors may send the students assignments by e-mail, which are then completed and returned via the tablet. An emerging trend in many college and academic programs is to issue tablet computers to their students that come preloaded with textbooks, online course materials, and other interactivities ready to use. Many instructors use tablets during lectures that connect to their cloud storage to access their developed media presentations.

Interactive Boards

An interactive board, typically mounted on the wall, uses touch detection for user input, much in the same way a personal computer does with a mouse (**FIGURE 6-7**). A projector is used to display a computer's video output on the interactive board, which then acts as a large touch screen. Interactive boards come with pens that allow the instructor to use "digital ink" to write on the board during a presentation. While using the system, a computer records the material, which can be saved and reviewed at a later time or emailed to students.

Dry-Erase Boards and Easel Pads

Low-tech, simple, and usually readily accessible, dry-erase boards (whiteboards) and easel pads remain

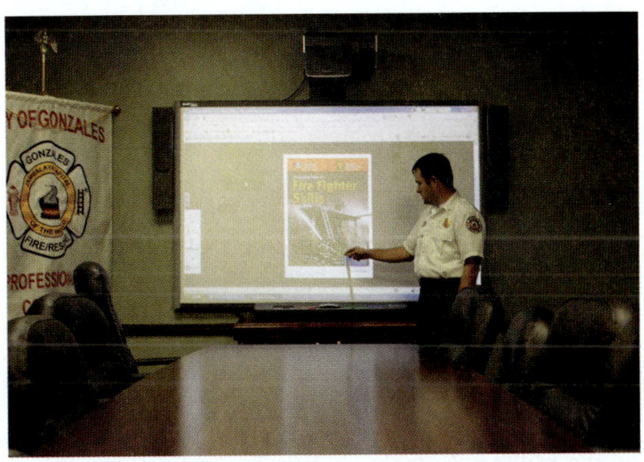

FIGURE 6-7 SMART Board® is brand of an interactive board that uses touch detection for user input.

a common and practical way to illustrate critical points in the learning environment.

Dry-erase boards use special markers. When using dry-erase markers, do not confuse them with permanent markers. Using a permanent marker on a dry-erase board will damage the whiteboard, so make sure you use the correct marker.

The easel pad can be developed before, during, or after a presentation, thereby becoming a flexible learning device. The greatest advantage to the easel pad is its flexible use in small-group settings. Members of each group can write their thoughts and ideas in response to the activity and post them for others to see, review, and discuss. Each group can write its responses to activities and post them for later discussion. The pads can also be used for later discussion to review information or to refer back to while clarifying a point or concept. Some brands provide a sticky side so that sheets in the pad can be torn off and stuck to a wall or other object to prevent the instructor from having to flip back and forth through the pages in the pad.

Virtual Reality and Simulation

Virtual reality devices allow students to interact with a computer-simulated environment. By displaying images either on a computer screen or via a headset, the goal is to immerse the student in an environment that can be controlled by the student and the programmer. This sensory experience is designed to force feedback from the student as he or she interacts with the environment. Although this technology is, in essence, a simulation, the visual, auditory, and tactile sensations create an artificial world wherein the student can make mistakes without causing injury.

The virtual environment can be designed to mimic a real-world scenario such as a burning grocery store, or it can be set up to resemble a video game. This technology is developing daily by quantum leaps, and it may become the standard means of training in the near future. Unfortunately, the currently available technology does not achieve the realistic look and feel instructors want for their students. In the future, as faster processors and more cost-effective systems emerge, instructors may be able to apply the best possible technology for the benefit of their students.

Like virtual reality systems, simulators allow students to interact safely with hazards in a controlled environment. This practical application was developed by the military to train soldiers for tactical operations during peacetime. Students today have the benefit of growing up with simplified simulators. With the advent of popular video games, many students are accustomed to being immersed in an imaginary world. Today, gaming has taken on new dimensions, as newer systems mimic the movements of the operator to accomplish a mission in the game. Simulations—no matter how simple or complex—allow students to be challenged and to learn from their mistakes.

Simulations have been developed both commercially and noncommercially. Commercially available simulators provide emergency responders with the opportunity to develop skills in command, control, coordination, and communications. Incidents faced in simulations may include structure and vehicle fire responses, aircraft accidents, terrorist acts, hazardous materials spills, fires, and natural disasters, with the programs being designed to test and validate students' understanding of emergency operations.

While this educational activity is not the same as live fire training, after a simulation the student walks away with concepts that can be applied and internalized long before he or she faces a live fire event. As with an actual live fire, replication of exact circumstances is difficult at best, yet with the simulator the same conditions can be repeated until the outcomes are acceptable. Simulators are no substitute for live fire training, of course.

Online certification courses such as Blue Card Hazard Zone Management use simulations for both instruction and evaluation purposes. Directed and distance learning opportunities can capture training opportunities with this technology and bring realism to a learning environment.

Audio Systems

Depending on the class size and the arrangement of the classroom, a microphone and audio system may be needed. Although this technology is not new, it is often misunderstood. Remember who your audience is. Can everyone see and hear your presentation? Do all of your students have the same hearing abilities? Just as some people don't like to wear bifocals when their vision begins to deteriorate with age, some do not want to admit that their hearing just isn't what it used to be.

When deciding which kind of audio system you will use, keep your presentation style in mind. Do you move around a lot, or do you stay at the podium with your notes? Wireless microphones offer you the most freedom to move around the classroom, but they have some problems, too. Wireless systems may have an issue with frequency usage, such that you might hear voices broadcast that are not supposed to be part of your program. Wireless microphones may also have limitations in terms of how far the microphone can be from the remote receiver and still operate properly.

The greatest limitation for wired systems relates to the cable. Is it long enough for you to move around effectively? Some wired microphones are permanently attached to the podium, in which case you lose the freedom to move around the classroom. Another disadvantage of wired systems is the potential for mishap if your feet become entangled in the wire.

Maintaining Technology

With any technology, maintaining its quality is an important consideration. Some vendors charge an additional fee to repair or replace damaged materials. When purchasing multimedia tools, get the maintenance contract in writing and understand what the contract covers in terms of repair and maintenance. Although this contract may seem to be just an additional step or an extra cost, it can pay dividends when you need it. Remember—like everyone else, fire fighters can and do break things.

Some multimedia products require less maintenance than others. A dry-erase board will not get a computer virus—but it also cannot transition from one slide to the next at the touch of a button. Be aware of the trade-offs between high technology and good traditional methods. You need to decide based on several factors (e.g., cost, ease in transportation, audience) what is appropriate for your event or presentation.

Instructional technology tools, like any other equipment, needs to be kept clean and in good order so that it will work when you need it. The simplest and safest way to make sure you are cleaning equipment properly is to follow the manufacturer's recommended maintenance practices, for any device. Most up-to-date equipment will simply need an occasional lens cleaning and dusting near the fan area to ensure reliable operation. Inspect cable connections regularly since they can become bent or frayed quite easily.

Another important maintenance item is to make sure your device has the latest software, as this factor can affect its ability to "talk" with other devices.

If your organization is considering building a training room or training center, consult with a reputable company with technical expertise in sound, lighting, and visual effects to develop an optimal and comfortable training environment. Many departments will build a new training room or space and have to go back later, at an increased cost, and retrofit sound systems, lighting, or audiovisual products because they were unaware of the deficiencies they would later experience.

Troubleshooting Common Multimedia Problems

Many things can go wrong when using multimedia applications. As a consequence, instructors need to know and practice a few alternatives in case problems crop up with this technology. **TABLE 6-1** can assist with some of the more common problems. The simplest things that can go wrong can often be easily fixed by taking a deep breath and thinking about the problem and potential solutions. Take the time to work with your equipment and know its limitations. Be prepared for the possibility that something may go wrong. Remember, always have a plan B.

Sometimes solving a problem is not as easy as referring to a simple chart. That is, sometimes you need to be able to diagnose the problem and verbalize it. This step is necessary to use the *help* files contained within most software programs. To find these files, look at the menu bar at the top of your screen. It typically lists options such as File, Edit, and View; at the very end of that list is Help. You can either double-click on the word Help or press the Alt and H keys simultaneously to open this script. Pressing the F1 key also brings up the help menu.

TABLE 6-1 Common Troubleshooting Procedures

Try each "solution" in order. There is no need to continue down the list if the first step solves your problem. If your problem remains unsolved, you may need more expert assistance.

Symptom	Solution
Presentation projector does not turn on/off	1. Point the remote directly at the projector and try again. 2. The remote may need new batteries.
No audio from podium	1. Make sure the audio system is turned on. 2. Make sure the microphone is turned on.
No audio from wireless microphone	1. Make sure the audio system is turned on. 2. Make sure the body pack is turned on. 3. The microphone may need new batteries.
No audio from DVD or computer	1. Check the volume controls to make sure they are not turned down. 2. Make sure the audio system is turned on. 3. Make sure connections are made to the audio output on the device and the input on the audio system.
No image from computer/laptop	1. Check that the correct input source has been selected. 2. Make sure the computer has not been turned off. 3. Change the video output from the computer (press the Alt and F5 keys simultaneously or other Alt Function keys, depending on the computer).
Projector light will not come on	1. If you hear a fan, make sure the lens cover is off. 2. If you hear a fan and the lens cover is off, you may need to replace the bulb.
Computer will not read media	1. Make sure the computer has the proper software needed for the media to work properly.

Training BULLETIN

JONES & BARTLETT FIRE DISTRICT
TRAINING DIVISION
5 Wall Street, Burlington, MA, 01803
Phone 978-443-5000 Fax 978-443-8000

Instant Applications: Technology in Training

Drill Assignment

Apply the chapter content to your department's operation, training division, and your personal experiences to complete the following questions and activities.

Objective

Upon completion of the instant applications, fire and emergency services instructor students will exhibit decision making and application of job performance requirements of the instructor using the text, class discussion, and their own personal experiences.

Suggested Drill Applications

1. Using the internet as your primary resource, research the best practices and recommendations for developing slide presentations. Using this information, develop a student handout outlining this information. In addition, take the information shared on the handout and develop a slide presentation for use in a classroom setting designed to introduce and familiarize students with PPT.
2. Select a current slide presentation and add additional graphics (photos, WordArt, illustrations) to better clarify or explain the topic of the original presentation.
3. Explore online fire incident simulator programs and determine the best of use of such technology, the cost of investing in the programs, and the ease of use of the respective programs.
4. Review the Incident Report for this chapter and be prepared to discuss your analysis of the incident from a training perspective and as an instructor who wishes to use the report as a training tool. Also discuss the technology options available to incorporate this Incident Report into a training session.

Incident Report: NIOSH Report F2001-38

Drill Assignment

Review the information in this incident report and prepare a practice presentation for class delivery at the direction of your instructor. Your presentation should include a summary of the incident facts and a review of the NFPA 1403 compliance and noncompliance findings. Use an outline to organize your thoughts. You may be evaluated on your communication skills during your presentation.

Lairdsville, New York—2001

The training evolution in Lairdsville, New York, involved a duplex that was to be razed. A search and rescue scenario with a rapid intervention crew (RIC) deployment was planned to simulate the entrapment of fire fighters on the second floor of one unit. For the purpose of the drill, the stairs to that unit would be considered impassable, so the RIC would have to enter from the other unit of the duplex and breach a second floor wall to reach the trapped fire fighters who were under light debris. Smoke from a burn barrel was used to obscure vision. The burn barrel was located in the back bedroom of the same unit as the trapped fire fighters, also on the second floor.

Neither of the two new fire fighters posing as victims had worn SCBA in fire conditions, and one (the deceased) was a brand new recruit fire fighter with no training. Both fire fighters wore full protective clothing and SCBA for this drill.

All of the crews assembled initially at the duplex. One engine was connected to a large water tanker on-site but no hose lines had been set up. A 1¾" (44.5 mm) hose line was supposed to be placed at the rear, with another at the front doors. An engine and heavy rescue were located off-site and would simulate a response to the scenario.

Safety officers were assigned and placed throughout both sides of the duplex. One officer was assigned to light the fire and place the new fire fighters in the front bedroom on the second floor. He was also instructed to guide the RIC if necessary. Another officer was assigned to a room on the second floor of the duplex unit, which the RIC was to enter first. He was assigned to guide the RIC if necessary, making sure they did not go through a wall opening that went to the outside. He was equipped with a 20-lb (9.1-kg) fire extinguisher. The 1st assistant chief was located on the first floor of the unit. The fire chief checked the scenario to make sure that accelerants were not used. He took command out front and the training was ready to begin.

The smoke barrel upstairs was ignited, but it was not creating the desired smoke conditions. Downstairs, the 1st assistant chief struck a road flare and ignited the foam mattress on a sleeper sofa that was located next to the open stairs (**FIGURE 6A**). The fire spread very rapidly across the ceiling, producing heavy smoke and flames, and flames quickly extended up the stairs and out the front windows.

The fire spread was so rapid that the officer in the adjoining unit could not enter to reach the new fire fighters, and he had to exit using a ground ladder. The 1st assistant chief exited the duplex and went to the rear exterior but he could not find a hose line. He then went to the pumper and pulled a 200' (61 m) preconnected hose line to the rear of the structure.

The fire fighter on the same floor as the trapped fire fighters had left his position to investigate the sound of another road flare being lit. Upon seeing the fire, he went back and reached the two new fire fighters. The flames were now entering the second floor windows. He led the

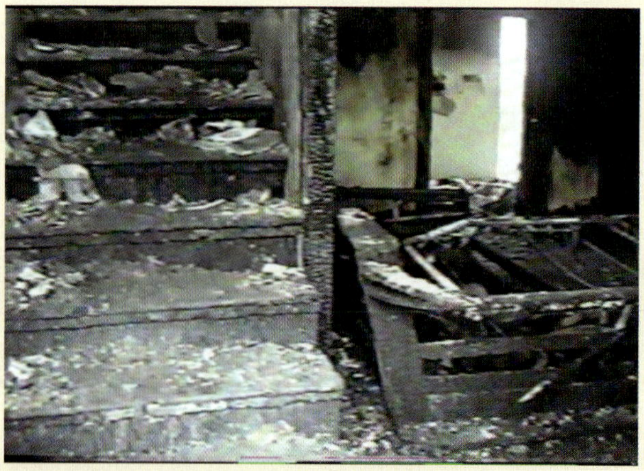

FIGURE 6-A A couch at the base of the stairs in the Lairdsville duplex.

From the NIOSH Fire Fighter Fatality Investigation and Prevention Program, Investigation Report F2001-38 NY.

new recruits to the stairwell, which was now fully engulfed in flames from the first floor. He lost his gloves and immediately burned his hands. At this point, he lost contact with the two recruit fire fighters. He was able to reach the back bedroom with heavy smoke and tenable heat. He searched for the boarded-up window and was able to break it open with his hands and jump from the second floor.

The 1st assistant chief advanced the hose line to the second floor, knocking down the fire. Arriving units were advised it was no longer a training and two RIC units were deployed to the second floor. One RIC forced entry through the involved unit's front door. One fire fighter was found and brought to the outside. The second RIC found the other fire fighter unresponsive. They removed him and transported him with advanced life support care to a local hospital, where he was later declared dead. The rescued fire fighter and the fire fighter who jumped from the window were both flown by EMS helicopters to a burn unit, due to the severity of their burn injuries.

During the ensuing investigation, the Lairdsville fire chief claimed he didn't know that a structure fire would be set as part of the training exercise, saying, "It was only supposed to be smoke." The 1st assistant chief was indicted and found guilty of criminally negligent homicide. He was sentenced to seventy-five days in jail and instructed to avoid contact with any fire department under a five-year term of probation. His attorney argued that the NFPA standard was not known by the department, and that it was the state's responsibility to distribute the guidelines to every volunteer fire fighter.

Postincident Analysis Lairdsville, New York

NFPA 1403 Noncompliant

- Students not sufficiently trained to meet job performance requirements (JPRs) for Fire Fighter I in NFPA 1001
- Debris from the structure used as fuel material
- Students acting as victims within the structure
- Deviation from the preburn plan
- Fire ignited without charged hose line present
- Exterior hose lines not in place
- Rapid Intervention Crew (RIC) not in place (NOTE: This is not a requirement of 1403, but is an OSHA requirement and is referenced in NFPA 1500, NFPA 1710, and NFPA 1720.)

After-Action REVIEW

IN SUMMARY

- Although training aids are fundamental in assisting the instructor in the learning process, remember that they are still simply aids, designed to help you impart the knowledge your students need to know and understand.
- One of the most dynamic and fast-changing concepts in education and training is technology-based instruction (TBI), also known as e-instruction, internet-based instruction, or distance learning.
- TBI is a good example of student-centered learning because course materials can be delivered in a variety of methods, providing each student with the resources that appeal to them.
- Computer-based training (CBT) software enables instructors to prepare course materials and efficiently manage day-to-day teaching tasks. Many CBT programs offer features that allow you to facilitate collaborative learning, personalize content based on students' unique needs, and positively affect learning outcomes.
- A learning management system (LMS) is a web-based software application that allows online courseware and content to be delivered to learners, that also includes classroom administration tools such as activity tracking, grades, communications, and calendars.
- Using multimedia tools enhances the learning process for students and can make the instructor's job easier. At the same time, multimedia tools can be a distraction if they are poorly developed or used improperly.
- Professionally developed presentations are intended to enhance students' learning experience, but do not replace the experienced instructor. Instructors must review materials ahead of time and adapt them to the students who will use them.
- Digital audio players have become a mainstream technology for students at most universities. Students can carry these devices easily and download lectures or pictures that can be reviewed outside of class.
- Virtual reality devices allow students to interact with a computer-simulated environment. The goal is to immerse the student in an environment that can be controlled by the student and the programmer.
- Like virtual reality systems, simulators allow students to interact safely with hazards in a controlled environment.
- As with any technology, maintaining the quality of multimedia tools is important.
- Multimedia tools should be used to simplify complex theories or to assist instructors in reinforcing their message through exercises or images.
- Selecting the right media application is critical. When used as an instructional aid, the right tool allows you to clarify the information you present to students.

KEY TERMS

Access Navigate for flashcards to test your key term knowledge.

Asynchronous learning An online course format in which the instructor provides material, lectures, tests, and assignments that can be accessed at any time. Students are given a time frame during which they need to connect to the course and complete assignments.

Courseware Any educational content that is delivered via a computer.

Flipped classroom An instructional approach that reverses or "flips" the standard learning environment by delivering online content for self-study and reserving the physical classroom for mentored practice that traditionally would have been assigned as homework.

Hybrid learning Learning environment in which some content is available for completion online and other learning requires face-to-face instruction or demonstration; sometimes referred to as "blended" or "distributed" learning.

Instructor-led training (ILT) A learning environment in which a human instructor facilitates both the in-person sections and the online components of coursework. Instructors usually set deadlines for submission, create quizzes and assignments, and track student progress.

Learning management system (LMS) A web-based software application that allows online courseware and content to be delivered to learners, that also includes classroom administration tools such as activity tracking, grades, communications, and calendars.

Self-directed study A learning environment in which learners can stop and start as they desire, progress to completion of a module, and submit a final score to determine whether they passed or failed the module, all without an instructor's involvement.

Social learning An informal method of learning using technologies that enable collaborative content creation. Examples include blogs, social media, collaborative discussions, and wikis.

Synchronous learning An online class format that requires students and instructors to be online at the same time. Lectures, discussions, and presentations occur at a specific hour and students must be online at that time to participate and receive credit for attendance.

Technology-based instruction (TBI) Training and education that uses the internet or a multimedia tool.

Virtual classroom A digital environment where content can be posted and shared, and where instructors can create quizzes and assignments to be completed and tracked online via an internet-connected computer.

Webinar An online meeting, occurring in real time, which usually allows for participants to share their desktop screens, web browsers, and documents live as the meeting is occurring.

REFERENCES

Capterra. 2017. "The Top 20 Most Popular LMS Software." https://www.capterra.com/learning-management-system-software/#infographic. Accessed August 17, 2018.

National Fire Protection Association. 2018. *NFPA 1403: Standard on Live Fire Training Evolutions*. Quincy, MA: National Fire Protection Association.

National Fire Protection Association. 2019. *NFPA 1041: Standard for Fire and Emergency Services Instructor Professional Qualifications*. Quincy, MA: National Fire Protection Association.

U.S. Department of Education. 2010. "Evaluation of Evidence-Based Practices in Online Learning: A Meta-Analysis and Review of Online Learning Studies." https://www2.ed.gov/rschstat/eval/tech/evidence-based-practices/finalreport.pdf. Accessed August 17, 2018.

CHAPTER PRESENTATION EXERCISE

Instructions: Your course instructor will assign individual or group discussions on the key points and teaching tips of this chapter. You or your group will review the chapter teachings and identify the major learning points from the chapter. You should be able to discuss the points, why they are important, and how and where they apply to your responsibilities at your level of instructor training.

REVIEW QUESTIONS

1. Describe the main benefits of using a learning management system.
2. How can the instructor minimize the amount of content that a student reads from slide, instead focusing the students on the instructor's message?
3. What elements make a strong multimedia or slide presentation? What elements detract from the quality or effectiveness of the presentation?

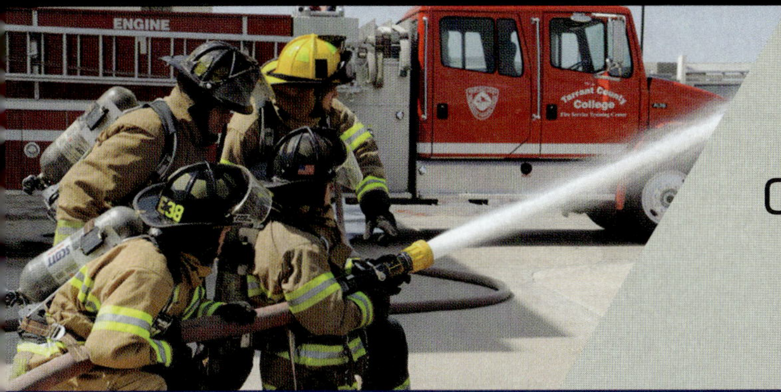

CHAPTER 7

Training Safety

NFPA 1041 JOB PERFORMANCE REQUIREMENTS

Note: An asterisk denotes that the 1041 standard contains further information in its annex section.

4.4.2 Organize the learning environment, given a facility and an assignment, so that lighting, distractions, climate control or weather, noise control, seating, audiovisual equipment, teaching aids, and safety are addressed.

(A) Requisite Knowledge.

Learning environment management and safety, advantages and limitations of audiovisual equipment and teaching aids, classroom arrangement, and methods and techniques of instruction.

(B) Requisite Skills.

Use of instructional media and teaching aids.

4.4.3 Present and adjust prepared lessons, given a prepared lesson plan that specifies the presentation method(s), so that the method(s) indicated in the plan are used and the stated objectives or learning outcomes are achieved, applicable safety standards and practices are followed, and risks are addressed.

(A)* Requisite Knowledge.

The laws and principles of learning, methods and techniques of instruction, lesson plan components and elements of the communication process, and lesson plan terminology and definitions; learner characteristics; student-centered learning principles; instructional technology tools; the impact of cultural differences on instructional delivery; safety rules, regulations, and practices; identification of training hazards; elements and limitations of distance learning; distance learning delivery methods; and the instructor's role in distance learning.

(B) Requisite Skills.

Oral communication techniques, methods and techniques of instruction, ability to adapt to changing circumstances, and utilization of lesson plans in an instructional setting.

4.4.5 Operate instructional technology tools and demonstration devices, given a learning environment and equipment, so that the equipment functions, the intended objectives are presented, and transitions between media and other parts of the presentation are accomplished.

(A) Requisite Knowledge.

Instructional technology tools, demonstration devices, and selection criteria.

(B) Requisite Skills.

Use of instructional technology tools, demonstration devices, transition techniques, cleaning, and field level maintenance.

KNOWLEDGE OBJECTIVES

After studying this chapter, participating in a structured learning environment, and completing assigned assessments, you will be able to:

- Discuss the relationship between training and fire fighter safety. (pp 158–159)
- Identify the life safety initiatives that relate to training activities. (p 159)

- Describe how to ensure safety in the learning environment. (**NFPA 1041: 4.4.2, 4.4.5**, pp 160–161)
- Describe how to promote and teach safety by example. (p 160)
- Describe the laws and standards pertaining to safety during live fire training. (pp 168–169)
- Discuss how to develop safety as part of your department's culture. (pp 169–170)
- Identify the legal considerations surrounding training safety. (**NFPA 1041: 4.4.2**, pp 170–173)

SKILLS OBJECTIVES

After studying this chapter, participating in a structured learning environment, and completing assigned assessments, you will be able to:

- Assess the level and use of personal protective equipment (PPE) necessary for hazards present during training. (p 161)
- Control safety hazards in the physical learning environment. (**NFPA 1041: 4.4.2**, pp 161; 167–168)
- Model safety conscious behaviors during lesson presentation. (**NFPA 1041: 4.4.3**, pp 160–162)
- Follow safety policies, practices, and procedures during training events. (**NFPA 1041: 4.4.3**, pp 162–167)

You Are the Fire and Emergency Services Instructor

Recently an instructor at a neighboring training facility was injured during a training drill that left the instructor unable to return to work. During the investigation, it was determined that the instructor had failed to wear all the correct personal protective equipment (PPE) and that this failure had caused his injuries to be more severe than if he had been wearing his PPE. This and other related incidents on a national level have prompted your training division staff to review your agency's policies and procedures—not only those dealing with PPE, but also those pertaining to instructor conduct during training.

1. As an instructor, how do you ensure the safety of fellow instructors working with you during training?
2. How do you ensure the safety of your students during training evolutions?
3. Which policies and guidelines do you have in place to ensure the safety of your fellow instructors and the students for whom you are responsible?

Introduction

Each year in the United States, countless fire fighters are injured and, on average, 10 fire fighters are killed during training-related activities. This trend has accelerated over the past few years and is a growing concern among fire service leaders. In addition to the higher number of injuries to students during training, the number of injuries to instructors who teach fire fighters has increased.

As an instructor, you must take measures to stop the preventable injuries and deaths that occur during training. Of course, for training to be effective, it has to be realistic and, therefore, a certain level of danger will exist

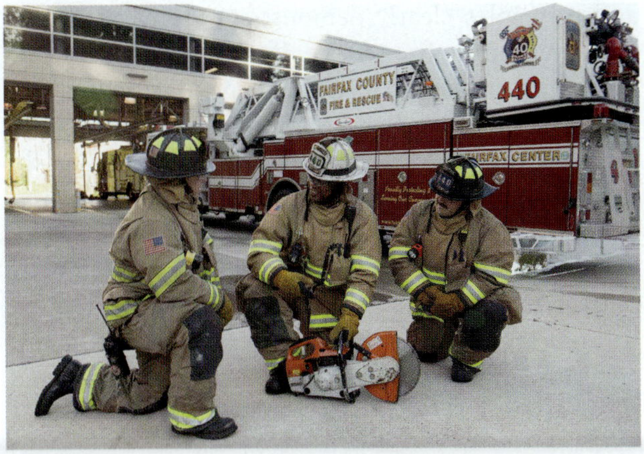

FIGURE 7-1 It is your responsibility to provide meaningful drills that allow fire fighters to apply their skills, knowledge, and abilities while keeping your students safe.

in all training events. Live fire training tops the list of high-risk training events, but this same high risk can be found in many other training activities (NIOSH, 2016).

You must always place students' safety ahead of any performance expectations for the training session. This mandate includes everything from assigning safety officers, to implementing rehabilitation protocols, to decreasing instructor–student ratios, to ensuring that enough trained eyes are watching out for the safety of all students. The standards, technology, and information needed to protect your personnel from training tragedies are readily available. You also need to apply relevant checklists, standards, and control measures to your training sessions correctly to keep your students safe. Fire fighters want meaningful drills that allow them to apply their skills, knowledge, and abilities. It is your responsibility to provide this training while keeping your students safe (**FIGURE 7-1**).

The 16 Fire Fighter Life Safety Initiatives

In 2004, the National Fallen Firefighters Foundation (NFFF) brought together fire service experts and leaders to discuss ways to slow the number of line-of-duty deaths (LODDs) experienced by the fire service. Their work culminated in 16 initiatives that were given to the fire service with the goal of reducing LODDs by 50 percent over a 10-year period (**TABLE 7-1**). These initiatives should provide both guidance and motivation to you while you are developing and conducting any training. They highlight the importance of training as a strategy that will help reduce the number of

TABLE 7-1 Sixteen Fire Fighter Life Safety Initiatives

1.	Define and advocate the need for a cultural change within the fire service relating to safety, incorporating leadership, management, supervision, accountability, and personal responsibility.
2.	Enhance the personal and organizational accountability for health and safety throughout the fire service.
3.	Focus greater attention on the integration of risk management with incident management at all levels, including strategic, tactical, and planning responsibilities.
4.	All fire fighters must be empowered to stop unsafe practices.
5.	Develop and implement national standards for training, qualifications, and certification (including regular recertification) that are equally applicable to all fire fighters based on the duties they are expected to perform.
6.	Develop and implement national medical and physical fitness standards that are equally applicable to all fire fighters, based on the duties they are expected to perform.
7.	Create a national research agenda and data collection system that relates to the initiatives.
8.	Utilize available technology wherever it can produce higher levels of health and safety.
9.	Thoroughly investigate all fire fighter fatalities, injuries, and near misses.
10.	Grant programs should support the implementation of safe practices and/or mandate safe practices as an eligibility requirement.
11.	National standards for emergency response policies and procedures should be developed and championed.
12.	National protocols for response to violent incidents should be developed and championed.
13.	Fire fighters and their families must have access to counseling and psychological support.
14.	Public education must receive more resources and be championed as a critical fire and life safety program.
15.	Advocacy must be strengthened for the enforcement of codes and the installation of home fire sprinklers.
16.	Safety must be a primary consideration in the design of apparatus and equipment.

fire fighter LODDs. As an instructor, you will be specifically charged with carrying out initiative 5, which states, "Develop and implement national standards for training, qualifications, and certification . . . that are equally applicable to all fire fighters based on the duties they are expected to perform." This initiative should be applied every time you instruct a course and in every drill-ground evolution you carry out.

Leading by Example

As an instructor, you will use many methods of delivery to teach. One of the most powerful methods is leading by example. Fire fighters, regardless of their rank, years on the job, or past experiences, will look to you and make mental notes on how the job *should* be done (**FIGURE 7-2**). As an instructor and mentor, you play an extremely influential role in determining the performance of your students. Given this responsibility, you must ensure that your own practices and principles clearly demonstrate the safety values employed in the fire service. If you do not correct an unsafe practice during training, your students will mistakenly believe that you condone the error. You must set a positive tone and embrace safety as the number-one priority of every lesson plan delivered. Both in the classroom and on the drill ground, use the controlled environment of the training arena to point out where things can go wrong in real-world applications. Prior to class, survey the classroom or teaching environment and correct any safety concerns that may exist.

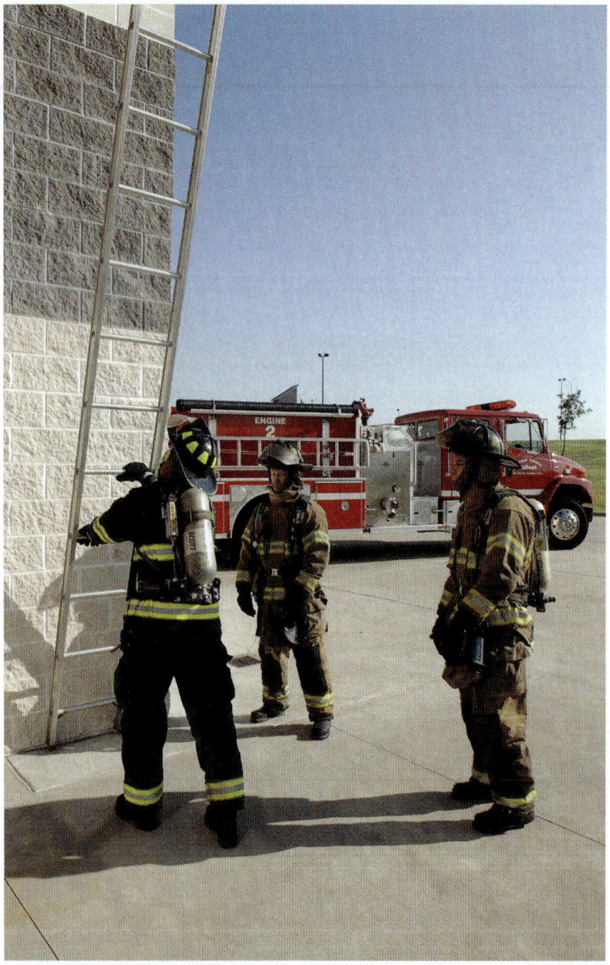

FIGURE 7-2 As the instructor, you will be demonstrating how the job should be done.

Safety in the Learning Environment

Safety during training begins with safety in the learning environment. First, consider the location of the classroom. While you may not have complete control over where the class is held, you can still affect some things. Survey the general learning environment. Are there inadequate fire exits or other unsafe conditions, such as remodeling in the area or icy steps leading to the classroom? If the classroom is in an engine bay, is the area subject to exhaust fumes, or is there oil on the floor? Evaluate the lighting conditions in the classroom. Not all students have good vision, and either low or high lighting may create eye strain. Excessive noise can be a problem as well—not only because it interferes with learning but also because it can cause unnecessary damage to students' hearing.

Next, review the physical arrangements of the classroom. Unsecured extension cords running throughout the classroom may trip either you or the students. Prior to each class, reroute or tape down extension cords. Also, be aware that fire stations may be the recipients of hand-me-downs from other city agencies. Often, chairs and tables that have outlived their usefulness in other areas are pressed into service in a fire department classroom and could be prone to collapsing. Make sure that each item is in good condition to prevent injuries to students.

At the beginning of class, be sure to raise safety awareness with the students. Go over the locations of the nearest fire exit and fire extinguishers. If you are teaching a class to an on-duty crew or a group of volunteer fire fighters, you should address what to do if an alarm sounds. For example, if some students in the class are on-call fire fighters, have them sit near an exit so that if they need to respond during class they can leave without interrupting the class. Explain the emergency plan to follow should a fire alarm activate or a severe weather event or natural disaster occur. It is important to emulate the behavior you teach to the general public and to remind your students that safety is paramount.

Hands-on Training Safety

Hands-on training includes all training activities conducted outside the classroom environment. Whether it consists of a simple tailboard chat on nozzles or a full-blown live fire training exercise, hands-on training is often the most powerful method of instruction for a student. Unfortunately, hands-on training also produces hazards that must be considered and mitigated. Slippery surfaces, sharp or jagged metal, and products of combustion need to be accounted for. Risk management practices need to be applied to limit, reduce, or eliminate risk exposure to students. Environmental factors—such as heat, cold, wind, rain, and storms—must be considered as well. Mother Nature can pose a significant risk to your students.

Personal Protective Equipment

Determine the appropriate level of PPE after reviewing the lesson plan. Lesson plans often specify the level of PPE required. However, local standard operating procedures (SOPs) may also exist that specify the level of PPE for training. A general statement of the PPE requirements for the training session needs to be part of your presentation. As an instructor, you must always wear the PPE required for the drill being conducted. The appropriate level of PPE depends on both the potential hazards and your department's SOPs.

The best practice is always to use the same PPE in training as you would in real-world incidents. In some departments, it may be acceptable to conduct ladder drills using helmets, gloves, and boots as opposed to full fire gear and self-contained breathing apparatus (SCBA), due to the skill being taught or reinforced. This modification to the PPE policy may make the drill safer by reducing the potential for heat stress. Another option may be to begin the training session in full levels of PPE and then to reduce the PPE required after signs of heat stress appear or when the skill has been performed properly. When these adaptations are implemented, you must make it very clear to your students that the modification is only allowable in the training session and should never be employed when responding to actual emergencies. If any level of hazard exists in the session, then the highest level of PPE available should be used.

Rehabilitation Practices and Hands-on Training

NFPA 1584: *Standard on the Rehabilitation Process for Members During Emergency Operations and Training Exercises* requires that rehabilitation protocols be established and practiced at training events that involve strenuous activities or prolonged operations. As an instructor, you must be aware of the content of this standard and apply it to these types of training sessions. These practices further reinforce the importance of following appropriate rehabilitation practices on the fire ground (**FIGURE 7-3**). Training should mirror as closely as possible the actual fire-ground operation. Medical care and monitoring, hydration, and cooling/warming materials are just a few of the rehabilitation considerations that NFPA 1584 requires to be available during training events.

COMPANY-LEVEL TRAINING TIP

Instructors should encourage training participants to begin hydrating for the training 24 to 48 hours prior to the training event. It is imperative for instructors who conduct live fire training to follow this guideline.

Not to be overlooked is the importance of instructors participating in the rehabilitation process. Too often, instructors will rotate students through the rehab station but neglect to rehab themselves. In reality, participation in rehabilitation is a safety factor as well as an important way to set the proper example for your students. All instructors must be monitored for dehydration, heat stress, and general fatigue. A rehab rotation for instructors should also be included in the training plan.

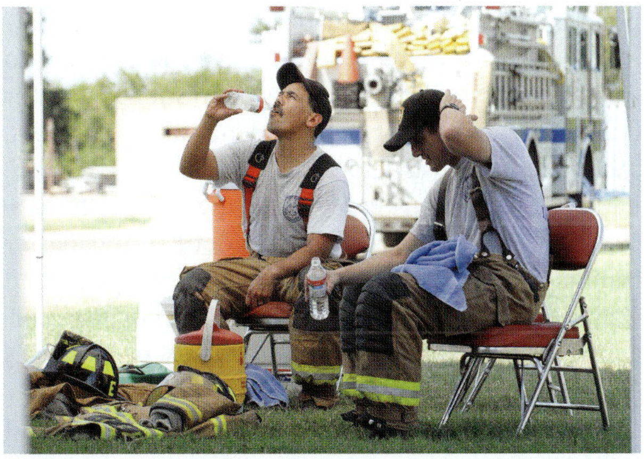

FIGURE 7-3 Rehabilitation is an important part of training.

Safety Policies and Procedures for Training

Your role as the instructor mandates that you have a firm grasp of the safety policies mandated by your fire department. All safety policies required on the fire ground must be reinforced and practiced during training. Indeed, one of the more common causes of injuries during training is failure to follow established safety practices. The instructor has a responsibility to ensure that all policies of the department are followed during training. Policies such as establishment of an incident command system, fire-ground accountability, rehabilitation, and full use of PPE are followed on the emergency scene, and adherence to those policies must not be set aside in training. Enforce those policies in the same manner a safety officer or incident commander would at an emergency incident.

On occasion, personnel from another agency might train with you at your facility if you are conducting mutual aid training or a special course. It is important in these types of situations that all fire fighters know which policies will be followed during the training. If you are hosting the training, all visitors must follow your policies, and your visitors need to be aware of what they are expected to do and which policies they will follow. When conducting live fire training, fire fighters from other organizations participating in interior training evolutions should have a signed letter from their fire chief or employer stating that they have met the training requirements set forth by NFPA 1403: *Standard on Live Fire Training Evolutions* and health requirements set forth by NFPA 1582: *Standard on Comprehensive Occupational Medical Program for Fire Departments*. This documentation can reduce the liability on the lead instructor in the event of injury.

You are responsible for drafting and forwarding policies relating to training through the chain of command. At the minimum, a training policy relating to training safety will include procedures for instructor qualifications, PPE for both students and instructors, safe student-to-instructor ratios, and effective rehabilitation practices during high-risk/high-exertion exercises. All levels of instructors must develop and deliver training that adheres to applicable safety points and must enforce a strict, zero-tolerance policy for deviations from accepted safety standards or practices (**FIGURE 7-4**).

As an instructor, you must also be informed of and follow the manufacturer's recommendations for using equipment. Read the accompanying owner's manuals for equipment such as chainsaws and heavy hydraulic equipment. Often the limitations of these tools are assumed, and an injury occurs when the tool is used in a manner counter to its intended use. When new apparatus is delivered to your department, you should be present for the initial training by the apparatus builder. Essential information presented by the manufacturer needs to be recorded, practiced, and reinforced whenever that piece of equipment is used.

Influencing Safety Through Training

As an instructor, you play a vital role in setting a good example in terms of safe fire-ground practices. Constantly remind yourself that you serve as the role model of a safe and effective fire fighter. Everything from your fitness level to the way you wear your uniform should exemplify your values related to safety and adherence to rules. The example that you set sends a far more powerful message to your students than any theories and concepts you present in a lecture or drill.

You should be acutely aware of how influential a role the fire and emergency services instructor plays, especially with new fire fighters. New fire fighters are uncertain about what is expected of them—that is, what is considered right versus what is considered wrong. With these students, whatever you do or say will be construed as the right thing. If you use improper techniques or fail to follow safety protocols while teaching, students will perceive that as the right way to do things. This faulty knowledge becomes dangerous when students leave your protection and perform on the emergency fire ground.

Your primary responsibility during a drill or training session is to ensure the safety of all students attending the drill. The actions of a fire fighter on the fire ground are the result of training. If you allow students to use unsafe practices in training, they will repeat those same actions on the fire ground, because decisions and actions on the fire ground are based on previous training.

You have many responsibilities related to the safety of your students during training, but one that stands above all others is the responsibility to have students practice safe principles and practices during training so that they remain safe on the fire ground. As part of your duties as an instructor, you must correct poor skills or bad decisions as they occur. If you witness a skill being performed incorrectly or a safety procedure not being followed but you do not correct the student's error, then you are reinforcing the incorrect behavior. This constant monitoring and correction is important with new recruits but can be more difficult with

Training Safety Plan

Drill Date: Time: Shift:

Drill Location:

Type of Training: (check all that apply)

- ☐ Fire Suppression
- ☐ Live Fire Training
- ☐ Driver Training
- ☐ Apparatus Operation
- ☐ Physical Fitness Activity
- ☐ Other:
- ☐ EMS
- ☐ Vehicle/Machinery Extrication
- ☐ Other Acquired Structure Training
- ☐ Preplan Survey or Simulation
- ☐ Technical Rescue
- ☐ Hazardous Materials/WMD
- ☐ Water/Dive Rescue

Drill Risk Assessment: ☐ High ☐ Medium ☐ Low

Maximum Student/Instructor Ratio: to Safety Officer Needed: (Required on High-Risk Drills)

Instructor PPE Requirements:

☐ SCBA ☐ Full PPE ☐ Helmet ☐ Eye Protection ☐ Filter Mask ☐ Hearing

☐ Gloves ☐ Radio ☐ Lights ☐ High-Visibility Vest

Drill Objective(s): (brief explanation of objectives)

Description of Training: (e.g., extricate victim from vehicle, victim search in limited visibility)

PPE/Equipment Required for Each Participant: (check all that apply)

- ☐ Helmet
- ☐ Eye Protection
- ☐ Hearing Protection
- ☐ Gloves (Type):
- ☐ Bunker Coat
- ☐ Hood
- ☐ Bunker Pants
- ☐ Safety Boots
- ☐ Other (Specify):
- ☐ Personal Flotation Device
- ☐ Buoyancy Compensator
- ☐ Mask/Snorkel/Fins
- ☐ SCBA
- ☐ SCUBA
- ☐ Other Respiratory Protection (Type):
- ☐ Hazardous Materials CPC (Type):
- ☐ Radio

Department Related SOPs or Technical References: (list number and name)

FIGURE 7-4 A sample drill safety plan.

Courtesy of Forest Reeder.

Hazards and Control Measures: (check all Hazards AND write in control measure)

- □ Atmospheric (e.g., smoke, dust, low oxygen):
- □ Combustible/Flammable Environment:
- □ Confined Space:
- □ Electrical:
- □ Elevation:
- □ Hazardous Substances (e.g., asbestos, chemicals):
- □ Nighttime Conditions:
- □ Other:
- □ Sewage/Septic:
- □ Sharp Edges/Objects:
- □ Structural:
- □ Terrain:
- □ Traffic:
- □ Water:
- □ Weather:

Accountability: (check all that apply)

- □ Buddy System
- □ Visual
- □ Passport
- □ Dive Master Control Sheet
- □ Other:

Communications:

- □ Radio—Primary Frequency:
- □ Radio—Secondary Frequency:
- □ Hand Signals
- □ Rope Line
- □ Lights
- □ Other:

In Case of Emergency: (check all that apply)

- □ Code or Signal Used:
- □ RIT Assigned:
- □ ALS Standby:

Resources Assigned: (check all that apply AND fill in designated unit)

- □ Battalion Chief(s):
- □ Rehab Officer/Area:
- □ Rescue Unit(s):
- □ Safety Officer:
- □ Specialty Unit(s):
- □ Suppression Unit(s):
- □ Other Resources/Equipment:

Rehabilitation Plan: (describe rehabilitation plan and guidelines)

FIGURE 7-4 *Continued*

Training Event Safety Analysis

1. Identify level of required PPE for each participant.

2. List basic steps required to safely complete evolution.

3. Identify potential accidents or hazards that may occur.

4. Determine recommended safe procedures.

Safety Planning Notes: (e.g., site plan, drawings)

Lead Instructor:

Signature: Date:

Reviewed by (print):

Signature: Date:

FIGURE 7-4 *Continued*

experienced personnel. Correcting unsafe or poor behavior demonstrated by a veteran fire fighter can be very challenging—but it is a challenge you cannot ignore. Correcting an unsafe skill should be the same whether the fire fighter is a raw recruit or a seasoned veteran.

Planning Safe Training

You should begin to address safety at the earliest stages of course development and preparation, while formulating or modifying lesson plans. Analyze and critique your training to ensure that safety measures are correctly addressed and emphasized. It is too late to address safety issues after an injury has occurred. Preventing injury becomes much easier when the hazards are identified and addressed early in the planning process.

Many of the NFPA standards provide additional information concerning safety and training and should be consulted during the planning process. NFPA 1500: *Standard on Fire Department Occupational Safety, Health, and Wellness Program* would be an important document to review when planning a program of instruction. In general, almost all NFPA standards in the 1400 series relate to a training recommendation and focus on providing safe training sessions. NFPA 1584: *Standard on the Rehabilitation Process for Members During Emergency Operations and Training Exercises* is also a valuable resource that can assist in planning safe training evolutions.

Creating a safety-conscious student must be a primary goal of nearly all training in the fire service. While there are inherent dangers in their occupation, fire fighters should constantly strive to reduce those risks through good awareness and safety practices. When determining the appropriate level of protective gear to use during training, for example, the instructor should consider the exercise's safety implications for students:

- First, is PPE necessary to ensure students' safety during the training activity? If so, full PPE must be used and any inconveniences mitigated. For example, because full PPE is needed for live fire training, be sure to provide rehabilitation in such a scenario.
- Second, consider whether *not* using full PPE will make the training safer. For example, perhaps hoods need not be worn during ladder practice because of the potential for heat stress in July.

- Third, consider whether *not* wearing full PPE will create a false perception that real scenes can be safely mitigated without its use.
- Fourth, ask yourself if you are considering reduced PPE owing to peer pressure or if this decision is *truly* in the best interest of the student.

Each of these considerations should be evaluated prior to making a determination of the level of PPE to be used. Safety cannot be an afterthought or an unwanted formality: Instead, it must be the first and foremost consideration to ensure the lives and safety of all (**FIGURE 7-5**).

An important part of the planning process is determining how many instructors are needed to conduct the desired training. Two factors should be considered in making this decision: the type or risk level of the training and the skill level of the students.

Training can be classified based on risk as either high risk, medium risk, or low risk. An example of high-risk training would be live fire evolutions in an acquired structure or swiftwater rescue training. Medium-risk training would include fire extinguisher training or ladder evolutions. Low-risk training would include a classroom lecture or a knot-tying practice session (**FIGURE 7-6**).

The skill level of those being taught should also be considered. High-risk training of new recruits should generate different concerns than high-risk training involving veteran fire fighters.

Other areas of planning include assembling the equipment that may be needed. Sometimes outdated equipment or equipment that has been replaced by upgrades within the department is used when conducting drills. Using old or outdated equipment has long been an accepted practice in the fire service, but it has often led to injuries that could have been

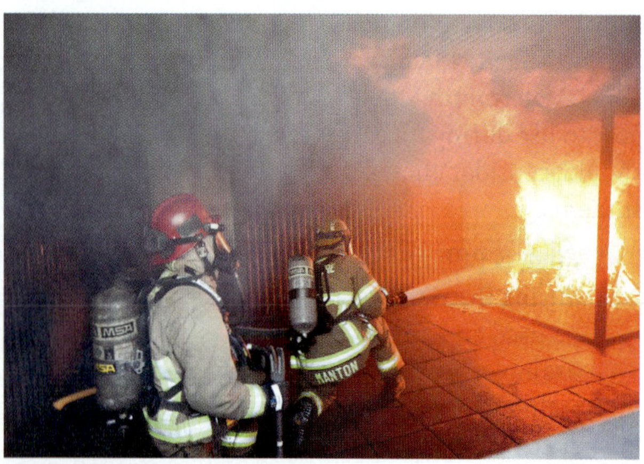

FIGURE 7-5 While there are inherent dangers in their occupation, fire fighters should constantly strive to reduce those risks through good awareness and safety practices.

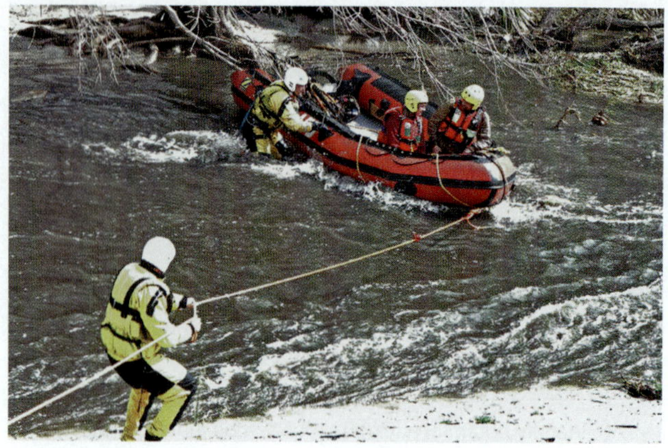

A

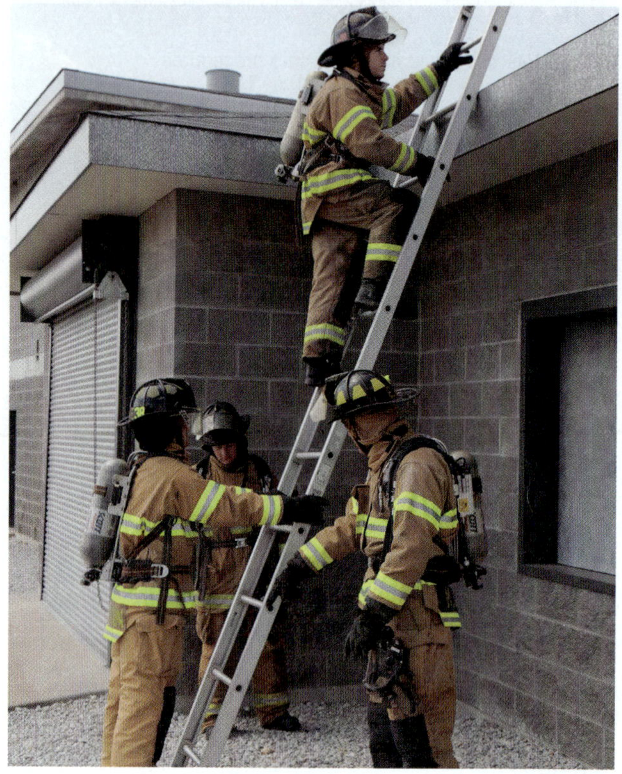

B

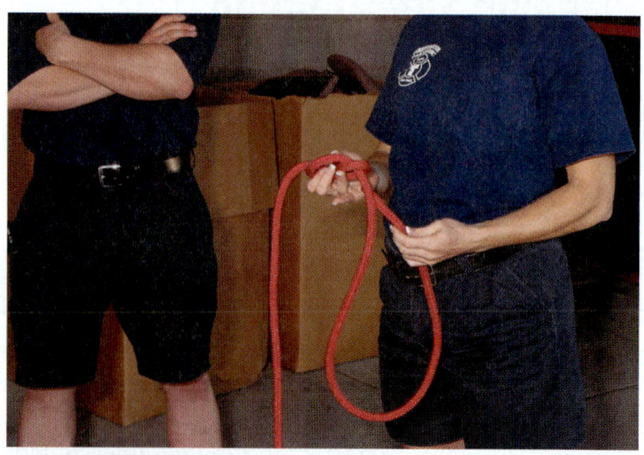

C

FIGURE 7-6 Examples of high-risk **(A)**, medium-risk **(B)**, and low-risk **(C)** training evolutions.

prevented. If the tool or apparatus does not meet the accepted performance standards, then it should not be used in training. You should also question whether using an outdated power saw, for example, is beneficial to students given that this type of saw is not used on current apparatus.

The instructor is also responsible for inspecting all equipment being used in the training to ensure that it meets the required standards prior to the drill. Do not assume that the equipment is in safe and operable condition. If your department does not have the equipment available to make the training safe, then it needs to find alternative equipment—perhaps by borrowing items from a neighboring fire department or the state fire training academy. Acquisition of the appropriate equipment should be arranged prior to the drill.

As the instructor, you are responsible for protecting students from physical and emotional harm in the classroom and on the drill ground. Most of this chapter focuses on means to protect students from physical injury. Nevertheless, instructors cannot overlook the psychological dangers students encounter during training both in and out of the classroom.

Hidden Hazards During Training

During training, students are asked to perform various tasks, recall policies, or demonstrate the ability to perform. When placed in an environment of peers, most students realize that their performance is being evaluated—not only by the instructor but also by their fellow classmates. Failure to accomplish the task or answer the question correctly can label the student as not competent or someone who cannot be trusted on the fire ground. This situation is particularly dangerous because the typical personality of fire fighters is driven by the need to succeed, regardless of the conditions or situation.

This scenario sets the stage for disaster if a fire fighter is placed in an overwhelming situation, such as being asked to conduct a simulated rescue of another fire fighter or a rescue mannequin that may be twice the candidate's size or weight. If the fire fighter is asked to perform this task while fellow classmates are watching, it forces the student to attempt the impossible. Often, the student makes a valiant attempt, only to suffer an injury in the process. You have a responsibility to construct the learning environment so that situations such as these do not arise.

Do not minimize your levels of performance or drop your benchmarks so that every student can achieve success; this is not realistic. At the same time, it is unacceptable for you to stand idly by as a student is placed into a scenario where he or she cannot perform successfully without being exposed to physical harm.

COMPANY-LEVEL TRAINING TIP

Using theatrical smoke during an evolution instead of live smoke during search-and-rescue training might allow for a candidate to have more confidence in their early training sessions. Theatrical smoke provides a non-IDLH atmosphere where, in the event of an emergency, the student is never in a dangerous environment.

Overcoming Obstacles

Money may be an obstacle in the training process, because instructors often face demands to train students while using limited resources. In the past, the fire service has been creative in developing methods and practices to accomplish drills or tasks with minimal cost. For example, when an acquired structure is not available for training on overhaul, it is easy to construct a wooden simulator from scrap 2-in. by 4-in. (2 × 4) lumber and cover it with discarded gypsum board that can be obtained from a lumber supply shop, often at very little expense (**FIGURE 7-7**). When foam is needed for a fire stream training session and expired or surplus foam is not available, you can make a homemade solution using dish soap liquid and water. Of course, if you are using something other than equipment or products that would normally be used in the evolution, make sure that they will not produce a safety hazard.

One item that cannot be minimized is personnel: An adequate number of personnel must be present to conduct the training safely. This is particularly true

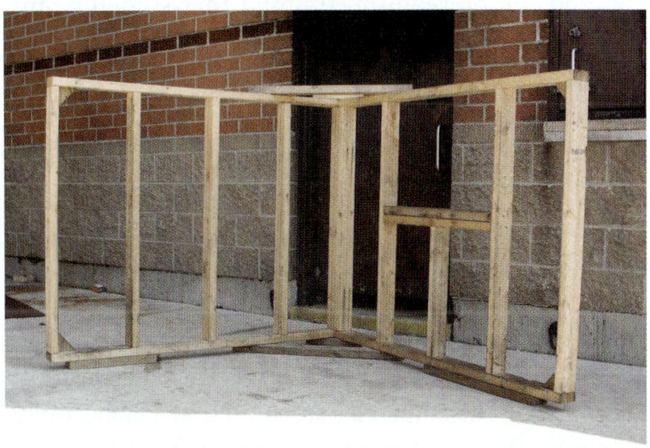

FIGURE 7-7 If an acquired structure is not available for training on overhaul, it is easy to construct a wooden simulator of scrap 2 × 4 lumber and cover it with discarded gypsum board.

Courtesy of Forest Reeder.

when conducting live fire training. Live fire training is the pinnacle of all firefighting training, but it is also one of the most hazardous drills. The hazard becomes even more pronounced when the drill occurs with fewer personnel than are acceptable to ensure a safe environment.

Analysis of your audience will help you select the best method of instruction for your training session. Some training sessions will require you to demonstrate the proper techniques in a step-by-step fashion, pausing to allow for questions and to provide clarification. This method may be appropriate for entry-level or new-skills training. Other sessions will require you to review the objectives or desired outcomes of the training session along with key safety behaviors. This approach may be applied to training sessions for experienced fire fighters or when doing evaluations of skill levels.

Live Fire Training

Perhaps one of the most hazardous but exciting portions of training involves live fire training evolutions. Safety considerations during live fire training should be the highest priority for all instructors involved with this type of high-risk training. NFPA 1041 now contains language on live fire training instructor requirements. This is an example of the emphasis on training safety in high-risk training activities, such as live fire evolutions.

As a result of past fire fighter fatalities involved with live fire training, the NFPA developed a standard that is to be followed during all live fire training evolutions. NFPA 1403: *Standard on Live Fire Training Evolutions* describes all aspects of the training process involving live fire training. It identifies the positions that must be staffed when conducting live fire training and the prerequisite training that students must complete before they can participate in any live fire exercises addressed by this standard. This standard applies to all types of live fire training, including acquired structures, gas-fired and non-gas-fired live fire props, and exterior live fire props. It includes the permit process, pre/post training, and documentation of the training process. NFPA 1403 must be consulted before the live burn exercise and followed to the letter when conducting live fire drills. As an instructor, you have a responsibility to ensure that all positions required by this standard are staffed at your training sessions. Do not attempt the drill with anything less than a full complement of trained and qualified staff.

Positions that must be filled during live burn activities include a designated **safety officer**, who has received training and background in the responsibilities of this position during live fire training. This safety officer is responsible for intervention in and control of any aspect of the operation that he or she determines to present a potential or actual danger at all live fire training scenarios. An **instructor-in-charge** is required to plan and coordinate all training activities and is responsible for following NFPA 1403. The instructor-in-charge must meet the requirements of NFPA 1041, Instructor II, while all other instructors must meet the Instructor I requirements. An additional position identified in this standard is the **ignition officer**, who is responsible for igniting and controlling the material being burned. The ignition officer coordinates all fire-lighting activities with the instructor-in-charge, the safety officer, and the fire control team. Note that an instructor cannot serve as an ignition officer for more than one evolution in a row (NFPA 1403, 4.7.6.1). Specific detail should be applied to the acquired structure to prepare it for the live fire training evolution. NFPA 1403 maintains a check-off sheet to assist the instructor with all aspects of preparation and execution of the live fire training exercise.

The proper student-to-instructor ratio when conducting training involving live fire is recommended to be 5:1. In some training sessions involving multiple fire departments, you will need a large pool of instructors to assist you and maintain the 5:1 ratio of crew members to instructors. This 5:1 ratio must be maintained throughout the evolutions and is set so that the typical span of control is not exceeded.

NFPA 1403 states that the agency conducting the live fire training is responsible for identifying the qualifications for instructors who direct live fire training, but experience has demonstrated over time that senior instructors and fire fighters should staff each of the positions as identified in the standard. 1403 also requires the instructor-in-charge to meet Instructor II, while all other instructors meet Instructor I. In addition to being qualified, each person who carries out these functions should be properly trained.

NFPA 1403 identifies specific positions to be staffed during live fire training due to the nature of the risks involved while working around fire. This same "safety" mindset should apply during any type of high-risk hazard training, such as high-angle, swiftwater, or confined-space training. Having an experienced instructor-in-charge with appropriate safety officer(s) and a low student-to-instructor ratio will enhance a safe training environment and promote a safety culture.

Other Training Considerations

In many fire-ground incidents, if a particular position is not filled, then the incident commander is responsible for completing all of the functions of that position. Although normal ICS procedures allow tasks not delegated to be performed by the IC, NFPA 1403 requires that "The safety officer shall not be assigned other duties that interfere with safety responsibilities." (NFPA 1403, 4.5.6). If company officers are available to assist with training, the responsibilities associated with these positions must be covered in depth before training.

You must pay attention to details when planning and conducting drills where students may face a risk of injury. With practical drills, many variables come into play and many things can go wrong, resulting in an injury to a student. One way in which you can minimize that possibility is to pay special attention to every detail of the drill. Mentally walking through the evolution during the planning session and drawing upon your own experiences or case reports of actual incidents can help develop your awareness of what might potentially go wrong. This review will allow you to create backup plans or, in the best case, to eliminate the hazard altogether.

When the drill includes large numbers of people whom you may not know (e.g., in disaster drills where many outside agencies are invited to participate), your preplanning skills will be put to the test. Asking for assistance from other instructors or agencies that have conducted similar exercises will help you in covering all the bases during the planning phase. As the instructor-in-charge, run through each aspect of the session, always asking, "What might go wrong here?" Aspects of the training to be considered include the weather, topography, equipment being used, and steps of the task.

Additional instructors should be employed at training sessions where the following conditions are present:

- Extreme temperatures are expected.
- The qualifications or skill level of the students are unknown, which could require more one-on-one time.
- Large groups of people will participate.
- Training will take place over a long duration.
- Training involves complex evolutions and procedures where additional instruction and safety oversight may be valuable.

Developing a Safety Culture

Fire and emergency services instructors are in a position to select personnel to assist with their training programs. Often company officers are used to help deliver the session or watch over a skill being evaluated. As an instructor, you have the responsibility to know about the people you are asking to help conduct this training. What are their qualifications? What are their values concerning fire service safety? Despite your best efforts to keep your training safe, you cannot be everywhere at all times. Thus, you must rely on other instructors to help supervise the drill.

Instructors who are not competent in or confident with the subject being presented should not be placed in a situation where they attempt to teach that material to others. The motivation of your subordinate instructors must be assessed as well. An instructor who has a propensity to show off or try to prove that he or she is superior to students is an accident waiting to happen. Often the focus of such an instructor is not on the students or their safety. Know your staff, their attitudes toward safety, the way they operate on the fire ground, their motivations for being instructors, and their teaching methods. All support personnel for the drill, including those who simply assist in prop construction, should be included in this assessment, because this information is essential to conduct training safely.

Anticipating Problems

As part of the preparation for instruction, you need to assess potential problems and rectify them before they result in an injury. You need to train your eye to pick out these hazards on first glance. It may be easy for a company to throw up a ladder and leave it unheeled; you should be able to foresee the potential consequences of that action and take steps to make sure the hazard is addressed. Most experienced instructors have this quality already. The more fire-ground experiences you have, the better you will become at recognizing the small details that might escalate into a full-scale disaster.

Your fire-ground experiences translate to the drill ground, and you should apply your firefighting experiences to every evolution you instruct. Tell your fire fighter students what can go wrong, what to watch out for, and how to be prepared for changing conditions throughout the training evolution. If a smoke generator will be used for the training session, let students know how it compares to smoke at a real incident, if the situation may be significantly different from the training experience.

Often training tragedies are not the result of a single catastrophic event, but rather represent the culmination of several small safety violations that combine to create a fire training tragedy. The instructor-in-charge may identify that an attack line of a smaller size is appropriate for the amount of fuel being used if it is advanced without delay. But hose lines can get kinked, water may be slow to reach the nozzle from the pump, and conditions may deteriorate and lead to a delayed attack that can bring the fuel load above the capacity of the slowly advancing attack line. Collectively, these elements are a prescription for disaster.

Changes in wind or weather, crew fatigue, or student motivation may also affect the evolution. Your guard must stay up until the evolution is complete. You might imagine that if just one thing goes wrong you can quickly correct it, but the escalation of events often occurs so rapidly that you cannot gain control of the one small mistake before an injury takes place. If you see a potential hazard, correct it immediately.

Accident and Injury Investigation

Despite all of your careful preparation, sometimes an accident might happen. In such circumstances, it is important to conduct a comprehensive investigation of the incident. A key factor in any investigation is the attitude held by those conducting the investigation. The purpose of such an investigation should be to find the reasons for and contributing factors to the accident or injury—not to assign blame. If the main focus is on finding the cause of the accident, then individuals will be more honest and open to this important process.

The investigation should include the date, location, events prior to and during the incident, equipment involved, PPE in use at the time of the accident, and personnel who were present when the incident occurred. Anyone who witnessed the incident should provide a written statement. This information will help the investigator determine the cause of the injury and enable the agency and training personnel to put control measures in place to prevent future occurrences. Keep all injury investigation notes, doctors' reports, and any information generated during the investigation on file. Periodically review these files for any emerging trends that might cue you to change a policy or procedure that is contributing to injuries. When types of injuries are compared over a period of time, trends in their incidence often become apparent. You should see that modifications are made to the training program based on this information.

COMPANY-LEVEL INSTRUCTOR TIP

Review the causes of accidents for the type of training you will be conducting to ensure you have taken all appropriate preventive measures.

Student Responsibilities for Safety During Training

Every student participating in training has a stake in ensuring his or her own personal safety. Each student is responsible for his or her actions as well as the actions of other crew members, training team members, and fellow students when it comes to addressing hazardous conditions. Students should be knowledgeable about the training to take place and should meet all of the prerequisites specified before participating in the drill. During high-risk training, this background becomes even more important because of how an unprepared student's performance can affect other students involved in the training. Several case studies have dealt with improperly prepared students contributing to the injury of fellow students.

Students should also adhere to all PPE requirements specified for the evolution and wear all other assigned safety devices or equipment. Observance of all safety instructions and safety rules throughout the training session will assist in maintaining the overall safety profile of the training session.

Each student should also be honest regarding his or her strengths and weaknesses. If a student is not prepared for the skill or evolution, he or she should notify you so that other students or instructors are not put at risk.

Legal Considerations

Instructors are held accountable for planning, lack of planning, adherence to standards and codes, and decision making during the training process. There are many types of liability that arise during training. As an instructor, you have a responsibility to stay informed about all laws and standards governing fire fighter training and safety. These laws and standards change over time, so you must keep up-to-date with the most current editions. Instructor networks, websites, and electronic bulletin boards are all popular methods of staying abreast of these ever-changing rules.

In many cases, the standard of care or best practices relating to training safety may be tied to your department's SOPs. As mentioned in earlier chapters, those SOPs must be referenced within the scope of training along with the application to the individual job description.

Another legal test that may be applied to training is the "reasonable person" concept. This standard tests your decisions against the decisions made by others with similar training and background, asking what your peers would do when faced with the same situation.

Negligence, Misfeasance, and Malfeasance

Negligence, **misfeasance**, and **malfeasance** are terms you are likely to encounter in cases where a civil wrong is alleged. Generally, two types of wrongs can be alleged in civil cases when an injury occurs:

- Unintentional conduct, which is best equated to the term *accident* (negligence, misfeasance)
- Conduct that includes an element of intent or knowledge that a wrong is being committed (malfeasance)

Which conduct constitutes negligence/misfeasance and which conduct constitutes malfeasance depend on the facts of each situation. This determination is based on the conduct involved, the fire department's rules and regulations, prior training, and national guidelines. In several LODD cases involving live fire training, there have been civil and criminal cases accusing instructors of these principles.

Negligence/Misfeasance

Negligence and misfeasance are kindred spirits: They are void of the element of intent and are based on a duty to prevent harm or injury to others by exercising a degree of care commensurate with the task being performed. Negligence exists when there is a breach of the duty owed to another, there is an injury, and the breach is the proximate cause of the injury.

Once these three elements are established, you can become legally liable for your conduct absent some type of immunity. **Liability** in its simplest form means responsibility. If a person or entity is found liable, that person or entity is responsible for paying for the damages caused by its actions or inactions.

An instructor's conduct is judged according to the reasonable person standard, which is an objective (not subjective) standard. In other words, the question is asked: What would a reasonable person have done in the same or similar situation? In the case of instructors, what constitutes "reasonableness" is gleaned from the department's policies and procedures, national standards, and federal and state law. For this reason, it is important that you remain apprised of changes in the laws that affect the fire service. It is also important that any changes in the law, technology, and the national guidelines be considered and incorporated into the policies and procedures of the fire department when appropriate.

Misfeasance is the most commonly encountered type of wrong in the performance of otherwise lawful acts. Simply defined, misfeasance consists of improper or wrongful performance of a lawful act without intent through mistake or carelessness. An example would be the hiring of a family member—a practice that, unbeknownst to you, is a violation of the department's nepotism policy.

Most states offer some level of protection to public employees against lawsuits premised on claims of negligence or misfeasance. These protections often take the form of immunity laws that bar certain causes of action outright or require a complainant to allege and substantiate a higher level of proof. The higher standard of proof usually requires that an element similar to intent be proved to prevail on a claim. Quite often, the highest standard requires proof of willful and wanton conduct or establishment of gross negligence. Gross negligence could be found, for example, if an instructor fails to follow a written protocol or a standing order. For example, a standing order might require personnel to wear protective equipment when dealing with a live fire; failure to do so could constitute gross negligence. The purpose of the higher standard of proof is to allow public employees to perform their jobs without fear that every little mistake will expose them to potential liability.

Willful and wanton conduct is defined by some courts as an act that, if not intentional, shows an utter indifference or conscious disregard for the safety of others. For example, it might include the failure to follow a written protocol or a standing order such that this omission creates a substantial risk to another person. That standard can be established if it is shown that, after having knowledge of an impending danger, a person failed to exercise ordinary care to prevent the injury. In addition, if, through recklessness or carelessness, a danger is not discovered by the use of ordinary care, the willful and wanton conduct standard may be satisfied.

Similarly, **gross negligence** is defined as an act (or a failure to act) that is so reckless it shows a conscious, voluntary disregard for the safety of others. Gross negligence involves extreme conduct but not intentional conduct. It falls somewhere between a mere inadvertent act that causes harm and acting with an intent to harm.

Whether a particular act constitutes willful and wanton conduct or gross negligence depends on the facts of the situation. The most common evidence considered when analyzing whether an act is willful and wanton are your departmental policies and procedures, surrounding departments' policies and procedures, training records, and national guidelines or standards. It is vital that your policies and procedures are reviewed annually to ensure that they are current and up-to-date with national standards set for the fire service. The same is true for the training evaluations used. Prior to revising an evaluation, it is important to verify that it still satisfies the standards of the fire service.

Legal exposures exist in many training sessions that you will teach or in which you will participate. In the event of almost any accident or injury, the training records and training history of the participants may be examined by attorneys and investigators in an attempt to identify any potential errors or omissions in the training and educational process. Many instructors fail to realize the importance of the documentation part of the training process. When shoddy records are reviewed during investigations, the professional reputation of the instructor may suffer—not to mention that such lackluster recordkeeping presents the potential for litigation under the heading of "failure to train" or "inadequate training." Training development from established reference sources based on up-to-date SOPs is fundamental to ensuring legally defensible training development.

COMPANY-LEVEL INSTRUCTOR TIP

There is no substitute for a consultation with an attorney who is knowledgeable in the law or for the applicable industry standards on training safety such as the NFPA.

Malfeasance

Malfeasance, unlike negligence and misfeasance, is more than a simple mistake or accident. Most often malfeasance is associated with public officials who partake in unlawful conduct even though they know that the conduct is illegal and contrary to their duties as public employees. Such conduct usually results in criminal charges but could be made part of a civil suit. An example of malfeasance would be the acceptance of a bribe by an instructor in return for a passing grade.

Many of the NFPA standards in the 1400 series provide guidance in the application of different types of training exercises. For example, NFPA 1451: *Standard for a Fire and Emergency Service Vehicle Operations Training Program* provides information about the development and delivery of a vehicle training program. Within that standard and others such as NFPA 1500: *Standard on Fire Department Occupational Safety, Health, and Wellness Program*, it is required that training on vehicle driving take place before the fire fighter is allowed to respond to emergencies as a driver. If the department does not adopt that policy as a standard practice, the failure to do so might be held against the department in a lawsuit.

Most of the safety protocols that govern fire fighter training are embedded in laws that describe broader topics, such as Occupational Safety and Health Administration (OSHA) rules on respiratory protection (or SCBA) and hazardous materials. The NFPA standard specific to conducting live fire training safely is NFPA 1403: *Standard on Live Fire Training Evolutions*, which addresses conducting live fire training in acquired structures, gas-fired live fire training structures, non-gas-fired live fire training structures, exterior prop fires, and Class B fuel fires. Many of the requirements for these exercises must also be applied to skills training.

NFPA 1403 was developed as a result of fire fighter fatalities and injuries in live fire training accidents. This standard is almost entirely devoted to practices that must be followed to conduct live fire training safely. Although NFPA standards are not laws, you can be held accountable for adhering to them just the same. For example, a training officer was recently held criminally liable for a fire fighter fatality that occurred during live fire training because he did not follow the guidelines in NFPA 1403 when conducting the drill. Strictly adhering to all recognized standards and laws for the type of training you are conducting will ensure that such training is conducted in a manner that will be safe for all participants.

If the training will involve participants from other fire departments, additional documentation should be obtained for those fire fighters. Moreover, your fire department should enter into a **hold harmless** and **indemnification agreement** with any other department or agency involved in the program. Such an agreement provides that your fire department will not be held monetarily or legally liable for injuries or conduct of the other department or agency's employees. This document is necessary to protect your fire department from individuals over whom you have no control. As a representative of the hosting fire department, you should also verify that all outside participants are medically cleared to participate in the training, have met the necessary prerequisites, and possess the proper credentials.

Off-site training is filled with additional risks not encountered with on-site training. You should perform a site inspection well in advance of scheduling the training and prior to development of any handouts to identify any unusual or potentially unsafe conditions. In addition, contact should be made with all other entities (town, city, utility companies) to verify that the proposed training does not violate any law or create any unreasonable risks. For example, you should confirm that no ordinances or local laws prohibit the proposed activity. Document each conversation that you have with other entities as well as the steps you take after each conversation.

Laws and standards are intended to keep fire fighter training within a framework of safe practices. Some critics might suggest that the requirements place so many restrictions on the training that it is no longer realistic or relevant. This is simply not true. First and foremost, instructors have a responsibility to keep the training safe and to follow procedures (**TABLE 7-2**). The notion that you have to discard safety requirements to make the training realistic is contrary to the entire idea behind conducting training sessions. The standards, rules, and laws established for safe live fire activities must be adhered to during skills training, as well.

TABLE 7-2 General Training Safety Procedures

Training Location	Procedures
Classroom training	Make sure all applicable department standard operating guidelines (SOGs) are referenced within your lesson plan. Ensure all participants are aware of facility safety procedures (e.g., fire alarm, smoking, restricted access areas). Identify trip, slip/fall, and other facility hazards.
Hands-on training	Specify all learning objectives and performances. Use incident action plans as appropriate for high-risk training such as live fire evolutions. State all required PPE for instructors and students. Identify all department procedures for skills being performed (use the same incident command system as required during actual operations). Identify and demonstrate any hazard control activities that have been taken or are in place. Review all applicable safety procedures (e.g., emergency procedures, mayday, backup assignments, communications, rehab, emergency medical services [EMS] standby or aid, accountability, and rapid intervention teams). Check all communications equipment. Follow all applicable standards for the training session (NFPA 1403 for live fire training).
Keys to safe and successful training	Identify companies/members who are in or out of service. Identify and document the lead instructor. Notify supervising officers of all training events. Brief all participants on all training expectations. Monitor the previously mentioned practical training safety factors throughout (act as instructor/safety officer/incident commander). Immediately stop all unsafe acts or conditions; do not try to train through them. Debrief all participants on how training expectations were met and identify opportunities to improve individual and company performance. Return all equipment and personnel to service refueled, recharged, rehabbed, and ready for the next response.

Training BULLETIN

JONES & BARTLETT FIRE DISTRICT

TRAINING DIVISION

5 Wall Street, Burlington, MA, 01803

Phone 978-443-5000 Fax 978-443-8000

Instant Applications: Safety During the Learning Process

Drill Assignment

Apply the chapter content to your department's operation, its training division, and your personal experiences to complete the following questions and activities.

Objective

Upon completion of the instant applications, fire and emergency services instructor students will exhibit decision making and application of job performance requirements of the instructor using the text, class discussion, and their own personal experiences.

Suggested Drill Applications

1. Review local policies relating to safety in training.
2. Read NFPA 1403: *Standard on Live Fire Training Evolutions*, and review the sample checklists used for conducting live fire training exercises.
3. Research fire fighter line-of-duty deaths in training accidents and review the recommendations of the investigators regarding ways to prevent similar occurrences.
4. Review the Incident Report in this chapter and be prepared to discuss your analysis of the incident from a training perspective and as an instructor who wishes to use the report as a training tool.

Incident Report: NIOSH Report F2005-31

Drill Assignment

Review the information in this incident report and prepare a practice presentation for class delivery at the direction of your instructor. Your presentation should include a summary of the incident facts and a review of the NFPA 1403 compliance and noncompliance findings. Use an outline to organize your thoughts. You may be evaluated on your communication skills during your presentation.

Pennsylvania State Fire Academy—2006

The Pennsylvania State Fire Academy was conducting a Suppression Instructor Development Program (ZFID), an instructor development program for live fire training. The course covers instructional components including academy policies, NFPA 1403, building fires in the permanent live fire training facility, the instructor's role in student safety, emergency and rescue operations, and more. Instructors taking the course are already Instructor I and Fire Fighter II certified, and have completed the incident safety officer course. Candidates act as students, ignition officers, incident safety officers, incident commanders, and instructors, with an academy instructor evaluating each participant's performance.

The 2½-story residential non-gas-fired structure used for live fire training was built in 1993 and is used for structural firefighting training (**FIGURE 7-A**). The building has a basement, ground floor, second floor, and an attic space. Burn rooms are located on the second floor and in the basement, where this incident occurred (**FIGURE 7-B**). The burn room in the basement has only one entrance, which can be accessed by either the interior or exterior stairwell. Only wooden pallets and excelsior are used for fuel.

As part of the ZFID program, six scripted (planned) evolutions were organized in the burn building. Certain problems or emergencies were planned, and while the candidates had a basic understanding of the types of events, they did not know which event would occur during each evolution. The candidates were evaluated on their ability to handle the events.

The fire fighter who lost his life in this incident had already served as the evaluator of an instructor candidate in previous evolutions that day. On this last evolution, he was assigned to be the ignition officer for the burn room in the basement. He had more than 30 years in the fire service and had been an adjunct instructor at the facility for 7 years. He was wearing full protective clothing, including coat, pants, helmet, hood, gloves, boots, and

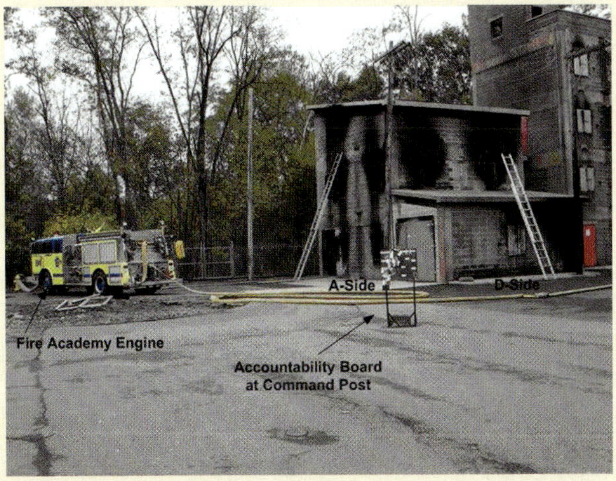

FIGURE 7-A The Pennsylvania State Fire Academy's non-gas-fired live fire training structure.

From the NIOSH Fire Fighter Fatality Investigation and Prevention Program, Investigation Report F2005-31.

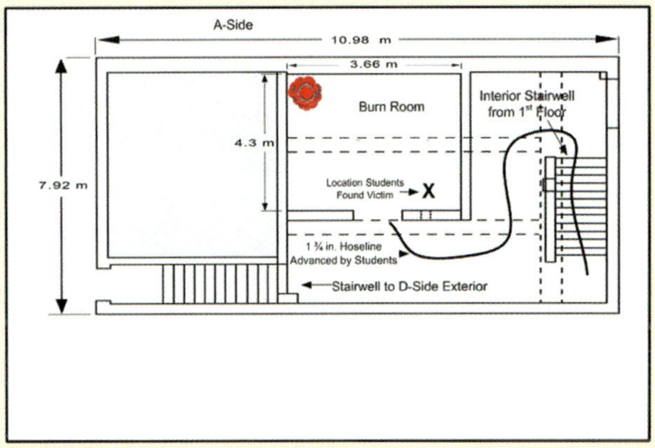

FIGURE 7-B The floor plan of the basement in the non-gas-fired live fire training structure at the Pennsylvania State Fire Academy.

From the NIOSH Fire Fighter Fatality Investigation and Prevention Program, Investigation Report F2005-31.

Incident Report continued

SCBA with integrated personal alert safety system (PASS), and he had a portable radio.

The fatal event occurred during the last evolution. The scenario was to simulate a fire that had not been knocked down enough from the previous evolution.

An instructor waiting to monitor the last crew was in the burn building. He reported good visibility with some smoke. While waiting, he heard the basement door open and saw the victim come out of the burn room and lie on the floor, pulling and moving his bunker gear about. The instructor asked the victim twice if he was okay. The victim answered, "It is hot as hell down there!" The instructor asked the victim if he was okay and if he wanted to go outside. Although the victim responded that he was okay, he was told to go outside. The victim declined, got up, and said that he was fine and would see the other instructor in the basement when the crew arrived. The victim went back down the basement steps. (Note: An estimated 1½ minutes elapsed from the time the victim came up the stairwell until he went back down to the basement.)

It is believed that the victim returned to the burn room and was carrying pallets to add to the fire. In NIOSH's report and following National Institute of Standards and Technology's (NIST) experiments, investigators hypothesized that excessive heat in the burn room caused a catastrophic failure of the lens of the victim's SCBA face piece. The face piece failure was a result of the heat conditions within the burn room and not a manufacturer's problem. The victim dropped the pallets and fell forward. The victim then struggled on the ground and crawled toward the exit.

As the next crew approached the burn room while advancing a hose line, they reportedly heard the victim moaning. They found him struggling on the floor in the right corner of the burn room. One of the candidates declared a mayday by radio, and the candidate serving as the incident commander deployed the rapid intervention crew (RIC). There was initial confusion whether this was part of the scenario or an actual emergency. The crew who found the victim immediately removed him from the burn room to outside, and emergency care was initiated. He was transported initially to a local hospital and then transferred by emergency medical services (EMS) helicopter to a regional trauma/burn unit, where he died 2 days later.

This was the first fatality of an instructor in a permanent live fire training prop, and only the second in such a facility. The fire fighters did not report the PASS device activating, as the victim was still moving. In this case, the PASS device did sound once removed from the victim; due to heat damage it could not be shut off, continuing to sound its alarm 2 days later.

Postincident Analysis Pennsylvania State Fire Academy

Key Recommendations

- Ensure that two training officers are present with a charged hoseline during the ignition or refueling of a training fire in accordance with NFPA 1403.
- Fire departments and training academies should use the minimum fuel load necessary to conduct live fire training (Ref 1403-7.3).
- An instructor shall not serve as an ignition officer for more than one evolution in a row (note, this is not in the report recommendations).

NFPA 1403 Compliant

- Structure in good condition
- Instructors had experience in the fire service and with live fire training
- RIC crew ready
- An ambulance staffed by two EMTs on scene

Other Contributing Factors

- Instructor working alone
- Repeated entries by instructor
- No monitoring of interior temperatures
- No method to rapidly ventilate building
- Basement with no "at grade" exit

After-Action REVIEW

IN SUMMARY

- You must always place students' safety ahead of any performance expectations for the training session.
- The 16 fire fighter life safety initiatives should provide both guidance and motivation to you while you are developing and conducting any training. They highlight the importance of training as a strategy that can help reduce the number of fire fighter line-of-duty deaths.
- As the instructor, you serve as a role model for students. For this reason, you should always reinforce safety policies as part of the teaching process.
- Safety during training begins with safety in the classroom.
- In hands-on training, risk management practices must be applied to limit, reduce, or eliminate risk.
- As an instructor, you must always wear the PPE required for the drill being conducted. The appropriate level of PPE depends on both the potential hazards and your department's SOPs.
- Training should mirror as closely as possible the actual fire-ground operation. Medical care and monitoring, hydration, and cooling/warming materials are just a few of the rehabilitation considerations that are required to be available during live fire training events.
- Knowledge of the department's safety policies and the manufacturer's recommendations for any equipment is the key to keeping students safe during training.
- The example that you set as an instructor sends a far more powerful message to your students than the theories and concepts you present in a lecture or drill.
- You are responsible for inspecting the equipment being used in training to ensure that it meets the required standards prior to conducting the drill. Do not assume that the equipment is in safe and operable condition.
- Live fire training is the pinnacle of all firefighting training, but it is also one of the most hazardous drills.
- NFPA 1403: *Standard on Live Fire Training Evolutions* is the nationally accepted standard for all live fire burn training.
- NFPA 1584: *Standard on the Rehabilitation Process for Members During Emergency Operations and Training Exercises* requires that rehabilitation protocols be practiced at training events that involve strenuous or prolonged operations.
- Instructors are responsible for both the physical and emotional well-being of students while in training.
- Instructors are held accountable for their planning and adherence to standards and SOPs during the training session.

KEY TERMS

Access Navigate for flashcards to test your key term knowledge.

Gross negligence An act, or a failure to act, that is so reckless that it shows a conscious, voluntary disregard for the safety of others.

Hold harmless An agreement or contract wherein one party holds the other party free from responsibility for liability or damage that could arise from the transaction between the two parties.

Ignition officer An individual who is responsible for igniting and controlling the material being burned at a live fire training.

Indemnification agreement An agreement or contract wherein one party assumes liability.

Instructor-in-charge An individual qualified as an instructor and designated by the authority having jurisdiction to be in charge of the live fire training evolution and who has met the requirements of an Instructor II in accordance with NFPA 1041 (NFPA 1403).

Liability Responsibility; the assignment of blame. It often occurs after a breach of duty.

Malfeasance Dishonest, intentionally illegal, or immoral actions.

Misfeasance Mistaken, careless, or inadvertent actions that result in a violation of law.

Negligence An unintentional breach of duty that is the proximate cause of harm.

Safety officer An individual appointed by the authority having jurisdiction as qualified to maintain a safe working environment at all live fire training evolutions (NFPA 1403).

Willful and wanton conduct An act that shows utter indifference or conscious disregard for the safety of others.

REFERENCES

National Fallen Firefighters Foundation. 2013. "16 Firefighter Life Safety Initiatives." Emmitsburg, MD: National Fallen Firefighters Foundation. http://www.lifesafetyinitiatives.com/.

National Fire Protection Association. 2015. *NFPA 1584: Standard on the Rehabilitation Process for Members During Emergency Operations and Training Exercises*. Quincy, MA: National Fire Protection Association.

National Fire Protection Association. 2018. *NFPA 1403: Standard on Live Fire Training Evolutions*. Quincy, MA: National Fire Protection Association.

National Fire Protection Association. 2018. *NFPA 1451: Standard for a Fire and Emergency Service Vehicle Operations Training Program*. Quincy, MA: National Fire Protection Association.

National Fire Protection Association. 2018. *NFPA 1500: Standard on Fire Department Occupational Safety, Health, and Wellness Program*. Quincy, MA: National Fire Protection Association.

National Fire Protection Association. 2018. *NFPA 1582: Standard on Comprehensive Occupational Medical Program for Fire Departments*. Quincy, MA: National Fire Protection Association.

National Fire Protection Association. 2019. *NFPA 1041: Standard for Fire and Emergency Services Instructor Professional Qualifications*. Quincy, MA: National Fire Protection Association.

National Institute for Occupational Safety and Health. 2017. "Preventing Deaths and Injuries of Fire Fighters During Training Exercises." Workplace Solutions, no. 2017-113. https://www.cdc.gov/niosh/docs/wp-solutions/2017-113/pdfs/2017-113.pdf?id=. Accessed October 12, 2018.

CHAPTER PRESENTATION EXERCISE

Instructions: Your course instructor will assign individual or group discussions on the key points and teaching tips of this chapter. You or your group will review the chapter teachings and identify the major learning points from the chapter. You should be able to discuss the points, why they are important, and how and where they apply to your responsibilities at your level of instructor training.

REVIEW QUESTIONS

1. Regarding the 16 Fire Fighter Life Safety Initiatives, which initiative(s) relate to training safety and live fire training? Explain the instructor's role in each one.
2. Name five conditions for which additional instructors should be employed at training sessions.
3. Explain why negligence and misfeasance are "kindred spirits."

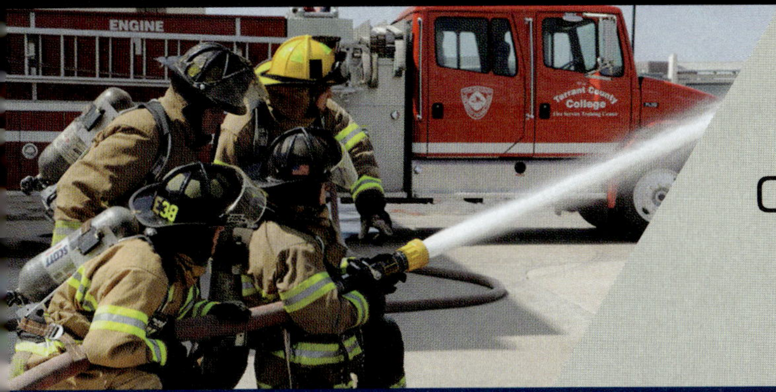

CHAPTER 8

Evaluating the Learning Process

NFPA 1041 JOB PERFORMANCE REQUIREMENTS

Note: An asterisk denotes that the 1041 standard contains further information in its annex section.

4.5.2 Administer oral, written, and performance tests, given the lesson plan, evaluation instruments, and evaluation procedures of the AHJ, so that bias or discrimination is eliminated, the testing is conducted according to procedures, and the security of the materials is maintained.

(A) Requisite Knowledge.

Test administration, laws and policies pertaining to discrimination during training and testing, methods for eliminating testing bias, laws affecting records and disclosure of training information, purposes of evaluation and testing, and performance skills evaluation.

(B) Requisite Skills.

Use of skills checklists and assessment techniques.

4.5.3 Grade student oral, written, or performance tests, given class answer sheets or skills checklists and appropriate answer keys, so the examinations are accurately graded and properly secured.

(A) Requisite Knowledge.

Grading methods, methods for eliminating bias during grading, and maintaining confidentiality of scores.

(B) Requisite Skills.

None required.

4.5.4 Report test results, given a set of test answer sheets or skills checklists, a report form, and policies and procedures for reporting, so that the results are accurately recorded, the forms are forwarded according to procedure, and unusual circumstances are reported.

(A) Requisite Knowledge.

Reporting procedures and the interpretation of test results.

(B) Requisite Skills.

Communication skills and basic coaching.

4.5.5* Provide evaluation feedback to students, given evaluation data, so that the feedback is timely; specific enough for the student to make efforts to modify behavior; and objective, clear, and relevant; also include suggestions based on the data.

(A) Requisite Knowledge.

Reporting procedures and the interpretation of test results.

(B) Requisite Skills.

Communication skills and basic coaching.

KNOWLEDGE OBJECTIVES

After studying this chapter, participating in a structured learning environment, and completing assigned assessments, you will be able to:

- Explain the reasons for conducting evaluations of learning. (**NFPA 1041: 4.5.1**, p 183)
- Describe the legal considerations for testing. (**NFPA 1041: 4.5.2**, p 183)
- Describe standard testing procedures. (**NFPA 1041: 4.5.2**, p 184)

- Describe common test administration procedures. (**NFPA 1041: 4.5.2**, pp 184–185)
- Identify considerations for maintaining test security. (**NFPA 1041: 4.5.2**, pp 184–190)
- Describe the methods used to grade evaluations. (**NFPA 1041: 4.5.3**, p 190)
- Explain the purpose of feedback. (**NFPA 1041: 4.5.5**, p 191)
- Identify the information that should be provided to students about their performance on evaluations. (**NFPA 1041: 4.5.5**, p 191)
- Explain the reasons that accurate reporting of evaluations is important. (**NFPA 1041: 4.5.4**, pp 190–191)

SKILLS OBJECTIVES

After studying this chapter, participating in a structured learning environment, and completing assigned assessments, you will be able to:

- Demonstrate methods of administering written, oral, and performance evaluations. (**NFPA 1041: 4.5.2**, pp 184–185)
- Demonstrate how to grade student evaluation instruments. (**NFPA 1041: 4.5.3**, p 190)
- Demonstrate how the results of an evaluation are recorded. (**NFPA 1041: 4.5.2, 4.5.4**, p 190)
- Demonstrate the methods for providing feedback on evaluation performance to students. (**NFPA 1041: 4.5.5**, p 191)

You Are the Fire and Emergency Services Instructor

As a fire instructor currently assigned to your fire training academy, you have been tasked by the academy director to administer and grade the next series of written examinations for the current schedule of classes. Your academy provides training for both recruit and incumbent fire fighters, so the curriculum used is quite broad and includes both classroom and drill-ground instruction.

1. Describe the different methods for administering written examinations.
2. Describe how written examinations are graded and how the results are recorded.
3. Describe methods for providing feedback on written examination results directly to the individual students.

JONES & BARTLETT LEARNING NAVIGATE 2 *Access Navigate for more practice activities.*

Introduction

Testing plays a vital role in training and educating fire and emergency services personnel. A sound testing program allows you to know whether students are progressing satisfactorily, whether they have learned and mastered learning objectives, and whether your instruction is effective. Without a sound testing program, there is no way to assess student progress or to determine which learning objectives have been mastered. In addition, it is impossible to determine the effectiveness and quality of training programs without evaluation.

Fire departments across the country continue to encounter problems with testing programs. Common problems in testing include the following issues:

- Lack of standardized test specifications and test format examples
- Confusing procedures and guidelines for test development, review, and approval

- Lack of consistency and standardization in the application of testing technology
- Failure to perform formal test-item and test analysis
- Inadequate instructor training in testing technology

This chapter is designed to provide the necessary information and training to help overcome these and other common weaknesses, thereby strengthening your testing program.

Legal Considerations for Testing

Testing for completion of training programs, job entry, certification, and licensure is governed by certain legal requirements and professional standards in the United States. These legal requirements and professional standards are readily available and should be important reference documents for anyone involved in the development of test items, construction of tests, administration of tests, analysis and improvement of tests, and maintenance of testing records. Because each state and municipality will have different laws and ordinances, be sure to establish a working knowledge of applicable laws and standards relating to testing and evaluation. As the instructor, you should be aware of laws and standards that apply to some of the following areas:

- Entry-level testing for new candidates for written and physical ability testing
- Certification testing rules and test candidate requirements
- Promotional testing criteria and the evaluation of promotional test results
- Continuing education testing requirements for emergency medical services (EMS), firefighting, and other certifications or licenses
- Recordkeeping, scoring, and test record storage

Among the most important reference documents are *Uniform Guidelines for Employee Selection*, published by the Equal Employment Opportunity Commission; *Standards for Educational and Psychological Testing*, published by the American Psychological Association (American Educational Resource Association, American Psychological Association, and National Council on Measurement in Education, 1999); and *Family Educational Rights and Privacy Act*, published by the U.S. Printing Office and other governmental organizations (U.S. Department of Education, 2011). Each of these references should be available in every fire department's training division library for instructors to study.

Purposes and Types of Tests

Tests should be used for the following three purposes:

1. To measure student attainment of learning objectives
2. To determine weaknesses and gaps in the training program
3. To enhance and improve training programs by positively influencing the revision of training materials and the improvement of instructor performance

The three basic types of tests are written, oral, and performance.

Written Tests

Written tests can be made up of the following types of test items:

- Multiple choice
- Matching (a form of multiple choice)
- Arrangement
- Identification
- Completion
- True/false
- Essay

The multiple choice exam is typically the most common form of written test because it is the most objective and thus the most reliable for testing; however, because there are many different learning styles, students should be given multiple formats in which to demonstrate their competency. The various types of written tests are discussed later in this chapter in the Written Test Items section.

Performance Tests

A **performance test**, also known as a **skills evaluation**, measures a student's ability to perform a task. This test category includes laboratory exercises, scenarios, and job performance requirements (JPRs).

Here is an example of a performance test item:

Perform a daily inspection of self-contained breathing apparatus (SCBA).

Any performance test should be developed in accordance with task analysis information and reviewed by a **subject-matter expert (SME)** to ensure technical accuracy in terms of the actual work conditions, and should be accompanied by a checklist detailing the steps of the skill in order.

Oral Tests

Oral tests, in which the answers are spoken either in response to an essay-type question (oral content)

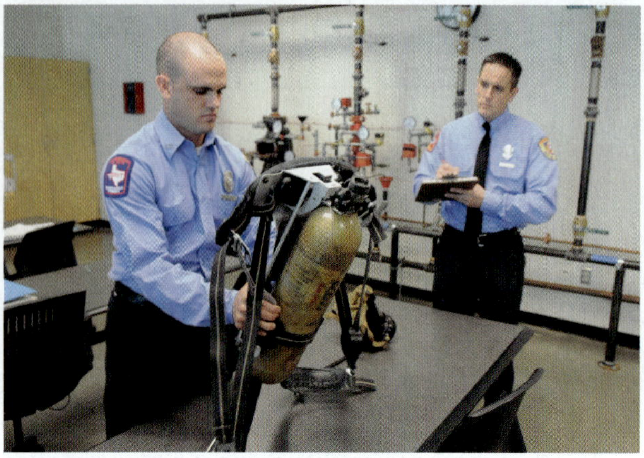

FIGURE 8-1 Oral tests assess knowledge, skills, and abilities before a performance test.

or along with a presentation or demonstration (oral presentation), are not widely used in the fire service specifically; however, this type of test has a place in technical and emergency services training. Oral tests are given in a structured and standardized manner to determine students' verbal response to assess knowledge, skills, and abilities important on the job (**FIGURE 8-1**). They primarily focus on safety-related skills to be performed. The oral test allows students to clarify answers and you to clarify questions. Oral tests are effective in ascertaining student knowledge and understanding when these aspects are not conveniently measured through other types of tests. An example of an oral test follows:

> *Describe the steps in the proper order that are required to properly engage a fire pump and begin the flow of water through a single 2½-in. port.*

Oral tests used in conjunction with performance tests should focus on critical performance elements and key safety factors. The overhead or directed questioning technique seems to work best when a group of students are preparing to take a performance test. Specific oral test questions can be used when a student is taking a performance test. Oral tests used in conjunction with performance tests are usually not graded, but rather are designed to reinforce key safety factors for students and to ensure critical safety factors are being confirmed by the instructor/proctor.

Standard Testing Procedures

Within a training department, the test development activities should adhere to a common set of procedures. These procedures should be included in standard operating procedure (SOP) or standard operating guideline (SOG) formats. These valuable documents should offer test development concepts, rules, suggestions, and format examples. You should use the procedures and guidelines specified in the SOP/SOG document throughout the test-item development, test construction, test administration, and test-item analysis processes.

Proctoring Tests

You will gain both knowledge and skills in test-item writing and test development when you complete the Instructor II requirements. Now, you should explore the other aspects of a solid testing program. Proctoring, or administering, tests encompasses much more than just being present in the testing environment; it requires specific skills to be performed professionally. Types of tests being proctored require different proctoring skills and abilities.

Proctoring Written Tests

The following are some suggested procedures for proctoring written tests:

- Arrive at least 30 minutes prior to the beginning time for the test to ensure the evaluation area is properly set up and everything is in order.
- Make sure the testing environment is suitable in terms of lighting, temperature control, adequate space, and other related items.
- During the arrival of test takers, double-check those who should be in attendance by checking identification documents and recording their presence. (You may develop a log or other means to document arrival time and departure time.)
- Provide specific written and oral guidance of test-taking rules and behavior guidelines for the testing period. Maintain order in the testing facility, discouraging any activities that might potentially be interpreted as cheating. Discipline anyone who becomes disruptive or violates the rules.
- Remain objective with all test takers. Do not show any form of favoritism.
- Answer questions about the testing process and the test itself.
- Do not answer an individual question about the content of the test unless that information is also shared with the entire group.
- Monitor test takers during the entire period of the test; never leave the testing environment for any reason.
- Require all test-item challenges to be made prior to test takers leaving the room. Advise that their challenge will be noted and addressed after all of the tests are scored.

- Collect and double-check answer sheets or booklets to ensure that all information is properly entered and that any supporting materials are returned before allowing test takers to leave the room.
- Maintain the security of testing materials at all times. Inventory all testing materials and return them to the designated person in the department when you are done with them.

Proctoring Oral Tests

Oral tests are generally given in conjunction with performance tests. Even so, there are preferred procedures that need to be followed to maximize the effectiveness of the oral test:

- Determine the oral test items to be used and the type of assessment technique that will be employed (e.g., overhead, direct).
- Make sure the oral test items are pertinent to the task to be performed.
- Focus on the critical safety items and dangerous steps within the performance.
- If the test taker misses the oral test item, redirect the question to another performer. If you are conducting a one-on-one oral test, then provide the test taker with on-the-spot instruction. Safety knowledge and dangerous task performance steps must be clear and mastered or corrected before performance begins.
- Use a scoring guide for the oral test and record any difficulties and lack of knowledge on the part of the test taker(s).
- If the group or individual has knowledge gaps regarding the critical safety items or dangerous performance steps, *do not* proceed to the performance test. More training and testing are required.
- Make a training record of oral test results using a prepared list of questions and including space for the evaluator to add comments and notes.

COMPANY-LEVEL INSTRUCTOR TIP

It is important to outline the required responses to oral test questions to ensure that proper feedback is given to the student.

Proctoring Performance Tests

Performance test proctoring requires considerably different skills than those needed to proctor the written and oral test. Proctors must have keen observational skills, technical competence for the task(s) being performed, ability to record specific test observations (including deficiency and outstanding performances), ability to foresee critical dangers that may lead to injury to the performer or others, and an objective relationship to the test takers (**FIGURE 8-2**). Following are some suggested procedures, including pre-test preparations:

- Arrive at the test site approximately 1 hour before the performance test to assess the test environment. Make sure all needed tools, materials, and props are present and in good working order.
- Determine whether the performance test will require an oral test before the actual performance of the task. (Obtain oral test items if required.)
- Check the test takers' identification as they arrive and record their presence.
- Review the test procedures and ask for questions from the test takers.
- Verify that all test takers know what will be expected during performance.
- Begin the performance test. Have the students tell you exactly what they will be doing before they undertake each step in the performance. (This is a critical step—it can help prevent an accident or unsafe performance before it happens.) In certification testing, missing safety-related steps or not knowing critical performances that may cause injury or damage to equipment is cause to terminate testing and refer the test taker for more training. This should also be true for the final performance test in a training program that leads to licensure.
- Remain silent and uninvolved in the task performance. Your job is to verify safe and competent performance.
- Record test results using standard protocols. You may provide technical information and critique the performance if your institution or agency permits proctor interaction after the test.
- Provide test results to the person(s) designated to receive them.

Written Test Items

Components of a Test Item

Test items are made up of components that create a testing tool. An important part of the question is the reference material that documents the standard the question is based on and the source of the information in a textbook.

Candidate: ______________________________ Date: ______________

ID#: ______________________________

Skill Drill 16-25

Fire Fighter I, 5.5.2

Performing an Accordion Hose Load					
Evaluator Instructions: The candidate shall be provided with a fire apparatus, supply hose, and gloves.					
Task: Performing an accordion hose load.					
Performance Outcome: The candidate shall demonstrate the ability to do an accordion hose load.					
Candidate Directive: "Properly perform an accordion hose load."					
No.	**Task Steps**	**First Test**		**Retest**	
		P	F	P	F
1.	Determines whether hose will be used for forward lay or reverse lay.				
2.	For forward lay, places male hose coupling in hose bed first. For reverse lay, places female hose coupling in hose bed first.				
3.	Starts hose lay with coupling at front end of hose compartment.				
4.	Lays first length of hose in hose bed on its edge against side of hose bed.				
5.	Doubles hose back on itself at rear of hose bed. Leaves female end extended so two hose beds can be cross connected.				
6.	Lays hose next to first length and brings it to front of hose bed.				
7.	Folds hose at front of hose bed so bend is even to edge of hose bed. Continues to lay folds of hose across hose bed.				
8.	Alternates lengths of hose folds at each end to allow more room for folded ends.				
9.	When bottom layer is completed, angles hose upward to begin second tier.				
10.	Continues second layer by repeating steps used to complete first layer.				
Retest Approved By:		Retest Evaluation:			

Evaluator Comments: ______________________________

Candidate Comments: ______________________________

Evaluator ________ Date ________

Candidate ________ Date ________

Retest Evaluator ________ Date ________

Retest Candidate ________ Date ________

FIGURE 8-2 A skills evaluation sheet can be a useful tool in evaluating a performance test.

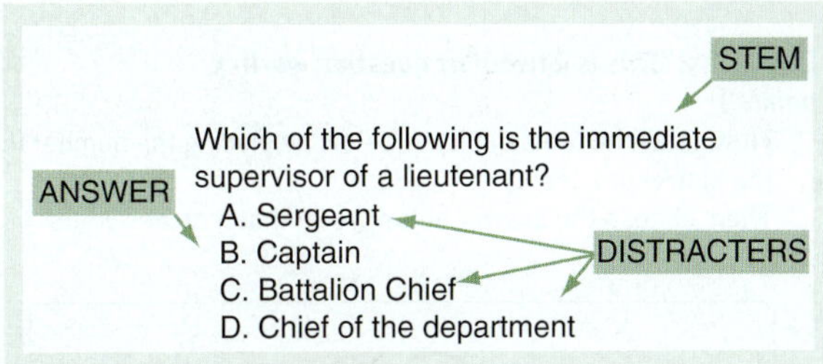

FIGURE 8-3 Multiple choice test items are made up of three components: the stem, the answer, and the distracter(s).

Fire department synthetic rope, new or used, should be kept

A. warm, dry, and in a sunlit place.
B. cool, moist, and in a sunlit place.
C. neatly coiled and stored out of sunlight.
D. damp and in a dark place.

FIGURE 8-4 An example of a properly formatted multiple choice test item.

Multiple Choice Test Items

In a multiple choice test item, the part of the question that asks the information is known as the stem (**FIGURE 8-3**). The choices are made up of a correct answer and distracters. The multiple choice test item is the most widely used in objective testing. This type of item also contributes to high test **validity** and **reliability** estimates. The multiple choice test item is a favorite among test-item developers because it comes nearer to incorporating the important qualities of a good test than any other type of test item. These qualities include content validity, reliability, objectivity, adequacy, practicality, and utility. Ease of grading of the test items and providing immediate feedback to students make multiple choice items extremely flexible for the instructor. The multiple choice test item is so versatile that it can be used to measure almost any cognitive information. The disadvantage is that it may take several well-written test items to cover the learning objective properly. Another disadvantage is the common occurrence of misleading or poorly written distractors. **FIGURE 8-4** provides an example of a properly formatted multiple choice test item.

While the multiple choice question is the most popular type of test item, it is essential to determine the testing method that best ensures competency related to the learning objective rather than to simply fall back on habit.

Matching Test Items

Matching test items are actually another form of multiple choice testing. This type of question is limited in use, but functions well for measuring such things as knowledge of technical terms and functions of equipment. Care should be taken during preparation of matching test items because all information must be factual. Typically, there are no more than four items to match with five choices when providing matches. **FIGURE 8-5** provides an example of a properly formatted matching test item.

Directions: Match the terms listed in column A with the definition provided in column B.

Column A	Column B
1. Oxidation 2. Conduction 3. Convection 4. Radiant heat	A. Rapid oxidation with heat and light B. Oxygen combining with other elements C. Heat energy carried by electromagnetic waves D. Heat transfer by circulation through a medium E. Heat transfer by direct contact

FIGURE 8-5 An example of a properly formatted matching test item.

The matching test item is particularly useful when a question requires multiple responses or when there are no logical distracters. The matching test item is very useful for low-level cognitive information measurement.

Arrangement Test Items

The arrangement test item is an efficient way of measuring the application of procedures for such things as disassembly and assembly of parts, start-up or shutdown, emergency responses, or other situations where knowing a step-by-step procedure is critical. An arrangement test requires the student to place things in the correct order, sometimes using photos or diagrams. These test items lose strength and efficiency steadily as time lags between the paper-and-pencil solution and the actual performance of the procedure. You should plan to administer an arrangement test shortly before an opportunity to perform the actual procedure, disassembly, or assembly.

One disadvantage of arrangement test items is inconsistent grading. A student may miss the order of one step and thus miss the order of all of the steps that follow, even though the remaining steps may be in the

Directions: (***This is a two-part question worth 3 points.***)
The six steps of the basic method that should be used in fire or explosion investigations appear out of order below. **First,** number the steps in the proper order by placing numbers (1–6) in the blanks beside the steps. **Next,** select the answer that matches yours from choices A–D.

_____ Conduct the investigation.
_____ Collect and preserve evidence.
_____ Receive the assignment.
_____ Analyze the incident.
_____ Prepare for the investigation.
_____ Report findings.

A. 1, 4, 5, 2, 3, 6   B. 2, 4, 5, 1, 3, 6
C. 6, 3, 4, 5, 1, 2   D. 3, 4, 1, 5, 2, 6

Answer: D

FIGURE 8-6 A properly formatted arrangement test item.

correct sequence after the error. Another potential issue is key steps that are included in the SOP or SOG being left out of the test item. The test item should be developed in agreement with actual procedures used on the job if such procedures are required. In cases where it is important to test procedures that are longer than 10 steps, consider grouping them at key points in the procedure. Knowledge of emergency procedures, fire drills, triage, or other related procedures where knowing exactly what to do under critical conditions can be measured with high reliability using an arrangement test item. **FIGURE 8-6** provides an example of a properly formatted arrangement test item that includes a multiple choice component.

Identification Test Items

The identification test item is essentially a selection-type test using a matching technique. Its major advantage over the matching test item is the ability of the student to relate words to drawings, sketches, pictures, or graphs. These test items do require reasoning and judgment, but basically focus on the ability to recall information. Identification test items can also be considered to be arrangement test items for assembly- and disassembly-type tasks.

Identification test items provide excellent content validity and contribute to high test reliability. With today's computer publishing capabilities, digital cameras, and other technologies, however, identification questions often can be easily developed using your own fire equipment and apparatus features as the basis for the identification test item. Using this technique

Directions: (***This is a two-part question worth 5 points.***)
First, label the tools depicted below by placing the number in the blanks provided.
Then, choose the answer below (A–D) that matches yours.

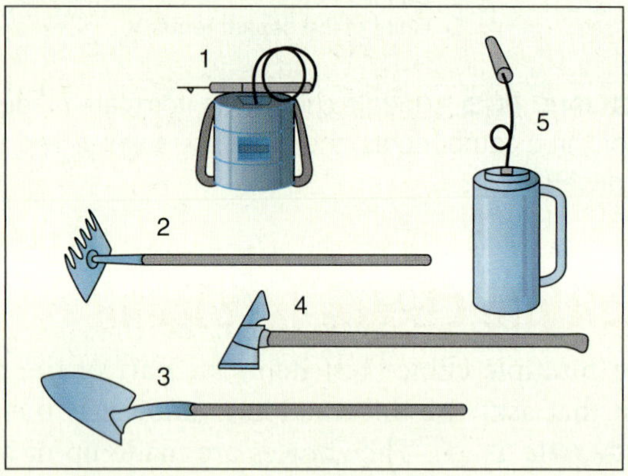

____ McLeod
____ Pulaski
____ Back pack pump
____ Shovel
____ Drip torch

A. 3, 5, 4, 2, 1
B. 2, 4, 1, 3, 5
C. 5, 3, 1, 2, 4
D. 4, 3, 1, 2, 5

Answer: B

FIGURE 8-7 An identification test item.

makes the test item more job related and makes it much easier to transfer required knowledge from the instructional setting to the job. **FIGURE 8-7** provides an example of a properly formatted identification test item.

Completion Test Items

The completion test item is easy to develop. Completion test items tend to be verbatim from the technical materials, thus they tend to encourage memorization and reinforce rote learning. These test items are appropriate for entry-level positions because they measure low-level cognitive knowledge. The best practice for developing and using completion test items is to follow specific procedures and to develop two test items for every one item that is expected to be included in the final group of test items.

Completion test items are of two types: supply and selection. The supply type requires the student being tested to supply the response that completes the test-item statement. The selection type requires the student being tested to select from a list of responses for completing the test item. The supply type primarily tests the recall capability of the student, whereas the selection type focuses on recognition and analysis.

True/False Test Items

True/false test items have been controversial for years. Test item developers have experimented with numerous ways to make true/false, right/wrong, and yes/no responses more valid and reliable. The major problem with two-answer selection tests such as the true/false is the guessing factor. A student who marks a response without reading the question has a 50 percent possibility of marking the correct response. Application of two or three rules for taking a true/false test could get the student a higher score than just by guessing alone. **FIGURE 8-8** is a typical true/false test item.

A more complex true/false test item can be developed that uses a multiple choice approach to the test item. **FIGURE 8-9** provides an example of a complex true/false test item.

Directions: Circle either "T" for true or "F" for false.

A forward lead-out takes place with a supply line being dropped at the fire area and the engine proceeding to a water supply. T F

Answer: F

FIGURE 8-8 Typical true/false test item.

Directions: Read the following statements regarding diversity programs and select your answer from choices A–D.

Statement 1: A diversity program creates an environmental and cultural change in an organization.

Statement 2: Achieving a culturally diverse organization is ethically and managerially a worthwhile accomplishment.

Statement 3: A diversity program is a single effort intended to integrate an organization to meet government mandates.

A. Statement 1 is true; statements 2 and 3 are false.
B. Statements 1 and 2 are true; statement 3 is false.
C. Statement 1 is false; statements 2 and 3 are true.
D. All three statements are true.

Answer: B

FIGURE 8-9 A complex true/false test item.

Essay Test Items

Modern test developers do not consider the **essay test** to be an objective form of testing. This position is based on research in which the major weaknesses of this testing method were examined. Some of the weaknesses that affect the objectivity of essay tests are listed here:

- Writing essay questions requires a lot of the instructor's time. Initial essay questions must be refined over several uses before they will function in a reasonably reliable manner.
- Students require much more time to prepare for and write answers to essay questions. Long tests tend to be fatiguing to students and can sometimes encourage lengthy responses containing extraneous information.
- The length of the student response tends to cloud the actual knowledge required by the question with extraneous knowledge closely related but not directed to the question. Students can "beat around the bush" without ever really addressing the question.
- Poorly prepared essay test items have been shown to reinforce negative learning. This means that the answer the instructor receives tends to support the wrong interpretation of facts and conditions, even among students considered to be outstanding.
- The order in which test papers are graded affects the grading. The first papers graded tend to receive lower grades than those graded last. This is especially true when tests are long and are graded one exam at a time. Grading one question at a time for all students tends to improve the consistency of grading on an essay test.
- Grading essay tests is time-consuming.
- Grading varies widely, even among instructors who are recognized SMEs.
- The "halo effect" influences the grading practices of some instructors. The more they know about a student, either favorable or unfavorable, the more the grade can be affected.

Research has revealed that an instructor can develop an objective test (questions based on objectives) in approximately the same amount of time that it takes to develop an essay test. However, the objective test will achieve higher content validity, comprehensiveness, discrimination, and reliability than is possible with an essay test.

Putting together a valid testing instrument may be one of the most challenging parts of the entire learning process. This process requires developing good questions where a student who knows the material is able to provide the correct response, whereas a student who does not know the material is not able to provide the correct response. It also should give those students who know the material the best chance to get more correct answers than those who know much less.

To accomplish this goal, take each learning objective and create questions that demonstrate competency for that learning objective. Use various styles of questions to discern the level of comprehension. For example, writing a scenario and having students apply the material concepts is much more difficult than developing questions where a student can recite rote information from the training materials.

Cheating During an Exam

With evaluations or exams, there is a risk of cheating. How cheating is addressed should be based on department policy developed by human resources personnel, the agency's legal advisor or attorney, and the chief of the department. Cheating by an individual reflects on the character of that individual and, in many departments, can affect employment status, raises, or promotions. Guidelines related to cheating should be established and communicated clearly before the testing occurs.

In general, a policy that addresses cheating will contain procedures to follow if a student has been observed cheating. In most cases, if you observe a student cheating, you should ask the student for an explanation of his or her conduct. If you determine that the student was indeed cheating, ask the student to leave the test site entirely or give a verbal warning and continue with testing. Again, the actions taken should follow department policy.

You must document what was observed, what the student said, and what you allowed the student to do next, ideally confirmed by a third-party witness. This information should be passed to a supervisor, who will review what happened and then follow up as necessary with additional interviews of the instructor and the student involved. The supervisor will determine what happens from this point. If it is determined that the student did cheat, then department policy will address the consequences. If it is determined that the student did not cheat, then arrangements should be made to allow the student to take the test again. Regardless of the consequences, the department should have a written policy to address how to handle possible cheating during an examination. Determine whether your organization has a policy on how to handle suspicions of cheating and follow it to the letter. Failure to do so is unfair to the student and can get you into trouble.

COMPANY-LEVEL INSTRUCTOR TIP

The proper handling of student information, including test grades, may be covered under laws that apply to you and your department. Know your responsibilities and play it safe by maintaining strict confidence of all student information.

Grading Student Oral, Written, and Performance Tests

The proper and accurate grading of oral, written, and performance tests is an essential function of the instructor. Students will desire feedback on their performance; likewise, instructors will want to know how successful their instructional efforts were. Class answer sheets or skills checklists will need to be carefully evaluated against master answer keys and then the answer keys will need to be properly secured for course validity purposes. Graded exams should be stored properly so that completed exams cannot compromise future offerings of the same test and the confidentiality of test scores remains in place. Elimination of bias in the grading process is necessary, especially when dealing with exam question types that do not have an objective format basis in their structure. After the exams are graded and scores are recorded, do not hesitate to secure the completed exam sheets and answer keys.

Reporting Test Results

Confidentiality of Test Scores

After the completion of the testing process, student scores must be maintained for various reasons. These test results should be protected using strict security measures. Electronic results should be password protected, and hard copies should be kept safe and secure. Test results should be released only with permission of the student who has completed the testing process.

When you release test scores to a class, you should do so on an individual basis. This sharing of the scores should be done in a private session, on a one-on-one basis, or in a personal letter to each student. The practice of posting scores on a bulletin board with Social Security numbers attached to them as identifiers is unsatisfactory and illegal.

Providing Evaluation Feedback to Students

Evaluation of examinations closes with feedback on the testing results with the students. This information must be considered confidential and should be completed in a timely manner using the evaluation data available to you. All feedback should be specific enough for the students to understand the following points:

- The overall score or grade
- Objectives that were missed and those that were met
- Skills that they did not complete to the learning objective standard
- What they may do to modify their behavior and performance in the future
- Any additional study areas or retesting requirements on missed items or failed skill evaluations

Grading scales should be part of the scoring process. When receiving feedback, the student may want access to score tables or percentage breakdowns for letter grades. A written policy should exist that deals with challenges to examination scores or practical skill failures to guide you on which actions should be taken during such a challenge.

Web-Based Training and Testing

In recent years, there has been a steady and significant increase in the use of computers for training and testing purposes. Many colleges and universities encourage students to take a portion of their program off campus, preferably online. Fire departments and EMS have made great strides in incorporating distance learning technology and continue to do so.

There are many options available for putting testing online 24 hours a day, 7 days a week, through computer hardware and professionally developed test banks. One of the primary benefits of online learning and testing is the convenience for people who work full-time jobs. An employer can also extend training and testing time into the available leisure time of willing employees. In addition to the convenience factors, the increasing costs of fuel, hotels, worker salaries, and other overhead costs indicates that web-based certification is here to stay.

Training BULLETIN

JONES & BARTLETT FIRE DISTRICT
TRAINING DIVISION
5 Wall Street, Burlington, MA, 01803
Phone 978-443-5000 Fax 978-443-8000

Instant Applications: Evaluating the Learning Process

Drill Assignment

Apply the chapter content to your department's operation, its training division, and your personal experiences to complete the following questions and activities.

Objective

Upon completion of the instant applications, fire and emergency services instructor students will exhibit decision making and application of job performance requirements of the instructor using this text, class discussion, and their own personal experiences.

Suggested Drill Applications

1. Review a recent written examination and compare the student responses to the answer key. Identify any test questions that were too easy (every student answered correctly) and ones that had poor success (high percentage of failures).
2. Review your local policy or practice on the posting of test scores and student completion records.
3. Develop a strategy to improve student performance based on a poor evaluation result.
4. Review the Incident Report in this chapter and be prepared to discuss your analysis of the incident from a training perspective and as an instructor who wishes to use the report as a training tool.

Incident Report: NIOSH Report F2003-28

Drill Assignment

Review the information in this incident report and prepare a practice presentation for class delivery at the direction of your instructor. Your presentation should include a summary of the incident facts and a review of the NFPA 1403 compliance and noncompliance findings. Use an outline to organize your thoughts. You may be evaluated on your communication skills during your presentation.

Port Everglades, Florida—2003

Note: This was the first U.S. fatality in a permanent live fire training structure.

A live fire training exercise was being conducted in a prop constructed from shipping containers to represent a seafaring vessel (**FIGURE 8-A**). This was the first live fire experience for the students in a class leading to state certification as Fire Fighter II. The students were all new employees of the same fire department.

Three evolutions took place, with no breaks in between the evolutions to allow the all-metal structure to cool. The participants were instructed not to crawl over the metal grating and to avoid holding the handrails, because the metal structure had gotten very hot and there was a possibility of getting burned through their gloves. They were told that failure to complete this evolution or getting injured would mean termination from the department. There was no preburn briefing or walkthrough.

Some members of the third squad received burn injuries during their rotation, and an instructor left during the evolution claiming he had problems with his gloves.

The fire fighter who later died was a member of the fourth squad of students performing the evolution on this particular day. Five students, three instructors, and an observer with a thermal imaging camera entered the enclosed structure on the second level. As in previous evolutions, the students were sent in one by one with the intention being that they would not be able to see or hear one another until arriving at the fire box. According to statements, the instructors did not monitor the students' movement or encourage their progress. Students followed the hose line through a series of three watertight hatches, and then crossed an open-grated catwalk over the gas-fueled fire in the engine room. At the end of the grated catwalk, a combustible materials fire burned in a corner. They then proceeded down a ladder and through the simulated engine room and into the "fire box." The fire box had a raised hearth, similar to a flashover simulator, and the fire was fueled primarily by wood pallets. The students gathered in the room and took turns operating a nozzle in various patterns. They were told to avoid getting water on the fire.

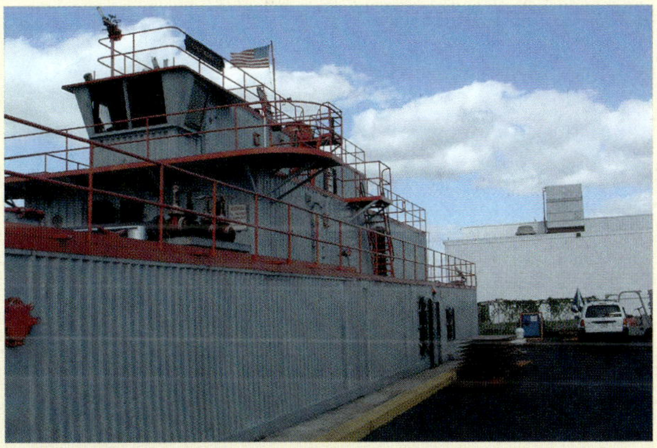

FIGURE 8-A Maritime training prop at Port Everglades, Florida.

The fire was knocked down, and an instructor in the burn room directed the crew to remain in the extremely hot area as the fire regained intensity. A "dead man" switch operated an open vent in the room, but it had been disabled so that it remained closed.

The instructor in the fire room was quoted by several trainees as saying the environment was too hot. He instructed the group to hurry up and "get out now." One set of students turned around to exit using the same route through which the group members had entered the room. Now out of sequence, the safety officer led the students up the ladder and over the metal grating in a very high heat environment. Meanwhile, two instructors exited through a side door directly from the fire box to an on-grade side exit, without advising the instructor-in-charge.

There are conflicting reports as to what occurred at the exit, but it was apparent that one student was missing. It is believed that he lost track of the hose, and ended up in a chase where heated gases and smoke were venting. Handprints on the walls indicated that he was trying to find a way out. While a search for him ensued, he collapsed. After seeing the downed student's

Incident Report continued

personal protective equipment (PPE), one officer entered to retrieve him, without protective clothing or SCBA, but had to abandon his attempt due to the heat. Another fire fighter wearing proper protective clothing and SCBA removed the victim to the outside. The victim's personal alert safety system (PASS) device did not sound while he was inside the structure; it is believed he was mobile until just before he was found.

The victim was unresponsive, with no pulse or respirations. After initial treatment by instructors, a medical rescue unit arrived and the victim was transported to a local trauma center, where he was pronounced dead. He reportedly had severe burns on both hands and sloughing of the skin to both knees and hands. He was described as cyanotic from the neck up. Several members of the same crew received second-degree burns to their hands and knees while they were attempting to exit the structure. One student lost consciousness after exiting and was initially cared for by other students. He and three other students were transported to the hospital.

Two separate investigations were conducted by the state fire marshal—one for criminal violations and an administrative investigation of state training codes. No criminal charges were filed, but the matter went to the state attorney. The fire department was cited by the state fire marshal for numerous code violations, and the reports cited 36 specific findings including almost total failure to follow NFPA 1403.

Postincident Analysis Port Everglades, Florida

NFPA 1403 Noncompliant

- No written, preapproved plan
- No previous live interior firefighting training
- Safety crews did not have specific assignments
- No preburn walkthrough for the trainees
- No designated safety officer
- No communication plan
- No emergency medical services on site
- Not all instructional personnel had specific live fire training or instructor certification
- Instructors did not monitor the trainees' movement
- Noncompliance with NFPA 1402 and 1403 (both required by state code)
- No temperature monitoring
- Multiple fires inside structure burning simultaneously, including polypropylene rope and other nonorganic materials
- Lead instructor determined the environment was excessively hot, but evolution was not terminated; also failed to identify and correct safety hazards

NFPA 1403 Compliant

- Three to four instructors per squad of five trainees

Other Contributing Factors

- No emergency plans in place
- No rapid intervention crew (RIC) assignment
- Command structure unknown to students and staff
- The fire box vent had been rendered unusable

After-Action REVIEW

IN SUMMARY

- Testing plays a vital role in training and educating fire and emergency services personnel.
- Testing for completion of training programs, job entry, certification, and licensure are governed by certain legal requirements and professional standards in the United States.
- Training and testing leading to hiring, promotion, demotion, membership in a group such as a union, referral to a job, retention on a job, licensing, and certification are all covered under the *Uniform Guidelines for Employee Selection* (Equal Employment Opportunity Commission).
- Tests should be developed for three purposes:
  - To measure student attainment of learning objectives
  - To determine weaknesses and gaps in the training program
  - To enhance and improve training programs by positively influencing the revision of training materials and the improvement of instructor performance
- Oral tests used in conjunction with performance tests should focus on critical performance elements and key safety factors.
- Any performance test should be developed in accordance with task analysis information and reviewed by subject matter experts to ensure technical accuracy in terms of the actual work conditions.
- Test development activities should adhere to a common set of procedures. These procedures should be included in standard operating procedure or standard operating guideline formats.
- Proctoring tests involves much more than simply being in the testing environment; it requires specific skills to be performed professionally.
- Performance test proctors must have keen observational skills, technical competence for the task(s) being performed, ability to record specific test observations, ability to foresee critical dangers that may lead to injury to the performer or others, and an objective relationship to the test takers.
- Performance testing is the single most important method for determining the competency of actual task performance.
- The multiple choice test item is the most widely used in objective testing.
- The arrangement test item is an efficient way to measure the application of procedures for such things as disassembly and assembly of parts, start-up or shutdown, emergency responses, or other situations where knowing a step-by-step procedure is critical.
- A major advantage of the identification test item over the matching test item is the ability of the student to relate words to drawings, sketches, pictures, or graphs.
- A major problem with two-answer selection test items, such as the true/false question, is the guessing factor. A student who marks a response without reading the question has a 50 percent possibility of marking the correct response.
- When cheating is suspected, the instructor must document what was observed, what the student said, and what the instructor allowed the student to do next.
- The proper grading of oral, written, and performance tests is an essential function of the instructor. Students will desire feedback on their performance, and instructors will want to know how successful their instructional efforts were.
- Release of test scores to a class should proceed on an individual basis. It should be done in a private session, on a one-on-one basis, or in a personal letter to each student.
- Evaluation of examinations closes with feedback on testing results being delivered to the students. This step must be considered confidential and should be completed in a timely manner using the evaluation data available to the instructor.
- Computer or web based testing is increasingly common in fire and EMS organizations.

KEY TERMS

Access Navigate for flashcards to test your key term knowledge.

Essay test A test that requires students to form a structured argument using materials presented in class or from required reading.

Oral test A test in which the answers are spoken in essay form in response to direct or open-ended questions. They may accompany a presentation or demonstration.

Performance test A test that measures a student's ability to do a task under specified conditions and to a specific level of competence. Also known as a skills evaluation.

Reliability The characteristic that a test measures what it is intended to measure on a consistent basis.

Skills evaluation A test that measures a student's ability to do a task under specified conditions and to a specific level of competence. Also known as a performance test.

Subject-matter expert (SME) An individual who is technically competent and who works in the field for which test items are being developed.

Validity The documentation and evidence that supports the test item's relationship to a standard of performance in the learning objective and/or performance required on the job.

Written test A test that may be made up of several types of test items, such as multiple choice, true/false, matching, essay, and identification questions.

REFERENCES

American Educational Resource Association, American Psychological Association, and National Council on Measurement in Education. 1999. *Standards for Educational and Psychological Testing*. Washington, DC: American Psychological Association.

Equal Employment Opportunity Commission. *Uniform Guidelines for Employee Selection*, 29 C.F.R. Part 1607. Washington, DC: Equal Employment Opportunity Commission.

National Fire Protection Association. 2018. *NFPA 1403: Standard on Live Fire Training Evolutions*. Quincy, MA: National Fire Protection Association.

National Fire Protection Association. 2019. *NFPA 1041: Standard for Fire and Emergency Services Instructor Professional Qualifications*. Quincy, MA: National Fire Protection Association.

National Fire Protection Association. 2019. *NFPA 1402: Standard on Facilities for Fire Training and Associated Props*. Quincy, MA: National Fire Protection Association.

U.S. Department of Education. 2011. *Family Educational Rights and Privacy Act*. Washington, DC: Family Policy Compliance Office.

CHAPTER PRESENTATION EXERCISE

Instructions: Your course instructor will assign individual or group discussions on the key points and teaching tips of this chapter. You or your group will review the chapter teachings and identify the major learning points from the chapter. You should be able to discuss the points, why they are important, and how and where they apply to your responsibilities at your level of instructor training.

REVIEW QUESTIONS

1. Describe the various types of test questions and discuss their main advantages and disadvantages.
2. What are the three main purposes for which tests are used, and what are the three basic types of tests?
3. Describe five of the important guidelines for proctoring written tests.

Appendix A

Resources for Fire and Emergency Services Instructors

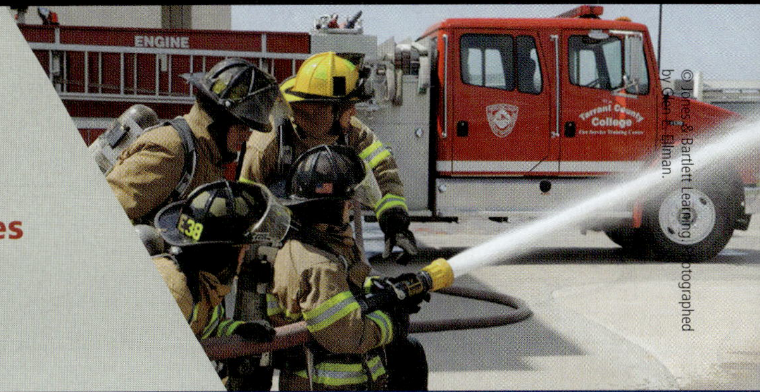

Contents

Training Record

Training Attendance Form

Date: ______________ Station(s): ______________ Description: ______________

Start Time: ______________ End Time: ______________ Credit Hours (Total Time): ______________

Method of Training: ☐ Classroom ☐ Practical ☐ Self-Directed ☐ Certification Credit: ☐ Yes ☐ No

Lead Instructor: ______________ Additional Instructor(s): ______________

Print Name	Dept ID #	Signature	Hours Attended

Objectives: ______________

Description of Training (Notes): ______________

____

____

______________ Instructor Signature

______________ Training Officer Approval

Type of Training *(ISO Category)*				
Company	Multi-Comp.	Officer	Mutual Aid	Night
Tower Burn	Classroom	Practical	Combo.	Driver

Equipment Used in Training Session	Feet of 1¾″ Hose Used	Feet of 2½″ Hose Used	Supply Hose Used/ Ft.	Feet of Ladders	Number of Engines	Number of Trucks	Gallons of Water	Number of SCBA	Total Number of Firefighters

Training and Education Report

Fire Department	Department Logo	Training Information Sheet

Name: ______________ ID#: ______________ Date of Birth: ______________

SS #: ______________ Date Entered Fire Service: ______________ Date of Hire: ______________

Driver's License #: ______________ Expiration Date: ______________ D/L Classification: ______________

Certification Record

Indicate Date of Certification in Boxes Below

Firefighter I (NFPA 1001)	Firefighter II (NFPA 1001)	Apparatus Operator (NFPA 1002)	HazMat Operations (NFPA 472)
HazMat Technician (NFPA 472)	HazMat Specialist (NFPA 472)	HazMat Specialist (NFPA 472)	HazMat Incident Command (NFPA 472)
NFPA 1006—Rope	NFPA 1006—Trench	NFPA 1006—Confined Space	NFPA 1006—Structural Collapse
NFPA 1006—Vehicle & Machinery	NFPA 1006—Wilderness Search	NFPA 1006—Water Rescue	NFPA 1006—Water Specialty
Instructor 1	Instructor 2	Instructor 3	Training Program Manager
Fire Officer 1 (NFPA 1021)	Fire Officer 2 (NFPA 1021)	Fire Officer 3 (NFPA 1021)	Fire Officer 4 (NFPA 1021)
Airport Firefighter (NFPA 1003)	Fire Inspector and Plan Examiner (NFPA 1031)	Fire Investigator (NFPA 1033)	Wildland Firefighter (NFPA 1051)
NIMS 100	NIMS 200	NIMS 300	NIMS 400
NIMS 700	NIMS 800	Command and General Staff	Incident Safety Officer
CPR/AED	EMS First Responder	EMT Basic	EMT Paramedic

Formal Education Record

High School Attended ________________ Year Graduated ________________ GED ________________

College Attended ________________ Credits Earned ________________ Degree ________________

Advanced Degree ________________ Credits Earned ________________ Degree ________________

Advanced Degree ________________ Credits Earned ________________ Degree ________________

Fire Department Administrative Directive/Policy/SOP

Department Training Program

Purpose and Scope:

This directive provides definition as to the training responsibilities of each rank within the department. This directive also establishes the basic format of the departments training program, including training requirements and documentation.

Responsibilities:

Training Officer

The training officer is responsible for the overall administration and management of the department's Training Division. Through working with the staff and line officers, the training officer is to develop and implement a comprehensive yearly training plan. The training officer has overall responsibility and accountability to ensure that department training activities are current and consistent with applicable standards and practices.

Instructor-In-Charge

The instructor in charge is the designated person who is responsible for the overall delivery of a specific lesson plan or training objective. All resources assigned to the training session are under the responsibility of the instructor in charge, including personnel, apparatus and facilities and equipment. The use of all required and best practice safety procedures throughout the training session will be the responsibility of the instructor in charge. All elements of documentation will also be overseen by the instructor in charge.

Instructor(s)

Instructors are responsible for assisting the instructor in charge at any high risk training event or routine training session where it has been determined that additional instructors are needed. This may be for the purpose of safety, accountability, or reduction in the student-to-instructor ratio. Instructors are responsible for delivering lesson plans, evaluating performance, providing feedback and documentation of the evolution or objectives as necessary. Instructors will be responsible for the safety of the members that are assigned to them during the evolution.

Shift Commanders

Shift commanders are responsible for administering and monitoring the department training plan within their assigned shift. This includes assisting in the coordination, presentation, and evaluation of specific department level training sessions. Shift commanders should make every attempt to attend high-risk training events, training events based on procedural operations where their presence is needed to simulate operations and any other training event where they can assist in the evaluation of member performance.

Through periodic evaluation of companies and/or individuals during training and emergency operations, the shift deputy commanders are responsible for identifying training deficiencies and providing recommendations to the training officer regarding the specific training needs of their shift.

Captains (or Other Mid-Level Shift Supervisors)

Captains are responsible for implementing and monitoring the department's training plan within their assigned area of authority (example—shift 2, west side). This includes reviewing monthly training reports to ensure company and individual compliance with training assignments. They also may be assigned by the training officer to assist in the coordination, presentation, and evaluation of specific department level training sessions. Captains are responsible for completing the training responsibilities of a company officer.

Company Officers/Acting Company Officers

The company officer is the key to the department's training program. They are the individuals most responsible for the training and readiness of their personnel. Company officers are required to complete each month's training assignments and submit all necessary documentation including training reports and skills checklists. Officers are to coordinate the various daily company activities so that training assignments are completed. They are responsible for coordinating company-level training so that all members receive the training regardless of time off, vacations, Kelly days, etc.

The monthly training assignments represent the minimum of what must be done.

The officer is not limited to this because each individual has strengths and weaknesses that must be addressed by the officer. It is the officer's responsibility to improve the performance of the personnel assigned to him or her. It is the officer's responsibility to foster an environment that encourages his or her company towards continuous improvement.

The monthly training calendar and company officer's packet lists the assigned training activities for the month. Some activities will have specific dates and/or time periods designated. For company level training assignments, the company officer has the authority to vary from the published schedule, if necessary for valid reasons. The company officer shall be responsible for scheduling and completing the training. The objective is for all training assignments to be completed by the end of each month.

Company officers are responsible for the safety of their personnel while training.

Company officers are responsible for maintaining the licensure required of their position. This includes EMT-B or Paramedic and appropriate driver's license classification.

Firefighters

Department firefighters are expected to maintain a high level of preparedness through regular training and individual study. This includes keeping current on both fire service and departmental changes and notifying their company officer of their training needs.

Firefighters are responsible to participate in an aggressive, safe and positive manner in all classroom and practical training. Firefighters are responsible for maintaining the licensure required of their position. This includes EMT-B or Paramedic and appropriate drivers license classification.

Monthly Training Assignments

The Training Division is responsible for providing monthly training assignments through the Training Bulletin, training calendar, and the Company Officers Training Packet issued at the beginning of each month. This shall specify the assigned and makeup dates for training (if applicable), who is required to attend and other necessary information.

Monthly training will be classified as follows:

Mandatory

This means training that must be accomplished by all members. This may also include 40-hour personnel. Mandatory training will include federally and state-mandated courses and courses deemed as mandatory by the Anytown Fire Department. These training sessions and make-up sessions will be scheduled by the Training Division and coordinated through the shift commanders.

Regular

Company level–Training that is to be completed by each company during the month. Company training designated as part of the Essential Skills program shall be completed by each company member. Other types of company-level training will specify whether make-up sessions are required for personnel who miss the training. Company officers are responsible for monitoring this and scheduling and conducting any necessary make-up training.

Department level–Training that is primarily scheduled and conducted through the Training Division. Department-level training that is designated as mandatory will have make-up sessions scheduled by the Training Division.

Documentation of Training

The training officer shall be responsible for providing to the shift commanders and captains a report as to the completion of training assignments from the previous month. The report shall be provided within the first 10 days of the next month. The shift commanders and captains are responsible for following up with their officers on the training that has not been completed.

The instructor of a specific training activity is responsible for completing and submitting the training report to the Training Division.

The company officer is responsible for ensuring that all skills checklists that may be required as part of a training assignment are completed and submitted to the Training Division.

For individual type training activities (i.e., independent study, reviewing fire service publications, physical fitness, etc.) the individual is responsible for completing the report and submitting it to his or her company officer for their signature.

Individuals attending classes outside of the fire department (i.e., fire officer classes, tactics seminars, etc.) are responsible for completing a training report upon returning from the course.

BY ORDER OF: ______________________________

DATE: ______________________________

Fire Department
Live Fire Training Instructor
Training and Experience Validation

Name: **Department:**

Years of Fire Service Experience: **Rank:**

Certification Levels

☐ Instructor 1 ☐ Instructor 2 ☐ Instructor 3 ☐ Training Program Manager ☐ TPM ☐ Advanced Degree

☐ Fire Officer 1 ☐ Fire Officer 2 ☐ Fire Officer 3 ☐ EFO ☐ Other

➢ Copies of certifications must be available upon request

Previous Live Fire Training Educational Experience

☐ ISFSI Fixed Facility Instructor credential

☐ ISFSI Acquired Structure credential

☐ ISFSI Instructor-in-Charge credential

☐ NFPA 1403 course/class at state training facility, local academy or agency

☐ Attended FDIC Live Fire Training programs

☐ Attended other national conference live fire training courses

➢ Copies of course/class completion certificates are available upon request

Previous Live Fire Training Practical Experience

Approximate # of Live Fire Training Exercises Conducted at:

☐ **Training Tower (Class A)** ☐ **Training Tower (Gas Fired)**

☐ **Acquired Structures** ☐ **Container/Simulator/Portable Unit**

☐ **Exterior Burn Prop** ☐ **Class B/Gas Fuel**

☐ **Approximate # of Years of Live Fire Training Experience**

Validation/Attestation Statement

I have read and understand all components of NFPA 1403, Standard on Live Fire Training and agree to abide by all requirements specified for the positions/roles that I am assigned for this training event. I understand and accept responsibility for the position requirements for the activities I am assigned to complete and do so knowing the hazards & dangers associated with these assignments.

________________________ ________________________

Signature *Date*

Fire Department
Firefighter Skill Performance Ratings

- **Unskilled (0)**
  - Member failed evolution or skill (Mandatory Re-evaluation will take place)
    - Exceeded time limit
    - Missed step in procedure
    - Created safety hazard to self or other member
    - Unable to perform task
    - Repeated failure of task attempt
  - Requires Personal Improvement Agreement and formal documentation on standard evaluation form
  - No credit is given for purpose of progress reporting or evaluation towards applicable certification

- **Moderately Skilled (1)**
  - Performance meets the minimum requirement for the task and is performed on first attempt. With additional practice, improved performance levels can be attained
  - Members performance of skill may require supervision on fireground in order to perform
  - Time performance near minimum requirement
  - All appropriate safety precautions are taken
  - Instructor/evaluator determines need for additional training or repeat of skill

- **Skilled (2)**
  - Performance is above the minimum level because:
    - The time was above average
    - Skill meets all performance levels and could be performed on fireground without supervision
    - No serious/critical errors were committed
    - All appropriate safety practices were observed and performed

- **Highly Skilled (3)**
  - Performance is at a high level of competence because:
    - It was error free
    - It was the fastest time
    - Member could supervise others doing same task and identify errors or suggest improvements
    - Member knows the role and importance of this task in relation to other fireground operations

Example

Subject	Skill	Subset	Equipment	Performance Rating
Forcible Entry	Force an Inward Swinging Door	Hand Tools	Halligan Bar/Flat Head Axe	3

Examples of Verbs Used to Write Learning Competencies

AFFECTIVE DOMAIN				
Levels of Learning				
Receiving	Responding	Valuing	Organization	Value Complex
ask	answer	complete	adhere	act
choose	assist	describe	alter	discriminate
describe	comply	differentiate	arrange	display
follow	conform	explain	combine	influence
give	discuss	form	compare	listen
hold	greet	initiate	complete	modify
identify	help	invite	defend	perform
locate	label	join	explain	propose
name	perform	justify	identify	qualify
point to	practice	propose	integrate	question
select	present	read report	modify	revise
set erect	read	select	order	serve
reply	recite	share	organize	solve
use	report	study	synthesize	use
	select	work	verify	
	tell			
	write			

Examples of Verbs Used to Write Learning Competencies

COGNITIVE DOMAIN					
Levels of Learning					
Knowledge	Comprehension	Application	Analysis	Synthesis	Evaluation
define	acquire	apply	break down	categorize	appraise
describe	convert	change	correct	combine	compare
identify	defend	compute	diagram	compile	conclude
label	distinguish	create	differentiate	compose	contrast
list	estimate	demonstrate	discriminate	create	criticize
match	explain	develop	discuss	devise	diagnose
name	extend	discover	distinguish	design	discriminate
outline	generalize	manipulate	identify	explain	enhance
provide	give	modify	illustrate	generate	justify
reproduce	examine	operate	infer	modifier	interpret
select	infer	predict	outline	organize	relate
state	paraphrase	prepare	point out	plan	research
	predict	produce	program	process	summarize
	rewrite	relate	relate	rearrange	support
	summarize	show	review	reconstruct	
		solve	select	relate	
		use	separate	reorganize	
			study	revise	
			subdivide	rewrite	
				sequence	
				summarize	
				tell	
				write	

Examples of Verbs Used to Write Learning Competencies

PSYCHOMOTOR DOMAIN			
Levels of Learning			
Imitation	**Manipulation**	**Precision**	**Articulation**
adjust	arrange	administer	conduct
apply	code	book	document
assemble	control	clip	encircle
build	design	derive	graph
calibrate	dismantle	draw	pull
change	display	focus	push
clean	drill	handle	regulate
combine	encapsulate	identify	sculpt
compose	expand	introduce	set
compute	fasten	locate	sketch
connect	fix	manipulate	slide
construct	follow	mend	start
correct	frame	mix	stir
create	graph	modify	transfer
debug	grind	nail	use
display	hammer	paint	vend
insert	heat	preserve	vocalize
install	input	point	weigh
map	interface	sand	work
operate	loop	transport	
probe	maintain		
repair	organize		
shade	punch		
transform	support		
troubleshoot	switch		
	transmit		
	work		

Division of Training
Personal Improvement Agreement

Agreement Initiated By: **Today's Date:**

Member's Name: **Department ID#:**

I. **Concerns/Area Needing Improvement:** (Description of behavior, situation or objective causing PIA)

II. **Standard Reference:** (What is the acceptable level of performance, attitude, conduct or ability?)

III. **Shift Commander/Station Officer Action Plan:** (What the officer will do to help improve the performance.)

IV. **Personal Action Plan:** (Written by the member describing what they will do to improve themselves.)

V. **Document Action Plan Progress:** (How we are doing and progress check dates.)

Initial Follow-Up Date

VI. **Has the area of concern been corrected?** (Has improvement been seen in this area?)

Yes: ☐

No: ☐

Completion Date

VII. **On-Going Monitoring:** (Describe how monitoring of issue will take place and for what duration.)

Firefighter Name (print): ______________________

Agreement Date: ______________________

Station Officer Name (print): ______________________

Shift Commander Name (print): ______________________

Training Division Review: ______________________

Outside Training Request Form

Out of Department School Request Form

Training Division Only	☐ *Approved*	☐ *Denied*	☐ *Hold*	*Comments*
	Training Officer Signature			

Attach Class Registration Form to Request

Payment Information/Registration Tracking (Training Division Use)		
Department Purchase Order #	Reimbursable (Y/N)	Method of Payment
Other Members Attending (Yes #/No)	Registration Completed	Member Notification Date/Method
FireHouse Class Code Created	Member Instructions Issued	Attendance Confirmation Received
Certificate Received	Certification Received	Monthly Report Entry

Member Information		
Member Name	Date of Request	Shift
Station	Company Officer Name	Dates of Course
Course Title	Course Location	Course Sponsor
Class Fee	Hours of Program	Is This a Certification Course?
Member Signature	Signature	

Training School Request Acknowledgements		
Company Officer Signature	Battalion Chief Signature	Special Teams Leader* (*if applicable)

Out of Town/Overnight Travel Information (Completed by Training Division)

Transportation		
Department Vehicle Authorized	Personal Vehicle Use	Mileage Reimbursement Eligible* *Reimbursement for mileage at approval of Chief
Rental Car Agency	Payment Method	Airfare, Rail, Other
Reimbursements to Employee	Secondary Billing	

Equipment Issued			
	Helmet		Personal Flotation Device
	Eye Protection		Buoyancy Compensator
	Hearing Protection		Mask/Snorkel/Fins
	Gloves (*Type*):		SCUBA
	Bunker Coat		Other Resp. Protection (*Type*):
	Hood		HazMat CPC (*Type*):
	Bunker Pants		SCBA
	Safety Boots		Spare Cylinders
	Radio/Spare Batteries		

Out-of-Town Arrangements		
Hotel Name	Confirmation Number	Direct Billing Arranged (Method)
Hotel Address	Hotel Phone	Check-in/Check-out Dates
Meals in Conference Fee	Per Diem Rate/Days/Total	TOTAL EXPENSES (Estimated)

Firefighter Performance Expectations

Work Ethic

- Actively seeks academic and technical knowledge for self-improvement
- Completes tasks assigned without shortcuts and without repeating of tasks
- Work is complete, thorough, and done in a professional manner
- Actively seeks out additional work as it improves the team's ability to thrive
- Accomplishes tasks or goals with a "safety-first" attitude
- Keeps commitments and meets deadlines
- Can be trusted with confidential information
- Can be trusted with the property of others
- Is committed to help at fire department events off duty as necessary

Judgement & Problem Solving

- Makes reasonable and safe decisions when attempting to accomplish a task or solve a problem
- Approaches problems in a safe, logical and well-thoughtout fashion
- Seeks pro-active solutions to problems
- Applies critical thinking skills to complex and varied situations

Time Management

- Consistently punctual and completes assignments on time
- Manages work so that quality of work is satisfactory and not hurried, incomplete, or overwhelming to self and team

Teamwork/Interpersonal Skills

- Places the success of the team above self-interest
- Effectively works with others in order to accomplish tasks or solve problems
- Offers to help other company members
- Understands and follows chain-of-command
- Is courteous and respectful of peers and supervisors
- Does not undermine team
- Helps and supports other team members

Adaptability/Stress Management

- Remains calm in stressful situations
- Adapts behavior in order to deal with changing situations in a safe manner
- Adapts behavior in order to accomplish individual and department goals
- Recognizes symptoms of stress in self and others and seeks to deal with stress appropriately
- Communicates with others to resolve problems
- Remains flexible and open to change

Practical Competence/Physical Ability

- Demonstrates a desire to develop skills that are above minimal performance levels
- Can accomplish multiple tasks in succession
- Can retain and recall previously mastered skills
- Strives to improve practical abilities
- Knows all applicable safety behaviors and actions related to practical skills
- Maintains a high level of physical fitness, dexterity, flexibilty and strength through on-going fitness program participation

Communication

- Uses appropriate tone of voice
- Articulates in a clear, logical and understandable manner
- Displays confidence in message
- Is persuasive and makes a positive impression
- Demonstrates appropriate non-verbal communication techniques
- Avoids letting stress control a communication process or method
- Writes legibly using correct grammar and punctuation
- Listens actively

Initiative/Motivation/Decisiveness

- Accomplishes tasks or goals without being ordered, coerced, or motivated by others
- Demonstrates desire for personal and professional development
- Makes decisions definitively and consistently

Empathy

- Shows compassion for others and responds appropriately to heightened emotional responses
- Demonstrates a calm, compassionate and helpful demeanor towards those in need
- Mindful of the impact of his/her demeanor on those in need, family, bystanders, and other members of the public

Community Awareness

- Exercises compassion and willingness to help persons in varied situations with varied backgrounds
- Is sensitive to individual and cultural differences
- Knows the role a member of DPFD represents to the community

Appearance and Personal Hygiene

- Always clean, neat, well-groomed, and in good personal hygiene
- Always wears appropriate uniforms in excellent condition

XYZ Fire Department/Academy **In-Service Training Program** ***JPR Skill Sheet***	DESCRIPTION: This JPR Training Guideline references the format identified in NFPA Professional Qualification Standard series. Knowledge, skill, performance and topic description are referenced from the applicable state and local certification objectives to meet the JPR. Local application of each training guideline should be made by instructors utilizing department procedures or guidelines.

Duty Area	Level	Subject	JPR #
Text Reference		Training Module	

Job Performance Requirement:

Objective Number	Skill/Knowledge/Performance/ Topic Description	Reference	Standard	Validated
			Pass/Fail	
			Pass/Fail	
			Pass/Fail	
			Pass/Fail	
			Pass/Fail	
			Pass/Fail	
			Pass/Fail	

Critical Safety Points	Required Equipment
▪ ▪ ▪	▪ ▪ ▪

Instructor Notes:

No.	TASK STEP	FIRST TEST		RETEST	
		Pass	Fail	Pass	Fail
1.					
2.					
3.					
4.					
5.					
6.					
7.					
8.					
9.					
10.					

TABLE AA-1 Resources for Training Officers

SCBA Training	
FF Near-miss incidents involving SCBA	www.firefighternearmiss.com
OSHA Standard 1910.134	www.osha.gov
SCBA training ideas	www.firehouse.com
Driver Training	
USFA Emergency Vehicle Driver Training program	www.usfa.fema.gov—publications section of Web site
Driver/Operator lesson plans	www.firehouse.com—training section of Web site
Fire apparatus and traffic safety related information	www.respondersafety.com
Driver safety information	www.drivetosurvive.org
Sample apparatus driving SOGs	www.vfis.com
Company Officer Development	
IAFC Officer Development Handbook	http://www.iafc.org/associations/4685/files/OffrsHdbkFINAL3.pdf
Wildland Fire Leadership Development	http://www.fireleadership.gov
Long Beach (CA) Fire Department	http://www.lbfdtraining.com/index.html

Miscellaneous Resources	
National Fire Academy library	www.lrc.fema.gov 1-800-638-1821
Fire Fighter Close Calls	www.firefighterclosecalls.com
National Fire Fighter Near Miss Reporting System	www.firefighternearmiss.com
Everyone Goes Home	www.everyonegoeshome.org
With the Command	www.withthecommand.com
Training Resources and Data Exchange (TRADE)	https://www.lsu.edu/feti/municipal/nfstrade.php
Regulatory Agencies	
OSHA	www.osha.gov
U.S. Environmental Protection Agency	www.epa.gov
NIOSH Fire Fighter Fatality Reports	www.cdc.gov/niosh/fire
NFPA Standards	
National Fire Protection Association (NFPA)	www.nfpa.org
Organizations	
Illinois Society of Fire Service Instructors	www.ill-fireinstructors.org
International Association of Fire Chiefs (IAFC)	www.iafc.org
International Association of Fire Fighters (IAFF)	www.iaff.org
International Society of Fire Service Instructors (ISFSI)	www.isfsi.org
National Volunteer Fire Council	www.nvfc.org
Fire Service Publications	
Fire Engineering Magazine	www.fireengineering.com
Firehouse Magazine	www.firehouse.com
FireRescue Magazine	www.firefighternation.com/
Online Magazines	
Vincent Dunn	www.vincentdunn.com

Appendix B

An Extract from: NFPA 1041, Standard for Fire and Emergency Services Instructor Professional Qualifications, 2019 Edition

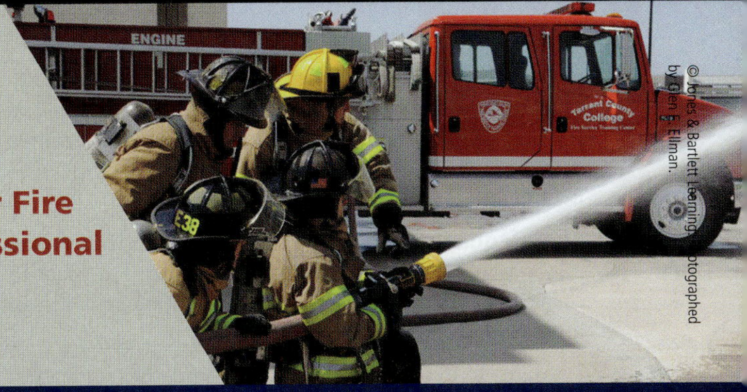

Chapter 4 Fire and Emergency Services Instructor I

4.1 General.

4.1.1 The Fire and Emergency Services Instructor I shall meet the JPRs defined in Sections 4.2 through 4.5 of this standard.

4.2 Program Management.

4.2.1 Definition of Duty. The management of basic resources, records, and reports essential to the instructional process.

4.2.2 Assemble course materials, given a specific topic, so that the lesson plan and all materials, resources, and equipment needed to deliver the lesson are obtained.

4.2.2(A) Requisite Knowledge. Components of a lesson plan, policies and procedures for the procurement of materials and equipment, and resource availability.

4.2.2(B) Requisite Skills. None required.

4.2.3 Prepare requests for resources, given training goals and current resources, so that the resources required to meet training goals are identified and documented.

4.2.3(A) Requisite Knowledge. Resource management, sources of instructional resources and equipment.

4.2.3(B) Requisite Skills. Oral and written communication, forms completion.

4.2.4 *Schedule single instructional sessions, given a training assignment, AHJ scheduling procedures, instructional resources, facilities and timeline for delivery, so that the specified sessions are delivered according to AHJ procedure.

4.2.4(A) Requisite Knowledge. AHJ scheduling procedures and resource management.

4.2.4(B) Requisite Skills. Training schedule completion.

4.2.5 Complete training records and reports, given policies and procedures, so that required reports are accurate and submitted in accordance with the procedures.

4.2.5(A) Requisite Knowledge. Types of records and reports required, and policies and procedures for processing records and reports.

4.2.5(B) Requisite Skills. Report writing and record completion.

4.3 Instructional Development.

4.3.1 *Definition of Duty. The review and adaptation of prepared instructional materials.

4.3.2 *Review instructional materials, given the materials for a specific topic, target audience, learner characteristics, and learning environment, so that elements of the lesson plan, learning environment, and resources that need adaptation are identified.

4.3.2(A) Requisite Knowledge. Recognition of student learner characteristics and diversity, methods of instruction, types of resource materials, organization of the learning environment, and policies and procedures.

4.3.2(B) Requisite Skills. Analysis of resources, facilities, and materials.

4.3.3 *Adapt a prepared lesson plan, given course materials and an assignment, so that the needs of the student and the objectives of the lesson plan are achieved.

4.3.3(A) *Requisite Knowledge. Elements of a lesson plan, selection of instructional aids and methods, and organization of the learning environment.

4.3.3(B) Requisite Skills. Instructor preparation and organization techniques.

4.4 Instructional Delivery.

4.4.1 Definition of Duty. The delivery of instructional sessions utilizing prepared course materials.

4.4.2 Organize the learning environment, given a facility and an assignment, so that lighting, distractions, climate control or weather, noise control, seating, audiovisual equipment, teaching aids, and safety are addressed.

4.4.2(A) Requisite Knowledge. Learning environment management and safety, advantages and limitations of audiovisual equipment and teaching aids, classroom arrangement, and methods and techniques of instruction.

4.4.2(B) Requisite Skills. Use of instructional media and teaching aids.

4.4.3 Present and adjust prepared lessons, given a prepared lesson plan that specifies the presentation method(s), so that the method(s) indicated in the plan are used and the stated objectives or learning outcomes are achieved, applicable safety standards and practices are followed, and risks are addressed.

4.4.3(A) *Requisite Knowledge. The laws and principles of learning, methods and techniques of instruction, lesson plan components and elements of the communication process, and lesson plan terminology and definitions; learner characteristics; student-centered learning principles; instructional technology tools; the impact of cultural differences on instructional delivery; safety rules, regulations, and practices; identification of training hazards; elements and limitations of distance learning; distance learning delivery methods; and the instructor's role in distance learning.

4.4.3(B) Requisite Skills. Oral communication techniques, methods and techniques of instruction, ability to adapt to changing circumstances, and utilization of lesson plans in an instructional setting.

4.4.4 *Adjust to differences in learner characteristics, abilities, cultures, and behaviors, given the instructional environment, so that lesson objectives are accomplished, disruptive behavior is addressed, and a safe and positive learning environment is maintained.

4.4.4(A) *Requisite Knowledge. Motivation techniques, learner characteristics, types of learning disabilities and methods for dealing with them, and methods of dealing with disruptive and unsafe behavior.

4.4.4(B) Requisite Skills. Basic coaching and motivational techniques, correction of disruptive behaviors, and adaptation of lesson plans or materials to specific instructional situations.

4.4.5 Operate instructional technology tools and demonstration devices, given a learning environment and equipment, so that the equipment functions, the intended objectives are presented, and transitions between media and other parts of the presentation are accomplished.

4.4.5(A) Requisite Knowledge. Instructional technology tools, demonstration devices, and selection criteria.

4.4.5(B) Requisite Skills. Use of instructional technology tools, demonstration devices, transition techniques, cleaning, and field level maintenance.

4.5 Evaluation and Testing.

4.5.1 *Definition of Duty. The administration and grading of student evaluation instruments.

4.5.2 Administer oral, written, and performance tests, given the lesson plan, evaluation instruments, and evaluation procedures of the AHJ, so that bias or discrimination is eliminated, the testing is conducted according to procedures, and the security of the materials is maintained.

4.5.2(A) Requisite Knowledge. Test administration, laws and policies pertaining to discrimination during training and testing, methods for eliminating testing bias, laws affecting records and disclosure of training information, purposes of evaluation and testing, and performance skills evaluation.

4.5.2(B) Requisite Skills. Use of skills checklists and assessment techniques.

4.5.3 Grade student oral, written, or performance tests, given class answer sheets or skills checklists and appropriate answer keys, so the examinations are accurately graded and properly secured.

4.5.3(A) Requisite Knowledge. Grading methods, methods for eliminating bias during grading, and maintaining confidentiality of scores.

4.5.3(B) Requisite Skills. None required.

4.5.4 Report test results, given a set of test answer sheets or skills checklists, a report form, and policies and procedures for reporting, so that the results are accurately recorded, the forms are forwarded according to procedure, and unusual circumstances are reported.

4.5.4(A) Requisite Knowledge. Reporting procedures and the interpretation of test results.

4.5.4(B) Requisite Skills. Communication skills and basic coaching.

4.5.5 *Provide evaluation feedback to students, given evaluation data, so that the feedback is timely; specific enough for the student to make efforts to modify behavior; and objective, clear, and relevant; also include suggestions based on the data.

4.5.5(A) Requisite Knowledge. Reporting procedures and the interpretation of test results.

4.5.5(B) Requisite Skills. Communication skills and basic coaching.

Appendix C

Correlation to NFPA 1041: Standard for Fire and Emergency Services Instructor Professional Qualifications, 2019 Edition

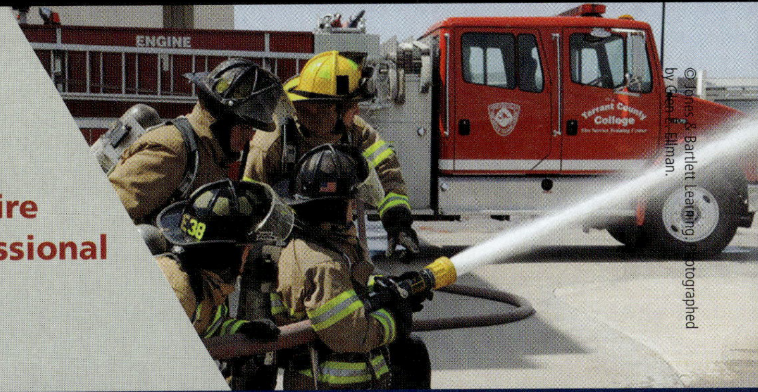

NFPA 1041, Fire and Emergency Services Instructor I, 2019 Edition	Corresponding Chapters	Corresponding Pages
4.2.2	5	124–129
4.2.2 (A)	5	124–129
4.2.3	5	128–129
4.2.3 (A)	5	128–129
4.2.3 (B)	4, 5	103–111; 129
4.2.4	5	128–129
4.2.4 (A)	5	128–129
4.2.4 (B)	5	128–129
4.2.5	1	14–19
4.2.5 (A)	1	18–19
4.2.5 (B)	1	14–19
4.3.1	5	129–132
4.3.2	2, 3, 5	37; 51–60; 83–92; 128–132
4.3.2 (A)	2, 3, 5	39–44; 51–52; 83–90; 128–132
4.3.2 (B)	3, 5	89–90; 128–132
4.3.3	3, 5, 6	83–92; 129–132; 143–148
4.3.3 (A)	3, 5, 6	76–92; 129–132; 143–148
4.3.3 (B)	3, 5	75–80; 129–132
4.4.2	1, 3, 6, 7	9–10; 79–90; 143–149; 160–170

NFPA 1041, Fire and Emergency Services Instructor I, 2019 Edition	Corresponding Chapters	Corresponding Pages
4.4.2 (A)	1, 3, 6, 7	9–10; 79–90; 143–149; 160–170
4.4.2 (B)	1, 3, 6	9–10; 73–77; 143–149
4.4.3	2, 3, 4, 5, 7	39–43; 73–82; 91–92; 101–110; 160–173
4.4.3 (A)	2, 3, 4, 5, 7	39–43; 73–82; 91–92; 101–110; 160–173
4.4.3 (B)	2, 3, 4, 5	39–43; 73–82; 91–92; 101–110
4.4.4	2, 3	37–61; 80–82
4.4.4 (A)	2, 3	37–61; 80–82
4.4.4 (B)	2, 3	37–61; 80–82
4.4.5	6, 7	140–149; 160
4.4.5 (A)	6	140–148
4.4.5 (B)	6	149
4.5.1	8	183–190
4.5.2	8	183–185; 190–191
4.5.2 (A)	8	183–191
4.5.2 (B)	8	185–190
4.5.3	8	190–191
4.5.3 (A)	8	190
4.5.4	8	190–191
4.5.4 (A)	8	184; 190–191
4.5.4 (B)	8	190–191
4.5.5	8	190–191
4.5.5 (A)	8	190–191
4.5.5 (B)	8	190–191

Appendix D

An Extract from: NFPA 1401, Recommended Practice for Fire Service Training Reports and Records, 2017 Edition

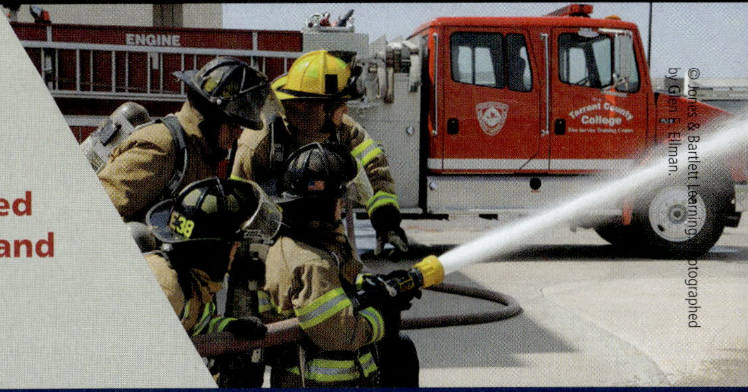

Chapter 4 Elements of Training Documents

4.1 General.

4.1.1 Training records and reports should be utilized by the training officer and line officers for analysis of the effectiveness of the training program in terms of time, staffing, individual performance rating, and financing.

4.1.2* Training records and reports should be utilized to develop specific training objectives and to evaluate compliance with, or deficiencies in, the training program.

4.1.3 Compliance with mandated training requirements should be documented.

4.1.4 The management of training functions should be performed in a closed-feedback loop.

4.1.5 The training functions should not operate as an open-ended cycle.

4.1.6 The closed-feedback loop should consist of the following:

- **(a)** Planning
- **(b)** Organization
- **(c)** Implementation
- **(d)** Operation
- **(e)** Review
- **(f)** Feedback/alteration

4.1.7* In each phase of the cycle, information should be provided for management to perform effectively.

4.1.7.1 The information is provided through various types of records, reports, and studies; therefore, records should be designed to fit into the overall training management cycle.

4.1.8 In order to be most effective, these records should contribute to the overall organization information cycle.

4.2 Elements of Information.

4.2.1* Training documents, regardless of their intent or level of sophistication, should focus on content, accuracy, and clarity.

4.2.2* These documents should relay to the reader at least five specific elements of information as follows *(see Annex B for examples of training record forms)*:

- **(1)** Who
  - **(a)** Who was the instructor?
  - **(b)** Who participated?
  - **(c)** Who was in attendance?
  - **(d)** Who is affected by the documents?
  - **(e)** Who was included in the training (individuals, company, multi-company, or organization)?
- **(2)** What
  - **(a)** What was the subject covered?
  - **(b)** What equipment was utilized?
  - **(c)** What operation was evaluated or affected?
  - **(d)** What was the stated objective, and was it met?
- **(3)** When
  - **(a)** When will the training take place? or
  - **(b)** When did the training take place?
- **(4)** Where
  - **(a)** Where will the training take place? or
  - **(b)** Where did the training take place?
- **(5)** Why
  - **(a)** Why is the training necessary? or
  - **(b)** Why did the training occur?

4.3 Additional Information. Additional information or detail, which should include but not be limited to the following, should be included to explain or clarify the document as necessary:

- **(1)** Source of the information used as a basis for the training
  - **(a)** Textbook title and edition
  - **(b)** Lesson plan title and edition
  - **(c)** Policy name and reference number
  - **(d)** Videotapes, CDs, and DVDs
  - **(e)** Distance learning sources
  - **(f)** Internet address
  - **(g)** Industry best practices
  - **(h)** Post-incident analysis (PIA)
  - **(i)** Other
- **(2)** Method of training used for delivery
  - **(a)** Lecture
  - **(b)** Demonstration
  - **(c)** Skills training
  - **(d)** Self-study
  - **(f)** Video presentation
  - **(g)** Mentoring
  - **(h)** Drill(s)
  - **(i)** Other
- **(3)** Evaluation of training objectives
  - **(a)** Written test
  - **(b)** Skills examination
  - **(c)** Other

Chapter 5 Types of Training Documents

5.1 Training Schedules.

5.1.1 Need for Training Schedules.

5.1.1.1 All members of a fire department should receive standardized instruction and training.

5.1.1.2 Standardized training should include considerable planning; however, standardization can be improved through the preparation of training schedules for use by department personnel.

5.1.1.3 Standardized training schedules should be prepared and published for both short-term scheduling (considerable detail), intermediate-term scheduling (less detail), and long-term scheduling (little detail) to facilitate long-term planning by the training staff, instructional staff, company officers, and personnel.

5.1.2* Types of Training Schedules. Training schedules should be prepared for all training ground and classroom sessions.

5.1.2.1 Periodic Training Schedule — Station Training. The station training schedule, which is prepared by the training officer, should designate specific subjects that are to be covered by company or station officers in conducting their station training.

5.1.2.1.1 The company officers should use this schedule to set their own in-station training schedule.

5.1.2.1.2 A balance between manipulative skills training and classroom sessions should be considered in the preparation of training schedules.

5.1.2.1.3 Such training schedules should include all of the topics necessary to satisfy job knowledge requirements and to maintain skills already learned.

5.1.2.2* Periodic Training Schedule — Training Facility Activities. The training facility activities schedule details when companies should report to the training facility for evolutions or classes.

5.1.2.2.1 Days also should be set aside for make-up sessions.

5.1.2.2.2 Training activities conducted outside the training facility or by outside agencies also should be shown on this schedule.

5.1.3* All Other Training. Schedules should be prepared for all training, including, but not limited to, the following:

(a) Recruit or entry-level training
(b) In-service training
(c) Special training
(d) Officer training
(e) Advanced training
(f) Mandated training
(g) Medical training
(h) Safety training

5.2* Training Reports.

5.2.1* Logical Sequence. A training report should be complete and should follow a logical sequence.

5.2.1.1 A report should clearly and concisely present the essentials so those conclusions can be grasped with a minimum of effort and delay.

5.2.1.2 Furthermore, a report should provide sufficient discussion to ensure the correct interpretation of the findings, which should indicate the nature of the analysis and the process of reasoning that leads to those findings.

5.2.2 Purpose. Each item of a report should serve a definite purpose.

5.2.2.1 Each table and chart in a report should be within the scope of the report.

5.2.2.2 The tables and charts should enhance the information stated or shown elsewhere, and they should be accurate and free of the possibility of misunderstanding, within reason.

5.2.3 Organization.

5.2.3.1* The process of writing reports should include five steps that are generally used in identifying, investigating, evaluating, and solving a problem.

5.2.3.2 These five steps, which should be accomplished before the report is written, are as follows:

(1) The purpose and scope of the report should be obtained.
(2) The method or procedure should be outlined.
(3) The essential facts should be collected.
(4) These facts should be analyzed and categorized.
(5) The correct conclusions should be arrived at and the proper recommendations should be made.

5.2.4* While there are differing needs among fire departments, certain reports should be common to most departments.

5.2.4.1 Typical recommended training reports should include the following:

(1) A complete inventory of apparatus and equipment assigned to the training division
(2) Detailed plans for training improvements that include all equipment and facility needs and cost figures
(3) A detailed periodic report on and evaluation of the training of all probationary fire fighters
(4) A monthly summary of all activities of the training division
(5) An annual report of all activities of the training division
(6) A complete inventory of training aids and reference materials available to be used for department training

5.2.4.2 The annual report should describe the accomplishments during the year, restate the goals and objectives of the training division, and describe the projected plans for the upcoming year.

5.2.5 Narrative Report. There are times when a narrative report should be necessary.

5.2.5.1 Before writing a narrative report, the writer should consider the audience for the report.

5.2.5.2 The comprehensiveness of the report should be determined by the recipients' knowledge of the subject.

5.3* Training Records.

5.3.1 Training records should be kept to document department training and should assist in determining the program's effectiveness. Information derived from such records should, for example, provide the supporting data needed to justify additional training personnel and equipment.

5.3.1.1 Training records can include paper or electronic media.

5.3.2 Performance tests, examinations, and personnel evaluations should contribute to the development of the training program if the results are analyzed, filed, and properly applied.

5.3.2.1 Training records should be kept current and should provide the status and progress of all personnel receiving training.

5.3.2.2 Frequent review of training records should provide a clear picture of the success of the training program and document lessons learned.

5.3.3 Properly designed training records should be developed to meet the specific needs of each fire department.

5.3.3.1 Training records should be detailed enough to enable factual reporting while remaining as simple as possible.

5.3.3.2 The number of records should be kept at a minimum to avoid confusion and duplication of effort.

5.3.4 Typical training records should include an evaluation of the competency of the student, as well as hours attended.

5.4* State Certification Records.

5.4.1 Minimum Information.

5.4.1.1 Information and documentation that should serve as a foundation for submission to state certification programs should include, as a minimum, the following:

(1) A single file that includes all training accomplished by the individual fire fighter during his/her career

(2) Dates, hours, locations, and instructors of all special courses or seminars attended

(3) Monthly summaries of all departmental training

5.4.1.2 These records should require the signatures of the instructor and the person instructed as a valid record of an individual's participation in the training.

5.4.2 The format used for state certification should be different from that utilized by an individual department. Otherwise, this is likely to cause considerable problems with accurate record submission and should be addressed on the state level by all parties concerned. Various state certification forms are contained in Annex B.

Chapter 6 Evaluating the Effectiveness of Training Records Systems

6.1 Evaluating Records of Individuals.

6.1.1 The evaluation of training records should be done at specified intervals by the local department training officer or training committee.

6.1.2 Each training record should be evaluated to determine the following:

(1) Has the individual taken all the required training?

(2) If not, has the individual been scheduled for missed classes?

(3) Do performance deficiencies show up on the individual's training record?

(4) If performance deficiencies exist, what kind of program is being developed to overcome them?

(5) Have companies met all the required job performance standards established by the department?

(6) If job performance standards have not been met, have the problems been identified and a program developed to overcome them?

(7) Are there areas of training that are being overlooked completely?

(8) Is the cycle of training sufficient to maintain skill levels?

6.2 Evaluating the Record-Keeping System.

6.2.1 All training records and the record-keeping system should be evaluated at least annually.

6.2.2 During the evaluation process, the following questions should be applied to each record:

(1) What is the purpose of the record?

(2) Who uses the information compiled?

(3) Is the record providing the necessary information?

(4) Do other records duplicate the material being compiled?

(5) How long should records be retained?

(6) Can training trends be determined from a compilation of the records?

(7) Is there a simpler and more efficient way of recording the information?

Chapter 7 Legal Aspects of Record Keeping

7.1 Privacy of Personal Information.

7.1.1* Employee training and educational records and other examination data included in an individual's training file should be disclosed only with written permission of the employee, unless required by law or statute, or by a court order.

7.1.2 The fire chief and the training officer should verify with legal counsel the federal, state, provincial, and local laws and ordinances regulating the disclosure of confidential information, and ensure adequate control measures are in place for the privacy of personal information.

7.1.2.1 Training records should not use the student's Social Security number for identification purposes.

7.1.2.2 The fire chief or training officer should ensure that training records do not include any confidential medical information.

7.1.2.3 All medical records should be kept in a completely separate file and not mixed with any other records or personnel files.

7.1.2.4 Access to any personally identifiable or proprietary information should be restricted.

7.1.3 Length of Time for Keeping Records or Reports.

7.1.3.1* Legal counsel should be contacted concerning the length of time records or reports, or both, need to be kept available and documented in a records retention schedule. *[See Figure B.1(m) for a sample schedule.]*

7.1.3.2 Documents should be maintained for a period of time as specified by law or as required by certain agencies and organizations.

7.1.4 Most training records should be maintained in their entirety in a computerized form, thus greatly reducing the amount of paper that needs to be stored.

7.1.4.1* Some training records should be maintained in their original hard-copy form, as required by certain agencies and organizations.

7.1.4.2* Computerized records should be backed up periodically and stored in an off-site location to avoid destruction.

7.2* Record Keeping and Risk Management. Agencies that conduct multijurisdictional training should have a signed release form for those individuals who participate in certain training activities.

Appendix E

An Extract from: NFPA 1500, Standard on Fire Department Occupational Safety, Health, and Wellness Program, 2018 Edition

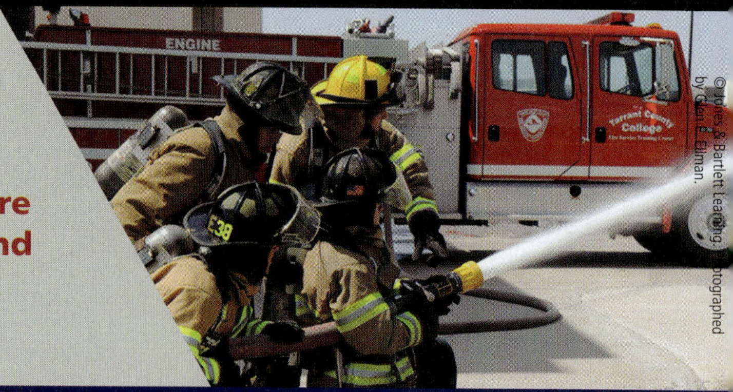

Chapter 5 Training, Education, and Professional Development

5.1 General Requirements.

5.1.1* The fire department shall establish and maintain a training, education, and professional development program with a goal of preventing occupational deaths, injuries, and illnesses.

5.1.2 The fire department shall provide training, education, and professional development for all department members commensurate with the duties and functions that they are expected to perform.

5.1.3 The fire department shall establish training and education programs that provide new members initial training, proficiency opportunities, and a method of skill and knowledge evaluation for duties assigned to the member prior to engaging in emergency operations.

5.1.4* The fire department shall restrict the activities of new members during emergency operations until the member has demonstrated the skills and abilities to complete the tasks expected.

5.1.5 The fire department shall provide all members with training and education on the department's risk management plan.

5.1.6 The fire department shall provide all members with training and education on the department's written procedures.

5.1.7 The fire department shall provide all members with a training, education, and professional development program commensurate with the emergency medical services that are provided by the department.

Δ 5.1.8* The fire department shall provide all members with a documented training and education program that covers all assigned personal protective equipment (PPE).

5.1.8.1 Training shall comply with applicable governing standards and follow the manufacturer's instructions and guidelines to include the following topics:

(1) The organization's overall program for the selection and use of protective ensembles, ensemble elements, and SCBAs
(2) Technical data package (TDP) where applicable
(3) Proper overlap and fit
(4) Proper donning and doffing (including emergency doffing)
(5) Construction features and function
(6) Usage and performance limitations (including physiological effects on user and effects of heat transfer on the protective ensemble)
(7) Recognizing and responding to indications of protective ensemble and SCBA failure
(8) Routine inspection cleaning, maintenance, and retirement
(9) Special incident procedure operation
(10) Proper storage

Δ 5.1.8.2 For maintenance of structural and proximity protective ensembles and ensemble elements, refer to NFPA 1851.

5.1.8.3 For maintenance of SCBA, refer to NFPA 1852.

5.1.8.4 For maintenance of protective ensemble for technical rescue incidents, refer to NFPA 1855.

5.1.9 As a duty function, members shall be responsible to maintain proficiency in their skills and knowledge, and to avail themselves of the professional development provided to the members through department training and education programs.

5.1.10 Training programs for all members engaged in emergency operations shall include procedures for the safe exit and accountability of members during rapid evacuation, equipment failure, or other dangerous situations and events.

5.1.11 All members who are likely to be involved in emergency operations shall be trained in the incident management and accountability system used by the fire department.

5.2 Member Qualifications.

5.2.1 All members who engage in structural fire fighting shall meet the requirements of NFPA 1001.

5.2.2* All driver/operators shall meet the requirements of NFPA 1002.

5.2.3 All aircraft rescue fire fighters (ARFF) shall meet the requirements of NFPA 1003.

5.2.4 All fire officers shall meet the requirements of NFPA 1021.

5.2.5 All wildland fire fighters shall meet the requirements of NFPA 1051.

Δ 5.2.6* All members responding to hazardous materials incidents shall meet the operations level as required in NFPA 472.

N **5.2.7** All members who engage in fire investigations shall meet the requirements of NFPA 1033.

N **5.2.8** All members who engage in fire inspections shall meet the requirements of NFPA 1031.

5.3 Training Requirements.

5.3.1* The fire department shall adopt or develop training and education curriculums that meet the minimum requirements outlined in professional qualification standards covering a member's assigned function.

5.3.2 The fire department shall provide training, education, and professional development programs as required to support the minimum qualifications and certifications expected of its members.

5.3.3 Members shall practice assigned skill sets on a regular basis but not less than annually.

5.3.4 The fire department shall provide specific training to members when written policies, practices, procedures, or guidelines are changed and/or updated.

5.3.5* The respiratory protection training program shall meet the requirements of NFPA 1404.

5.3.6 Members who perform wildland fire fighting shall be trained at least annually in the proper deployment of an approved fire shelter.

5.3.7 All live fire training and exercises shall be conducted in accordance with NFPA 1403.

5.3.8 All training and exercises shall be conducted under the direct supervision of a qualified instructor.

5.3.9* All members who are likely to be involved in emergency medical services shall meet the training requirements of the AHJ.

5.3.10* Members shall be fully trained in the use, limitations, care, and maintenance of the protective ensembles and ensemble elements assigned to them or available for their use.

5.3.11 All members shall meet the training requirements as outlined in NFPA 1561.

5.3.12 All members shall meet the training requirements as outlined in NFPA 1581.

N **5.3.13** All members shall be trained in the risks associated with workplace exposure to products of combustion, carcinogens, fireground contaminants, and other incident-related health hazards.

N **5.3.13.1*** Members shall be trained to recognize when a workplace exposure has occurred and to know the control methods for personal decontamination, decontamination of protective clothing and equipment, and the risks of cross-contamination.

5.4 Special Operations Training.

5.4.1 The fire department shall provide specific and advanced training to members who engage in special operations as a technician.

5.4.2 The fire department shall provide specific training to members who are likely to respond to special operations incidents in a support role to special operations technicians.

5.4.3 Members expected to perform hazardous materials mitigation activities shall meet the training requirements of a technician as outlined in NFPA 472.

Δ **5.4.4** Members expected to perform technical operations at the technician level as defined in NFPA 1670 shall meet the training requirements specified in NFPA 1006.

5.5 Member Proficiency.

5.5.1 The fire department shall develop a recurring proficiency cycle with the goal of preventing skill degradation and potential for injury and death of members.

5.5.2 The fire department shall develop and maintain a system to monitor and measure training progress and activities of its members.

5.5.3* The fire department shall provide an annual skills check to verify minimum professional qualifications of its members.

N **5.6 Training Activities.**

N **5.6.1*** All training and exercises shall be conducted under the direct supervision of a qualified instructor.

N **5.6.2*** All live fire training and exercises shall be conducted in accordance with NFPA 1403.

N **5.6.2.1** Emergency medical services shall be provided for live fire training exercises in accordance with Section 4.10 of NFPA 1403.

N **5.6.3*** For non-live fire training exercises, fire departments shall conduct a risk assessment to determine the appropriate emergency medical capabilities to be available at the training site.

Shaded text = Revisions. Δ = Text deletions and figure/table revisions. • = Section deletions. *N* = New material.

Appendix F

An Extract from: NFPA 1403, Standard on Live Fire Training Evolutions, 2018 Edition

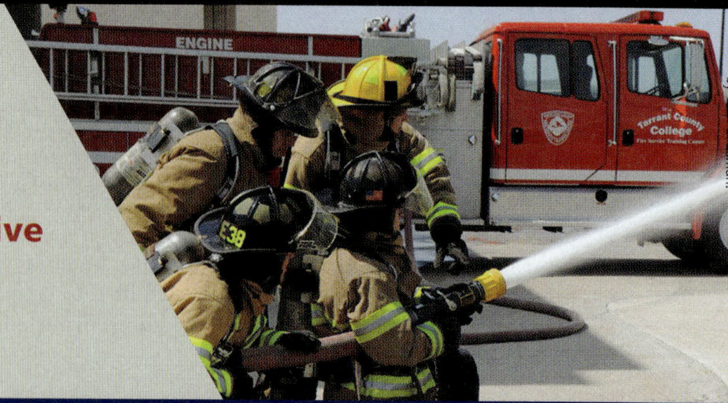

Chapter 5 Acquired Structures

5.1 Structures and Facilities.

5.1.1* Any acquired structure that is considered for a structural fire training exercise shall be prepared for the live fire training evolution.

5.1.1.1 Buildings that cannot be made safe as required by this chapter shall not be utilized for interior live fire training evolutions.

5.1.2 Adjacent buildings or property that might become involved shall be protected or removed.

5.1.3* Preparation shall include application for and receipt of required permits and permissions.

5.1.4* Ownership of the acquired structure shall be determined prior to its acceptance by the AHJ.

5.1.5 Evidence of clear title shall be required for all structures acquired for live fire training evolutions.

5.1.6* Written permission shall be secured from the owner of the structure in order for the fire department to conduct live fire training evolutions within the acquired structure.

5.1.7* A clear description of the anticipated condition of the acquired structure at the completion of the evolution(s) and the method of returning the property to the owner shall be put in writing and shall be acknowledged by the owner of the structure.

5.1.8* Proof of insurance cancellation or a signed statement of nonexistence of insurance shall be provided by the owner of the structure prior to acceptance for use of the acquired structure by the AHJ.

5.1.9 The permits specified in this chapter shall be provided to outside, contract, or other separate training agencies by the AHJ upon the request of those agencies.

5.1.10 A search of the acquired structure shall be conducted to ensure that no unauthorized persons, animals, or objects are in the acquired structure immediately prior to ignition.

5.1.11 No person(s) shall play the role of a victim inside the acquired structure.

5.1.12 Only one fire at a time shall be permitted within an acquired structure.

5.2 Hazards.

5.2.1 In preparation for live fire training, an inspection of the structure shall be made to determine that the floors, walls, stairs, and other structural components are capable of withstanding the weight of contents, participants, and accumulated water.

5.2.2* All hazardous storage conditions shall be removed from the structure or neutralized in such a manner as to not present a safety problem during use of the structure for live fire training evolutions.

5.2.3 Closed containers and highly combustible materials shall be removed from the structure.

5.2.3.1 Oil tanks and similar closed vessels that cannot be removed shall be vented to prevent an explosion or overpressure rupture.

5.2.3.2 Any hazardous or combustible atmosphere within the tank or vessel shall be rendered inert.

5.2.4 All hazardous structural conditions shall be removed or repaired so as to not present a safety problem during use of the structure for live fire training evolutions.

5.2.4.1 Floor openings shall be covered to be made structurally sound.

N **5.2.4.2** Fires shall not be ignited under exposed structural members.

5.2.4.3 Missing stair treads and rails shall be repaired or replaced.

5.2.4.4 Dangerous portions of any chimney shall be removed.

5.2.4.5 Holes in walls and ceilings shall be patched.

5.2.4.6* Roof ventilation openings that are normally closed but can be opened in the event of an emergency shall be permitted to be utilized.

5.2.4.7* Low-density combustible fiberboard and other highly combustible interior finishes shall be removed.

5.2.4.8* Extraordinary weight above the training area shall be removed.

5.2.5* All hazardous environmental conditions shall be removed before live fire training evolutions are conducted in the structure.

5.2.5.1 All forms of asbestos deemed hazardous shall be removed by an approved manner and documentation provided to the AHJ.

5.2.6 Debris creating or contributing to unsafe conditions shall be removed.

5.2.7 Any toxic weeds, insect hives, or vermin that could present a potential hazard shall be removed.

5.2.8 Trees, brush, and surrounding vegetation that create a hazard to participants shall be removed.

5.2.9 Combustible materials, other than those intended for the live fire training evolution, shall be removed or stored in a protected area to preclude accidental ignition.

5.3 Utilities.

5.3.1 Utilities shall be disconnected.

5.3.2 Utility services adjacent to the live burn site shall be removed or protected.

5.4 Exits.

5.4.1 Exits from the acquired structure shall be identified and evaluated prior to each training burn.

5.4.2 Participants of the live fire training shall be made aware of exits from the acquired structure prior to each training burn.

5.4.3 Fires shall not be located in any designated exit paths.

Δ **5.5 Rapid Intervention Crew (RIC).** A RIC trained in accordance with NFPA 1407 shall be provided during a live fire training evolution.

N **5.6 Water Supply.** For acquired structures the minimum water supply and delivery for the live fire training evolutions shall meet the criteria identified in NFPA 1142.

Chapter 6 Gas-Fired Live Fire Training Structures and Mobile Enclosed Live Fire Training Props

6.1 Structures and Facilities.

6.1.1 This section pertains to all interior spaces where gasfired live fire training exercises occur.

6.1.2 Live fire training structures shall be left in a safe condition upon completion of live fire training evolutions.

6.1.3 Debris hindering the access or egress of fire fighters shall be removed prior to the beginning of the training exercises.

6.1.4 Flammable gas fires shall not be ignited manually.

6.2 Inspection and Testing.

6.2.1* Live fire training structures shall be inspected visually for damage prior to live fire training evolutions.

6.2.1.1* Damage shall be documented and the building owner or AHJ shall be notified.

6.2.2 Where the live fire training structure damage is severe enough to affect the safety of the participants, training shall not be permitted.

6.2.3 All doors, windows and window shutters, railings, roof scuttles and automatic ventilators, mechanical equipment, lighting, manual or automatic sprinklers, and standpipes necessary for the live fire training evolution shall be checked and operated prior to any live fire training evolution to ensure they operate correctly.

6.2.4 All safety devices, such as thermal sensors, combustible gas monitors, evacuation alarms, and emergency shutdown switches, shall be checked prior to any live fire training evolutions to ensure they operate correctly.

6.2.5 The instructors shall run the training system prior to exposing students to live flames in order to ensure the correct operation of devices such as the gas valves, flame safeguard units, agent sensors, combustion fans, and ventilation fans.

6.2.6* The structural integrity of the live fire training structure shall be evaluated and documented annually by the building owner or AHJ.

6.2.6.1 If visible structural defects are found, such as cracks, rust, spalls, or warps in structural floors, columns, beams, walls, or metal panels, the building owner shall have a follow-up evaluation conducted by a licensed professional engineer with live fire training structure experience and expertise, or by another competent professional as determined by the building owner or AHJ.

6.2.7* The structural integrity of the live fire training structure shall be evaluated and documented by a licensed professional engineer with live fire training structure experience and expertise, or by another competent professional as determined by the AHJ, at least once every 10 years, or more frequently if determined to be required by the evaluator.

6.2.8* All structures constructed with calcium aluminate refractory structural concrete shall be inspected by a structural engineer with expertise in live fire training structures every 3 years.

6.2.8.1 The structural inspection shall include removal of concrete core samples from the structure to check for delaminations within the concrete.

6.2.9* Part of the live fire training structure evaluation shall include, at least once every 10 years, the removal and reinstallation of a representative area of thermal linings (if any) to inspect the hidden conditions behind the linings.

Chapter 7 Non-Gas-Fired Live Fire Training Structures and Mobile Enclosed Live Fire Training Props

7.1 Structures and Facilities.

7.1.1 This section pertains to all interior spaces where nongas- fired live fire training exercises occur.

7.1.2 Live fire training structures shall be left in a safe condition upon completion of live fire training evolutions.

7.1.3 Debris hindering the access or egress of fire fighters shall be removed prior to the beginning of the training exercises.

7.2 Inspection and Testing.

7.2.1* Live fire training structures shall be inspected visually for damage prior to live fire training evolutions.

7.2.1.1* Damage shall be documented, and the building owner or AHJ shall be notified.

7.2.2 Where the live fire training structure damage is severe enough to affect the safety of the participants, training shall not be permitted.

7.2.3 All doors, windows and window shutters, railings, roof scuttles and automatic ventilators, mechanical equipment, lighting, manual or automatic sprinklers, and standpipes necessary for the live fire training evolution shall be checked and operated prior to any live fire training evolution to ensure they operate correctly.

7.2.4 All safety devices, such as thermal sensors, oxygen and toxic and combustible gas monitors, evacuation alarms, and emergency shutdown switches, shall be checked prior to any live fire training evolutions to ensure they operate correctly.

7.2.5* The structural integrity of the live fire training structure shall be evaluated and documented annually by the building owner or AHJ.

7.2.5.1 If visible structural defects are found, such as cracks, rust, spalls, or warps in structural floors, columns, beams, walls, or metal panels, the building owner shall have a follow-up evaluation conducted by a licensed professional engineer with live fire training structure experience and expertise or by another competent professional as determined by the AHJ.

7.2.6* The structural integrity of the live fire training structure shall be evaluated and documented by a licensed professional engineer with live fire training structure experience and expertise or by another competent professional as determined by the AHJ at least once every 5 years or more frequently if determined to be required by the evaluator.

7.2.7* All structures constructed with calcium aluminate refractory structural concrete shall be inspected by a structural engineer with expertise in live fire training structures every 3 years.

7.2.7.1 The structural inspection shall include removal of concrete core samples from the structure to check for delaminations within the concrete.

7.2.8* Part of the live fire training structure evaluation shall include, once every five years, the removal and reinstallation of a representative area of thermal linings (if any) to allow inspections of the conditions hidden behind the linings.

7.3 Sequential Live Fire Burn Evolutions.

7.3.1 The AHJ shall develop and utilize a safe live fire training action plan when multiple sequential burn evolutions are to be conducted per day in each burn room.

7.3.2 A burn sequence matrix chart shall be developed for the burn rooms in a live fire training structure.

7.3.2.1 The burn sequence matrix chart shall include the maximum fuel loading per evolution and maximum number of sequential live fire evolutions that can be conducted per day in each burn room.

7.3.3* The burn sequence for each room shall define the maximum fuel load that can be used for the first burn and each successive burn.

7.3.4* The burn sequence matrix for each room shall also specify the maximum number of evolutions that can be safely conducted during a given training period before the room is allowed to cool.

7.3.5 The fuel loads per evolution and the maximum number of sequential evolutions in each burn room shall not be exceeded under any circumstances.

Shaded text = Revisions. Δ = Text deletions and figure/table revisions. • = Section deletions. *N* = New material.

Glossary

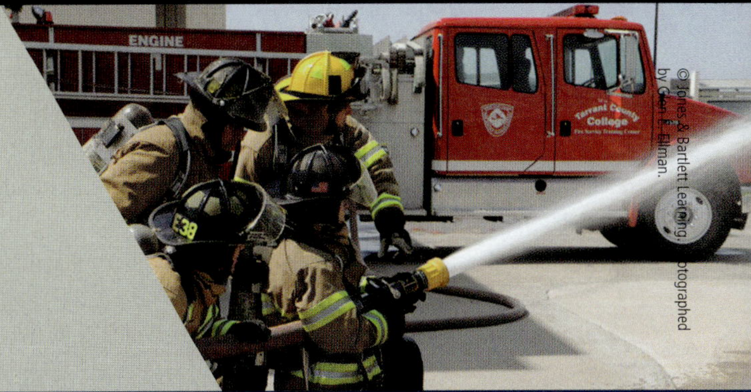

ABCD method A process for writing lesson plan objectives; it includes four components: audience, behavior, condition, and degree.

Active listening The process of hearing and understanding the communication sent; demonstrating that you are listening and have understood the message.

Adapt To make fit (as for a specific use or situation).

Affective domain The domain of learning that affects attitudes, emotions, or values. It may be associated with a student's perspective or belief being changed as a result of training in this domain.

Ambient noise The general level of background sound.

Andragogy The art and science of teaching adults.

Assignment The part of the lesson plan that provides the student with opportunities for additional application or exploration of the lesson topic, often in the form of homework that is completed outside of the classroom.

Asynchronous learning An online course format in which the instructor provides material, lectures, tests, and assignments that can be accessed at any time. Students are given a time frame during which they need to connect to the course and complete assignments.

Attention-deficit/hyperactivity disorder (ADHD) A disorder in which a person has a chronic level of inattention and an impulsive hyperactivity that affects daily functions.

Audience analysis The determination of characteristics common to a group of people; it can be used to choose the best instructional approach.

Audience Who the students are.

Baby boomers The generation born after World War II (i.e., 1946–1964).

Behavior An observable and measurable action for the student to complete.

Behaviorist perspective The theory that learning is a relatively permanent change in behavior that arises from experience.

Blended learning An instruction method that combines online/independent study with face-to-face meetings with the instructor.

Bloom's Taxonomy A classification of the different objectives and skills that educators set for students (learning objectives).

Certificate Document given for the completion of a training course or event.

Certification Document awarded for the successful completion of a testing process based on a standard.

Coaching The process of helping individuals develop skills and talents.

Cognitive domain The domain of learning that effects a change in knowledge. It is most often associated with learning new information.

Cognitive objective A statement that defines a learning outcome that is based on knowledge and understanding.

Cognitive perspective An intellectual process by which experience contributes to relatively permanent changes (learning). It may be associated by learning by experience.

Communication process The process of conveying an intended message from the sender to the receiver and getting feedback to ensure accuracy.

Competency-based learning Learning that is intended to create or improve professional competencies.

Condition The situation in which the student will perform the behavior.

Confidentiality The requirement that, with very limited exceptions, employers must keep medical and other personal information about employees and applicants private.

Continuing education Education or training obtained to maintain skills, proficiency, or certification in a specific position.

Courseware Any educational content that is delivered via a computer.

Degree Document awarded by an institution for the completion of required coursework.

Degree In reference to the ABCD method, the last part of a learning objective, which indicates how well the student is expected to perform the behavior in the listed conditions.

Delegation Transfer of authority and responsibility to another person for the purpose of teaching new job skills or as a means of time management. You can delegate authority but never responsibility.

Demographics Characteristics of a given population, possibly including such information as age, race, gender, education, marital status, family structure, and location of agency.

Direct threat A situation in which an individual's disability presents a serious risk to his or her own safety or the safety of his or her co-workers.

Disability A physical or mental condition that interferes with a major life activity.

Dyscalculia A learning disability in which students have difficulty with math and related subjects.

Dyslexia A learning disability in which students have difficulty reading due to an inability to interpret spatial relationships and integrate visual information.

Dysphasia A learning disability in which students lack the ability to write, spell, or place words together to complete a sentence.

Dyspraxia A lack of physical coordination with motor skills.

Enabling objective An intermediate learning objective, usually part of a series that directs the instructor on what he or she needs to instruct and what the learner will learn to accomplish the terminal objective.

Essay test A test that requires students to form a structured argument using materials presented in class or from required reading.

Ethics Principles used to define behavior that is not specifically governed by rules of law but rather in many cases by public perceptions of right and wrong. They are often defined on a regional or local level within the community.

Feedback The fifth and final link of the communication chain. It allows the sender (the instructor) to determine whether the receiver (the student) understood the message.

Flipped classroom An instructional approach that reverses or "flips" the standard learning environment by delivering online content for self-study and reserving the physical classroom for mentored practice that traditionally would have been assigned as homework.

Formal communication An official fire department communication. The letter or report is presented on stationery with the fire department letterhead and generally is signed by a chief officer or headquarters staff member.

Four-step method of instruction The primary process used to relate the material contained in a lesson plan to the students; the steps are preparation, presentation, application, evaluation.

General orders Short-term documents signed by the fire chief that remain in force for a period of days to 1 year or more.

Generation X People born after the baby boomers.

Generation Y People born immediately after Generation X.

Generation Z People born immediately after Generation Y, starting in the late 1990s.

Gross negligence An act, or a failure to act, that is so reckless that it shows a conscious, voluntary disregard for the safety of others.

Hold harmless An agreement or contract wherein one party holds the other party free from responsibility for liability or damage that could arise from the transaction between the two parties.

Hybrid learning Learning environment in which some content is available for completion online and other learning requires face-to-face instruction or demonstration; sometimes referred to as "blended" or "distributed" learning.

Identifying The process of selecting those persons whom the instructor would like to mentor, coach, and develop.

Ignition officer An individual who is responsible for igniting and controlling the material being burned at a live fire training.

Indemnification agreement An agreement or contract wherein one party assumes liability.

Independent study A method of distance learning in which students order the course materials, complete them, and then return them to the instructor.

Informal communications Internal memos, e-mails, instant messages, and computer-aided dispatch/mobile data terminal messages. Informal reports have a short life and are not archived as permanent records.

Instructor-in-charge An individual qualified as an instructor and designated by the authority having jurisdiction to be in charge of the live fire training evolution and who has met the requirements of an Instructor II in accordance with NFPA 1041 (NFPA 1403).

Instructor-led training (ILT) A learning environment in which a human instructor facilitates both the in-person sections and the online components of coursework. Instructors usually set deadlines for submission, create quizzes and assignments, and track student progress.

Interrogatory A series of formal written questions sent to the opposing side of a legal argument. The opposition must provide written answers under oath.

Kinesthetic learning Learning that is based on doing or experiencing the information that is being taught.

Learner characteristics Designating a target group of learners and defining those aspects of their personal, academic, social, or cognitive self that may influence how and what they learn (NFPA 1041).

Learning A relatively permanent change in behavior potential that is traceable to experience and practice.

Learning domains Categories that describe how learning takes place—specifically, the cognitive, psychomotor, and affective domains.

Learning environment A combination of a physical location (classroom or training ground) and the proper emotional elements of both an instructor and a student.

Learning management system (LMS) A web-based software application that allows online courseware and content to be delivered to learners, that also includes classroom administration tools such as activity tracking, grades, communications, and calendars.

Learning objective A goal that is achieved through the attainment of a skill, knowledge, or both, and that can be measured or observed.

Lesson outline The main body of the lesson plan; a chronological listing of the information presented in the lesson plan.

Lesson plan A detailed guide used by an instructor for preparing and delivering instruction.

Lesson summary The part of the lesson plan that briefly reviews the information from the presentation and application sections.

Lesson title The part of the lesson plan that indicates the name or main subject of the lesson plan. Also called the lesson topic.

Level of instruction The part of the lesson plan that indicates the difficulty or appropriateness of the lesson for students.

Liability Responsibility; the assignment of blame. It often occurs after a breach of duty.

Major life activity Basic functions of an individual's daily life, including, but not limited to, caring for oneself, performing manual tasks, breathing, walking, learning, seeing, working, and hearing.

Malfeasance Dishonest, intentionally illegal, or immoral actions.

Medium The third link of the communication chain, which describes how you convey the message.

Mentoring A relationship of trust between an experienced person and a person with less experience for the purpose of growth and career development.

Message The second and most complex link of the communication chain; it describes what you are trying to convey to your students.

Method of instruction Various ways in which information is delivered to student, both in a classroom and on the training ground (NFPA 1041).

Misfeasance Mistaken, careless, or inadvertent actions that result in a violation of law.

Motivation The activator or energizer for an activity or behavior.

Motivational factors States of the person that are relatively temporary and reversible and that tend to energize or activate the behavior of the individual.

Negligence An unintentional breach of duty that is the proximate cause of harm.

Networking An activity or process of like-minded individuals meeting and developing relationships for professional and personal growth through sharing of ideas and beliefs.

Oral test A test in which the answers are spoken in essay form in response to direct or open-ended questions. They may accompany a presentation or demonstration.

Organizational chart A graphic display of the fire department's chain of command and operational functions.

Passive listening Listening with your eyes and other senses without reacting to the message verbally.

Pedagogy The art and science of teaching children.

Performance test A test that measures a student's ability to do a task under specified conditions and to a specific level of competence. Also known as a skills evaluation.

Prerequisite A condition that must be met before a student is allowed to receive the instruction contained within a lesson plan—often a certification, rank, or attendance of another class.

Psychomotor domain The domain of learning that requires the physical use of knowledge. It represents the ability to physically manipulate an object or move the body to accomplish a task or use a skill.

Psychomotor objective A statement that defines a learning outcome that is based on increasing the learner's ability to perform a specified motor skill.

Reasonable accommodation An employer's attempt to make its facilities, programs, policies, and other aspects of the work environment more accessible and usable for a person with a disability.

Receiver The fourth link of the communication chain. In the fire service classroom, the receiver is the student.

Recommendation report A decision document prepared by a fire officer for the senior staff. The goal is support for a decision or an action.

Reliability The characteristic that a test measures what it is intended to measure on a consistent basis.

Safety officer An individual appointed by the authority having jurisdiction as qualified to maintain a safe working environment at all live fire training evolutions (NFPA 1403).

Self-directed study A learning environment in which learners can stop and start as they desire, progress to completion of a module, and submit a final score to determine whether they passed or failed the module, all without an instructor's involvement.

Sender The first link of the communication chain. In the fire service classroom, the sender is the instructor.

Sharing The basic concept of giving to others with nothing expected in return.

Skills evaluation A test that measures a student's ability to do a task under specified conditions and to a specific level of competence. Also known as a performance test.

Social learning An informal method of learning using technologies that enable collaborative content creation. Examples include blogs, social media, collaborative discussions, and wikis.

Standards A set of guidelines outlining behaviors or qualifications of positions or specifications for equipment or processes. Often developed by individuals within the regulated profession, they may be applied voluntarily or referenced within a rule or law.

Student-centered learning Educational methodologies that focus on student engagement and require students to be active, responsible participants in the learning experience (NFPA 1041).

Subject-matter expert (SME) An individual who is technically competent and who works in the field for which test items are being developed.

Succession planning The act of ensuring the continuity of the organization by preparing its future leaders.

Synchronous learning An online class format that requires students and instructors to be online at the same time. Lectures, discussions, and presentations occur at a specific hour and students must be online at that time to participate and receive credit for attendance.

Tailboard chat An informal gathering where fire fighters discuss various issues.

Technology-based instruction (TBI) Training and education that uses the internet or a multimedia tool.

Terminal objective A broader outcome that requires the learner to have a specific set of skills or knowledge after a learning process.

Validity The documentation and evidence that supports the test item's relationship to a standard of performance in the learning objective and/or performance required on the job.

Virtual classroom A digital environment where content can be posted and shared, and where instructors can create quizzes and assignments to be completed and tracked online via an internet-connected computer.

Webinar An online meeting, occurring in real time, which usually allows for participants to share their desktop screens, web browsers, and documents live as the meeting is occurring.

Willful and wanton conduct An act that shows utter indifference or conscious disregard for the safety of others.

Written test A test that may be made up of several types of test items, such as multiple choice, true/false, matching, essay, and identification questions.

Index

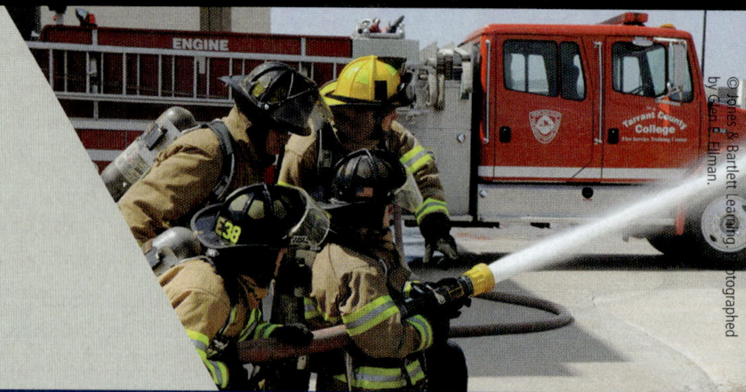

Note: Page numbers followed by '*f*' and '*t*' refers to figures and tables respectively.

M

N

O

P

U

V

W